Textbook of

Pharmacology
for
Nurses

THIRD EDITION

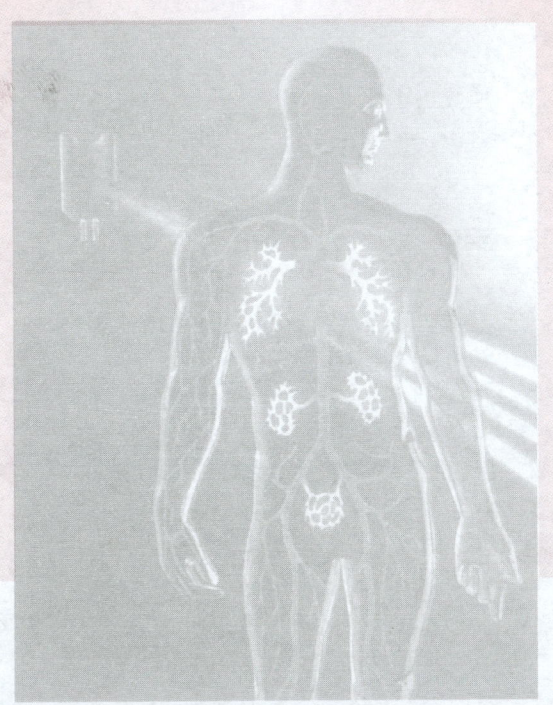

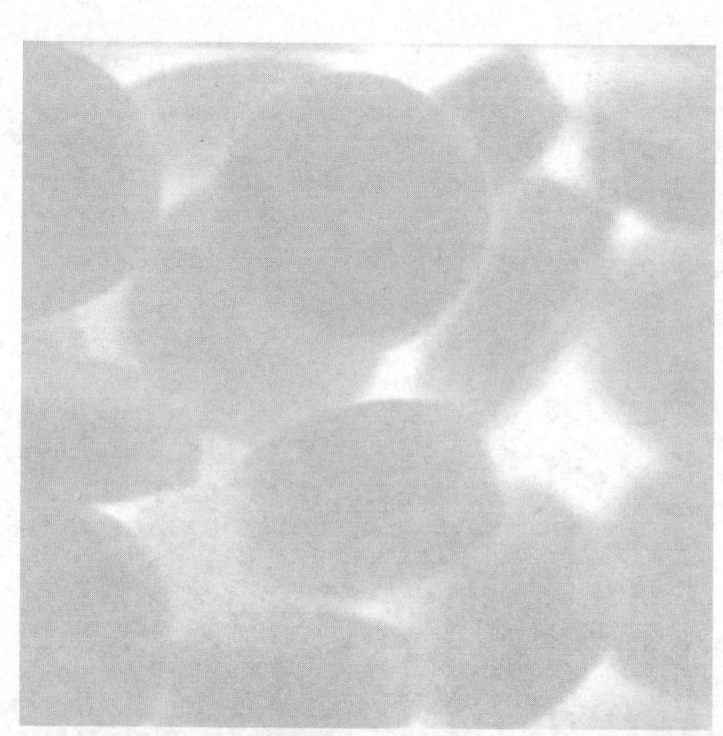

Textbook of
Pharmacology for Nurses

THIRD EDITION

JK Grover MBBS MD

Ex-Professor
Department of Pharmacology
All India Institute of Medical Sciences
New Delhi

Monica Malik MBBS MD

Assistant Professor
Department of Radiotherapy
Nizam's Institute of Medical Sciences
Hyderabad, AP

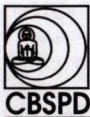

CBSPD

CBS Publishers & Distributors Pvt Ltd

New Delhi • Bengaluru • Chennai • Kochi • Kolkata • Lucknow • Mumbai
Hyderabad • Jharkhand • Nagpur • Patna • Pune • Uttarakhand

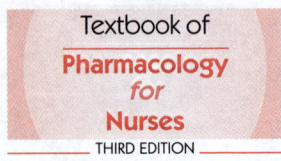

Textbook of
Pharmacology
for
Nurses
_____ THIRD EDITION _____

ISBN: 978-81-239-2254-6

Copyright © Authors and Publisher

Third Edition: 2013
  Reprint: 2015, 2018, 2023
First Edition: 1989
Second Edition: 2002

Published by Satish Kumar Jain and produced by Varun Jain for

CBS Publishers & Distributors Pvt Ltd
4819/XI Prahlad Street, 24 Ansari Road, Daryaganj, New Delhi 110 002, India
Ph: 011-23289259, 23266861   Website: www.cbspd.com
                                                e-mail: delhi@cbspd.com
Corporate Office: 204 FIE, Industrial Area, Patparganj, Delhi 110 092
Ph: 011-4934 4934   Fax: 011-4934 4935   e-mail: publishing@cbspd.com; publicity@cbspd.com

Branches

- **Bengaluru:** Seema House 2975, 17th Cross, K.R. Road, Banasankari 2nd Stage, Bengaluru 560 070, Karnataka, India
  Ph: +91-80-26771678/79   Fax: +91-80-26771680   e-mail: bangalore@cbspd.com
- **Chennai:** 7, Subbaraya Street, Shenoy Nagar, Chennai 600 030, Tamil Nadu, India
  Ph: +91-44-26680620, 26681266   Fax: +91-44-42032115   e-mail: chennai@cbspd.com
- **Kochi:** 42/1325, 1326, Power House Road, Opp KSEB, Power House, Ernakulam 682 018, Kerala, India
  Ph: +91-484-4059061-65   Fax: +91-484-4059065   e-mail: kochi@cbspd.com
- **Kolkata:** 147, Hind Ceramics Compound, 1st Floor, Nilgunj Road, Belghoria, Kolkata-700056, West Bengal, India
  Ph: 033-25633055, 033-25633056   e-mail: kolkata@cbspd.com
- **Lucknow:** Basement, Khushnuma Complex, 7-Meerabai Marg (Behind Jawahar Bhawan) Lucknow 226001, India
  Ph: 0522-4000032   e-mail: tiwari.lucknow@cbspd.com
- **Mumbai:** PWD Shed. Gala no. 25/26, Ramchandra Bhatt Marg, Next to JJ Hospital Gate no. 2, Opp. Union Bank of India
  Noorbaug Mumbai-400009, Maharashtra, India
  Ph: 022-66661880/89   e-mail: mumbai@cbspd.com

Representatives

- **Hyderabad**   0-9885175004
- **Patna**   0-9334159340
- **Jharkhand**   0-9811541605
- **Pune**   0-9923910676
- **Nagpur**   0-9421945513
- **Uttarakhand** 0-9716462459

Printed at Mudrak, Noida, UP, India

to

Late Shri HN Grover
and
Jai Devi Grover

Parents of first author
and
grandparents of second author

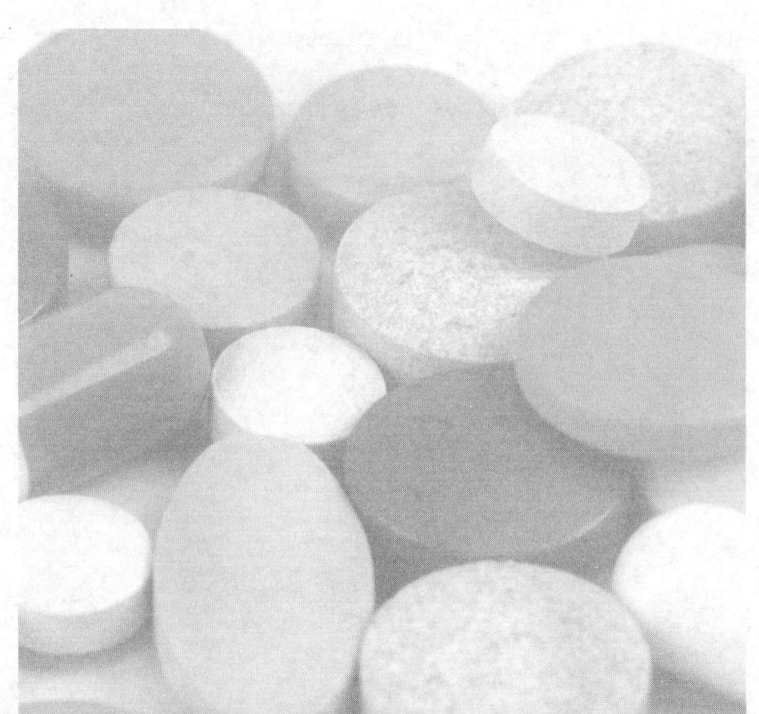

Foreword

We improve the efficiency of practice through the acquisition of information, whether this be thoughtfully accumulated or subconsciously absorbed. This accumulated or subconsciously absorbed knowledge has been passed on by Dr JK Grover in the book entitled *Textbook of Pharmacology for Nurses*. This book is both timely and useful, such an account has long been needed and the task has been most skillfully performed. Dr Grover has had the great advantages of also teaching the BSc (Hons) nursing students, apart from the medical graduates. Thus, this book reflects an understanding of pharmacological principles of nursing practice derived from day-to-day touch with these students, towards practical applications of their work. The author also acquired an appreciation of the necessity for a solid foundation in basic principles of pharmacology acquired during the twenty-two years of her teaching experience. I am delighted to have been asked to write the Foreword to this admirable book by a colleague. I wish it had been available to the students of nursing at early date.

Dr SD Seth
Ex-Professor and Head
Department of Pharmacology
All India Institute of Medical Sciences
New Delhi

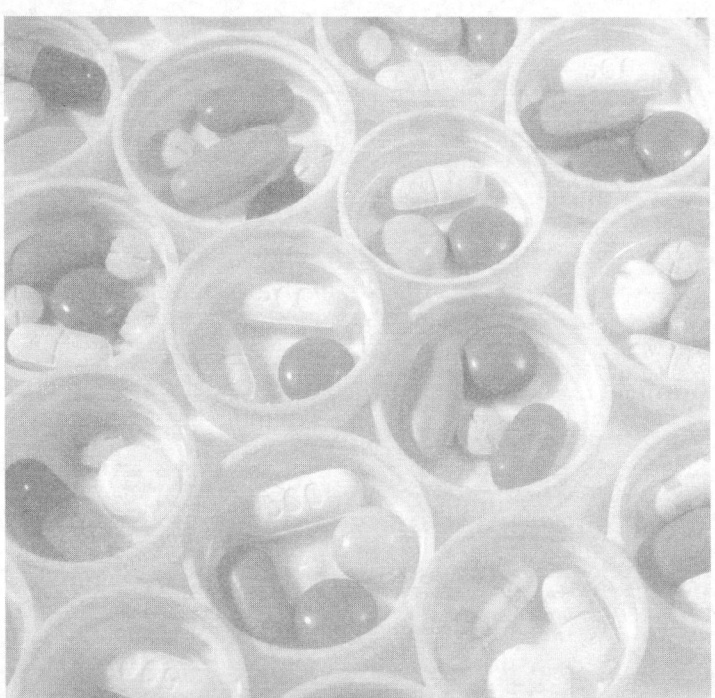

Preface to the Third Edition

Third edition has been thoroughly revised and updated to include latest developments in pharmacology. Special emphasis has been laid on meeting requirements of nurses in correctly handling the drugs.

The book has been designed to cater to the needs of nursing students and their teachers.

JK Grover
Monica Malik

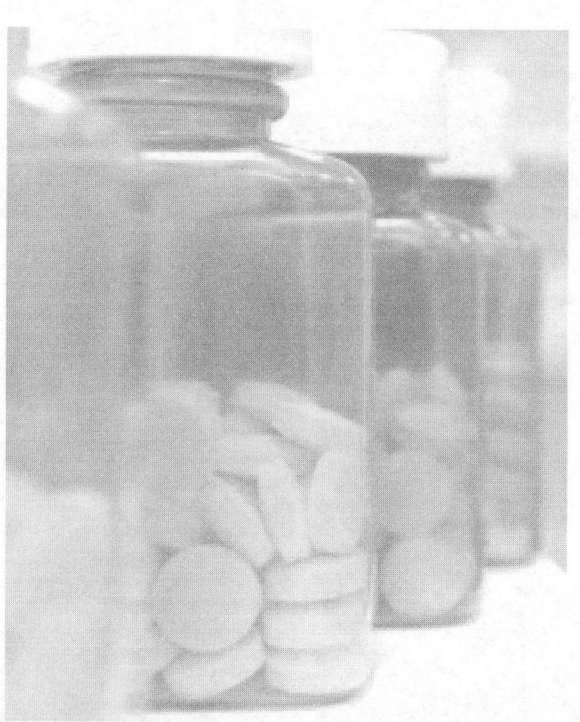

Preface to the Second Edition

With increase in knowledge in pharmacology, new concepts in therapeutics keep developing. Many new drugs with better therapeutic profile entered the market during the last few years. Therefore, a need was felt to impart this information (on new concepts and new drugs) to the students which necessitated introduction of a new edition. Significant additions in this edition include information on new drugs, update on clinical management, update on adverse drug reactions and interactions.

The present edition is, therefore, moderately enlarged.

JK Grover
Monica Malik

Preface to the Second Edition

Rapid growth in knowledge in pharmacology, new concepts in therapeutics keep developing. Keeping new drug with better therapeutic profile glorifies the understanding the last few years. Therapeutic agents were to improve this. To enhance their new dose standard new edition. In this, students which pharmacological reduction of have been. New updating matter in this edition. In this, information on new drugs, updated on clinical management keeping information keeping therapeutics caused.

Prospered is what machining learn in learn it is helps.

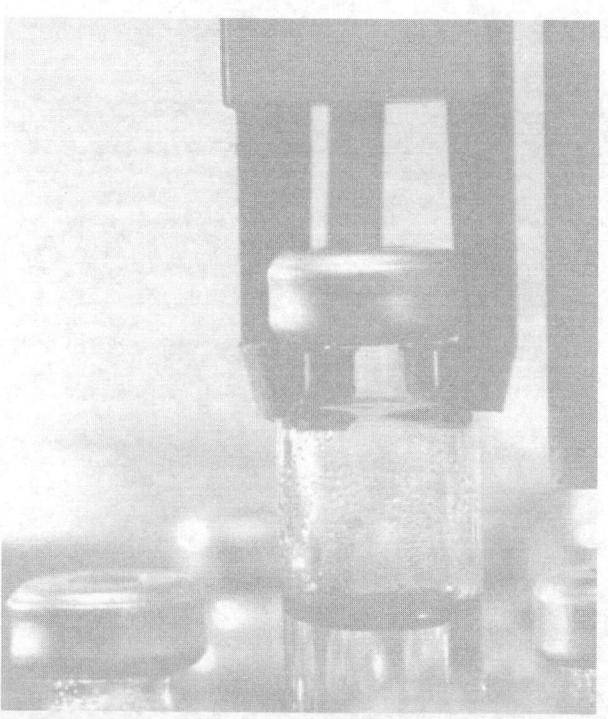

JK Glover
Monika Mulik

Acknowledgements

It is our pleasant duty to acknowledge the help received in the preparation of the manuscript of this book.

It was my father who encouraged me to write this book. We are grateful to Dr Vikrant Vats and Dr Geetanjali Uppal for their contribution. It is through the hard work of Miss Leela Pant, Shri Kuber Routela and Shri Anil that the typing of manuscript was completed in time.

JK Grover

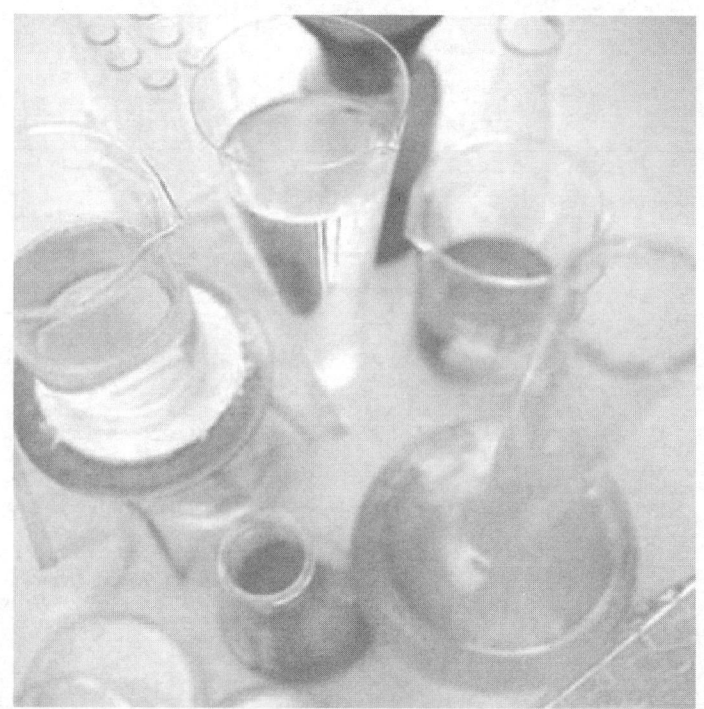

Contents

Section III: Central Nervous System

Section IV: Local Anaesthetic Agents

Section V: Cardiovascular System

Section VI: Drugs Acting on the Respiratory System

Section VII: Endocrinology

Section VIII: Digestive System

Section IX: Haemopoietic System

Section X: Drugs Acting on Urinary Tract

Section XI: Chemotherapy

General Pharmacology

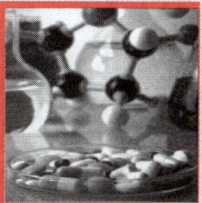

1

Introduction

Pharmacology is a study of effective and safe use of drugs in the **diagnosis, prevention or treatment** of disease.

HISTORY OF PHARMACOLOGY

Indian medicine is probably oldest. Sumerian tablet (2100 BC) describes ointments and medicines containing asafoetida, sodium chloride and potassium nitrate. Ebers papyrus (1550 BC) contains prescription of castor oil and opium.

In modern times Hippocrates (469–370 BC) is called **father of medicine**. He postulated the modern concepts of disease and separated it from ghosts.

Aristotle (384–322 BC) separated superstitle from fact.

Galen (131–201 AD) encouraged the idea of polypharmacy.

Paracelsus (1493–1541 AD) started using mercurials in the treatment of syphilis.

Francois Megendied (1783–1855) introduced the concept of scientific methods in studies on drugs.

Schmiedoerg (1838–1973), John Jabob Abel (1857–1938) and Sir Ram Nath Chopra (1882–1973) developed the modern concept of experimental pharmacology in Germany, USA and India respectively.

Sources of Drugs

1. **Plants:** Till the beginning of last century leaves, barks or roots were used to treat diseases. Quinine, morphine, ephedrine and digitoxin are still in use. Chemical purification of these products yield active ingredients like **alkaloids** (morphine, atropine, emetine and quinine), **glycosides** (digitalis), **fixed oils** (castor and peanut oil) and **volatile oils** (asafoetida, ginger and eucalyptus).

2. **Mineral oil:** liquid paraffin is used as purgative.

3. **Heavy metals and minerals:** Gold is used in rheumatoid arthritis. Magnesium trisilicate is used as an antacid in peptic ulcer. Radioactive minerals (^{133}I, ^{32}P) are used for diagnosis and treatment of cancer.

4. **Animal products:** Antitoxic sera and antivenom for toxins and snake bites are derived from animals and used in human.

5. **Synthetic:** Majority of the drugs these days are **synthetic**.

Advantages of Synthetic Preparations

(a) These are available in pure form and therefore quality is better controlled.

(b) Easy to manufacture in bulk.

(c) These are cheaper.

(d) Drugs can be chemically modified so as to possess more effective and more specific actions.

(e) Produce less allergic reactions.

Examples of synthetic drugs—aspirin, glucocorticoids, calcium channel blockers and sulfonamides.

6. Microorganism: Certain important drugs have been obtained from bacteria and fungi (penicillin and bacitracin). Lately insulin is also being developed from bioengineered microorganisms.

PHARMACOLOGY AND RELATED SUBJECTS

Pharmacology is a study of drugs about their actions (both advantageous and disadvantageous) on the living—man, animals, organs or tissues. It consists of:

(a) **Pharmacodynamics** is the qualitative study of the effects of drugs on tissues. This also includes mode of action of the drugs.

(b) **Pharmacokinetics** is the study of absorption, distribution, metabolism and excretion of drugs.

Clinical pharmacology is the study of effects of drugs in human beings.

Toxicology is the science that deals with poisons.

Chemotherapy is a branch of therapeutics with specific toxicity towards microorganisms, parasites and cancer cells in animals or human beings.

ALLIED SUBJECTS

Pharmacy is concerned with selection, preparation, standardisation, compounding, formulations and dispensation of drugs.

Pharmacognosy is the science of identification of drugs.

PROPERTIES OF DRUGS

Therapeutic actions are actions of drugs which are useful in management of diseases.

Side effects are effects of drugs which are not useful and are exerted by the drug at therapeutic dose level.

Toxic effects are produced by higher doses of drug.

The two together are referred to as **adverse drug reactions**.

SOURCES OF DRUG INFORMATION

Textbooks which give out the details about the drugs.

Materia medica deals with source, physical and chemical properties, preparations and uses of drugs.

Pharmacopoeia is an official document containing list of drugs which have established their use. It contains description of physical properties and tests for identification, purification and potency of the medicinal preparations of these drugs. **However, it does not contain any information on nursing.**

Drug formulary is an official book containing formulations used therapeutically

1. Indian pharmacopoeia: It is published by the Ministry of Health and Family Welfare, Government of India.

2. **National Formulary of India:** This too is published by Ministry of Health and Family Welfare, Government of India.

3. **Monthly Index of Medial Specialities** (MIMS) is published every month. It contains information on drugs, their trade names, along with name of the manufacturing company with indications and contraindications of each drug, price of the product, container size and the dosage.

Journals: These are an important sources of information when a specific topic is to be researched in details.

Nomenclature of the drugs: Drugs can be listed according to their chemical name, generic name, official name and trade name.

Chemical name: When drugs are identified according to their chemical nature, the description of the drug composition is listed alone with the actual formulation of its constituents. This is of particular interest to the chemist and medical student, e.g. acetyl salicylic acid.

Generic name is proposed by the company that first develops the drug. It usually represents an abbreviation of the chemical name of the drug, e.g. aspirin is the generic name for acetyl salicylic acid.

Official name: Pharmacopoeia and National Formulary contain official names of the drugs.

Trade name or brand name is the name given by the company and designates the manufactures ownership of that trade name, e.g. different companies sell aspirin under different trade names by, e.g. Aspro, Disprin, Wimprin, etc.

Significance of Pharmacology in Nursing:
In the present day, nurse is expected to exercise judgement in the management of drug therapy. This requires an understanding of drug action and the ability **to detect both therapeutic and adverse reactions**.

Nurses are expected to advise patients regarding:
   (a) Storage of drugs.
   (b) Planning of drugs schedule for optimal effects.
   (c) In selected conditions nurse may be involved in prescribing drugs.
   (d) Her role is of great significance in poison control, non-medicinal use of drugs and drug abuse.
   (e) Record keeping of drugs.

It is the duty of the nurse to promote responsible use of chemicals to enhance health. She must try to minimise the detrimental effects of use. This needs knowledge about practical and technical procedures in handling, controlling and administering drugs.

DRUG REGULATIONS IN INDIA

Manufacturing, sale, import and export of drugs are controlled by the Government. The central drug authority is based at Nirman Bhawan, New Delhi. The drug authorities of respective states are mostly based in their respective capitals. Central drug authority formulates the policy and the peripheral authorities implement these policies.

Implementation is under **Drug Controller.**

1. **Advisory agency** includes Drug Technical Advisory Board (DTAB) and drug consultative committee. DTAB frames and modifies rules regarding drugs.

2. **Analytical agency** includes **Central Drug Laboratory** (situated at Calcutta) and Drug Laboratories in respective states. These laboratories test and analyse the samples of drugs and cosmetics.

3. **Executive agency** is an authority which grants license to various organisations for manufacturing, storing, recapping, selling, importing and exporting of drugs.

Drug inspectors inspect the premises of companies licensed for production of drugs. Inspectors can collect samples of drugs suspected to be misbranded, adulterated or banned.

Any new drug has to be cleared by drug controller.

Drugs are also classified according to safety and availability of the drugs.

Prescription drugs: Requires a prescription for purchase because that drug is judged to be unsafe except under medical supervision. Examples: morphine, pethidine and barbiturates.

Official drugs are preparations adopted by government and listed in pharmacopoeia.

Over the counter drugs are a non-prescription drugs sold directly to the public without requiring a prescription. These are usually either a well known substance or mixture judged safe for use without medical supervision and are taken for minor symptoms.

Placebo: It is an inert substance that causes biological response due to power of suggestion.

Dangerous drugs: Coca leaf, opium, hemp and manufactured products from these sources are dangerous drugs as these are addicting and fall under the Dangerous Drugs Act of 1930.

(a) Cultivation and collection of opium plant is prohibited except under government control.

(b) Manufacture of opium products (imports, exports, transport and possession) is prohibited.

(c) Sale of dangerous drugs is prohibited.

(d) Production and supply of opium is controlled by central government and state traffic is controlled by state governments.

Drug Standards

Medicine can vary considerably in their purity, strength, bioavailability, efficacy and safety or toxicity.

Standards are the yardsticks by which drug preparations are judged. Standard for drug quality are generally established and enforced by the government. Standards are outlined in the Pharmacopeia and National Formulary.

NURSE AND THE DRUGS

Number of drugs used in therapeutics is so large that it is impossible for any human to remember the details of all drugs. It is therefore necessary for the nurse to familiarise herself with the drugs that are commonly used.

The features to be remembered regarding drugs.

1. **Name of the drug** by its generic name or by generally recognised abbreviations, e.g. APC.

   All popular names by which commonly used drugs are known in the health community should be recorded and remembered.

2. **Drug family:** Drugs are classified either according to the action that they produce, e.g. (analgesic, antipyretic, antiepileptics, etc.) or by the route of their administration, e.g. inhalational anaesthetics or intravenous anaesthetics, etc. or by their mechanism of action, e.g. anticholinergic drugs, CNS stimulants, etc.

3. **Desired therapeutic effects:** It is important to remember the main action of the drug that forms the basis of its use. It is desirable to understand the mechanism by which the drug produces its pharmacological action.

4. **Side effects and toxic effects:** These are not intended for any medical benefit. For example, atropine is given to relieve intestinal colic. It relieves colic by relaxing the intestine through its anticholinergic activity. At the same time this anticholinergic action produces dryness of mouth which is not a desired effect. Hence, difficulty in passing urine and dryness of mouth are labelled as side effects or adverse effects.

5. **Contraindications:** These are conditions in which the drug should not be used because drug is likely to worsen the condition of the patient, e.g. atropine is contraindicated in glaucoma because atropine precipitates glaucoma in the patients prone to it and aggrevates glaucoma if it is already present.

Nurse must decline to administer any drug, she believes will cause harm to the patient.

2

Weights and Measures

Metrology is a science of measurements. There are two systems of weighing and measuring drugs.

1. Metric system
2. Apothecaries system

Metric system is based on the decimal system and accepted all over the world and is commonly used though some people continue to write prescriptions in apothecaries system.

Advantages

1. Tables are simple
2. Tables of weights, volume and measure are correlated.

Length is measured in meters, weight in gram (g) and volume in litres.

Gram is defined as weight of 1 ml distilled water at 4°C in vacuum.

Table of weights

1000 nanogram (ng)	=	1 microgram (mcg)
1000 microgram	=	1 miligram (mg)
10 mgms	=	1 decigram (dg)
1000 mg	=	1 gm
1000 gms	=	1 kilogram (kg)

Table of volumes

1000 microlitres (ul)	=	1 millilitre (ml)
1000 millilitres	=	1 litre (l)
1000 litres	=	1 kilolitre (kl)

Table of length

1000 millimetres	=	1 metre
10 millimetres	=	1 centimetre
100 centimetre (cm)	=	1 metre (m)

Apothecaries System

Table of volumes

60 minims	=	2 fluidram
3 fluidram	=	1 fluid ounce
16 fluid ounces	=	1 pint
2 pints	=	1 quart
4 quarts	=	1 gallon

Apothecaries system and its equivalents in metric system

60 mgms	=	1 grain
1 ounce	=	30 grams
1 fluid ounce	=	30 ml
1 pint	=	500 ml

Household measures

1 drop	=	0.1 ml
1 teaspoonful	=	5.0 ml
1 table spoonful	=	15.0 ml
1 water glass	=	250 ml
1 milk bottle	=	500 ml

Concentration of the solutions can be expressed in various ways.

1. Percent weight in volume   %   w/v   gms per 100 ml (e.g. 1% solution contains 1 g of substance in 100 ml of solvent)

2. Percent volume in volume   %   v/v   no. of ml per 100 ml (1% v/v = 1 ml of active substance in 100 ml of vehicle)

3. Percent weight in weight   %   w/w   no. of grams of active drug in 100 gms of the total.

4. Molar concentration is number of moles of a substance in one litre of a solution.

Mole of a particular substance is the number of grams equal to the molecular weight of the substance (1 mole = 1 gm mol weight) per 1000 ml.

3

Types of Preparations

Pharmaceutical preparations are available in variety of forms to facilitate the administration of drug.

Tablets are compressed powders or granulated ingredients of drugs.

Advantages

1. Easy to swallow.
2. Drug is released in stomach.

Enteric coated tablets: Cellulose — acetate, phthalate, gluten, etc. are used to cover tablets so that the active drug is not destroyed by gastric acidity. The coating gets disintegrated in alkaline medium of intestine from where the drug gets absorbed.

Capsules: These are gelatin containers used to enclose drugs. The drugs in the form of powder or granules are released from the capsule and are absorbed. **Enteric coated granules** can also be put in the capsule and dispensed. Absorption from these granules is slow.

Sustained releasing preparations are similarly made to prolong the duration of active of drugs.

Disadvantages: These preparations are expensive.

Pills are mixtures of powdered drug and a liquid. These are rarely used as they have short shelf life.

Powders are single or mixed powders wrapped in paper and dispensed.

Fillers: Solid medications (powders and tablets) often contain fillers which are added to active drug. Fillers are chemically as well as pharmacologically inert substances. These may however influence the absorption of active drug.

Mixtures are liquid preparations meant for internal use. These may be of substances soluble in water or suspensions or effervescent mixtures (quinine mixture).

Emulsions are mixtures of two **immiscible liquids** (water and oil) uniformly dispersed.

Liniments are emulsions meant for local use, e.g. liniment turpentine.

Solutions are solutions of water soluble drugs.

Suspensions are combinations of a solid (insoluble) and a fluid in which the particles of the former are mixed with but not dissolved in it.

Oils are viscous liquids that are insoluble in water. Oils may be volatile or fixed. **Volatile oils** leave no greasy stain, evaporate easily and emit aroma. **Fixed oils** do not evaporate at room temperature and leave stain.

Aromatic waters are saturated aqueous solutions of volatile substance (e.g. peppermint oil, etc.).

Syrups are mixtures of water and sugar and the drug is contained in this mixture, e.g. ipecac syrup.

Elixirs are mixtures of alcohol, volatile oils and sweeteners (e.g. elixis of iodine).

Spirits are high concentrations of alcohol (50% or higher) and volatile substances (e.g. camphor spirit).

Tinctures are mixtures of vegetables or chemical substances contained in high alcohol (50% or above) e.g. tincture digitalis or tincture iodine. They are meant for systemic as well as local use.

Fluid extract is highly concentrated preparation (100%) of the alcoholic solutions of vegetable drugs (e.g. cascara sagrada).

Gels are mixtures of insoluble drugs and water, e.g. milk of magnesia.

Mucilages are viscous mixtures of gums or starch in aqueous solutions.

Ointments are semisolid preparations intended for local application to the skin or mucus membranes.

Lotions are suspended particles in aqueous solutions for local applications, e.g. lotion calamine.

Suppositories are molded mixtures of the drug in a firm base for rectal, vaginal or urethral insertion, e.g. glycerine suppositories.

Flavouring agents and dyes: These are added to foods, cosmetic and the drugs to improve the aesthetic value. Common flavouring additives such as cherry, raspberry, chocolate and licorice syrups are used to disguise unpleasant tastes.

4

Storage of Drugs and Drug Containers

Chemical deterioration is hastened by heat, moisture and in few cases by light. Sterile substance must be protected from bacterial contamination. All drugs should be kept in a separate place meant only for drugs.

Stocks of drugs should be inspected regularly. Any drug whose shelf life has expired or has changed in appearance should be discarded.

1. Drugs should be kept in their original containers with their original labels.
   Advantages of original containers.
   (a) Containers which protect them from deterioration, e.g. amber coloured bottles are used to protect drug liable to be spoilt by light.
   (b) Transfer of sterile substance to another container adds risk of infection.
   (c) Handling of the container should not spoil the label as original label is important.
2. Storage areas should be kept clean, cool and dry.
3. Medicines should bear accurate labels at all times.
4. Medicines meant for internal use should be stocked separately from those meant for external use.
5. In hospital practice, a locked cabinet is necessary for storing drugs. Narcotics and legally restricted drugs must be kept in a special locked compartment.
6. Key of the medicine cupboards should be with senior sister.
7. Insulin, serums, vaccines and certain antibiotics should be kept in refrigerator.
8. Food should not be stored in the medicine refrigerator.

CARE AND KEEPING OF DRUGS

For taking proper care of drugs records are kept handy for interpretation. Depending on the level of stock and expiry date of product the product is ordered for replenishment. The value of the product determines its stock. Drugs can be classified according to its value:

(a) Products which are very costly
(b) Moderately costly
(c) Some are inexpensive.

These can also be classified according to their utility, e.g.

(a) Some products are vital (V)
(b) Some are essential (E)
(c) Some are desirable (D).

According to availability their records can be maintained in the following way:

1. Some easily available (d).
2. Some are scarcely available (s).

According to rate of consumption

Some products are consumed at rapid rate (E) and some are medium (M) running and some are slow (S) in their consumption.

Stocks of drugs should be inspected regularly. **Any drug whose shelf life has expired or have changed in appearance indicates possible deterioration.** These drugs should be discarded.

Documentation of Drug Administration: All data pertaining to drug must be recorded. All drugs, their doses, route of administration and the exact time of administration must be recorded in the chart. This serves three purposes:

1. Chart is a legal document.
2. This helps in establishing the relationship between drug and the symptoms of adverse reactions.
3. Time of drug administration influences its effect.

For best results the appropriate drug must be given in right dosage by the correct route at the right time.

Drug failure occurs

1. When the dose administered is not correct.
2. It has not been absorbed due to vomiting or diarrhea.
3. There is altered state of health due to associated diseases.

All these factors must be looked into before changing the drug.

5

Routes of Drug Administration

Drug can be used either to produce a local or systemic effect.

For Local (Topical) Effects

(a) Tinctures	(b) Ointments
(c) Lotions	(d) Sprays
(e) Drops	(f) Plaster
(g) Dusting powders	(h) Pastes

Topical applications may be for the mucous membranes and for various body cavities, e.g. irrigation and instillation of eyes, ears, nose, throat, mouth, bladder and vagina. Lozenges are given by mouth, suppositories through urethra, rectum or vagina.

Nursing care

Self medication is a rule with these drugs therefore a nurse must educate her patients regarding their toxicity.

Only small amounts of these drugs should be prescribed and dispensed at one time.

Each container should be used only by one individual.

Before use the appearance of preparation should be checked.

Drops are better tolerated if they are administered at body temperature.

Eye Medications: Eye drop should be instilled into the lower eye lid pouch.

Dropper should not come in contact with the eyeball.

During infection separate containers of medicines should be used for each eye.

Ointment should be extruded from the tube along the inner edge of lower eyelid.

If crusts are present on eyelids, these should be removed before instillation of drugs or ointment application.

Ear Medications: At the time of instillation ear drops should be at body temperature.

Asceptic technique should be employed if the eardrum is perforated.

Nose Drops and Sprays: Nasal decongestants are frequently applied. Avoid excess of drug as it may get aspirated.

Transdermal route: Lipid soluble drugs when applied on skin get absorbed, e.g. nitroglycerin in angina. Skin should be cleaned before any application.

Patches can be applied but they tend to produce inflammation.

Vaginal medications: These are often given at bedtime and the patient should be instructed to remain lying down for a short time after administration.

Inhalation: This route is used for local as well as systemic actions.

Nurse is asked to handle oxygen inhalation for systemic use and aerosols for local effects. Educate the patient to the use of atomiser. Instruct patient to place dispenser in his mouth and inhale while activating atomiser.

General anaesthesia is given through inhalational route. Response is immediate and toxic reactions appear immediately hence, **this route is left for doctors to handle**.

FOR SYSTEMIC EFFECTS

Oral route: Drugs are given by mouth more frequently than by any other route. Powders, tablets, pills, capsules, mixtures are administered through this route.

Advantages

1. This route is safer and pleasanter and convenient.
2. It is economical.
3. Complications of parenteral therapy are avoided.

Disadvantages

1. Onset of action is slower than with parenteral route.
2. This route cannot be used in unconscious patients.
3. Drugs cannot be orally administered during diarrhoea and vomiting.
4. Certain drugs (enzymes, insulin, etc.) cannot be given through this route as they are destroyed in stomach or during passage through liver.
5. Absorption of certain drugs is erratic and unreliable.

Nursing care

Sufficient water or fluid should be given with drug:
  (a) to prevent sticking of drug in oesophagus.
  (b) to reduce irritant effect of the drug.
  (c) hydrophilic softeners require fluids to perform action.
  (d) in elderly patients tablets can be crushed and given mixed with fruit juice. Enteric coated tablets/capsules should not be crushed before giving.

Hydrochloric acid (given in achlorhydria) is administered through straw placed in mouth. This is done to prevent contact with teeth.

Patients who have difficulty in swallowing should get medicines in liquid form (suspensions, mixtures).

Medication through feeding tube:
Nasogastric or gastrostomy feeding tubes are put in for oral feeds in certain conditions.

Nursing care

1. Pinch the tube so as to avoid entry of air.
2. One ounce of water must be administered before giving drug. This rinses the tubing.
3. Administer drug in liquid or powder form.
4. Additional water should follow the drugs to propel them into stomach.

Sublingual: A tablet containing the drug is placed under the tongue. It is allowed to dissolve in the mouth. The active agent gets absorbed and reaches circulation without passing through the liver. Nitrites for treatment of angina are given through this route.

Advantages

1. Onset of action is quick.
2. Patient can monitor the dose by spitting the drug when either relief occurs or there is toxicity.
3. Destruction of the drug in the stomach and intestine is avoided. Metabolic degradation in liver is also avoided as drug directly reaches site of action (heart and lungs).

Following drugs are given through sublingual route:

(a) Nitroglycerin tablets in angina.

(b) Isoprenaline sulfate in bronchial asthma.

Lozenges and trouches are designed to dissolve gradually in the mouth for local effect.

Nursing care

These drugs must be kept separate from the drugs generally given orally or through other routes.

RECTAL MEDICATIONS

Suppositories are medicines incorporated in waxy basis that melt at body temperature. These have to be stored in refrigerator, e.g. suppositories of indomethacin for rheumatoid arthritis and aminophylline for bronchial asthma and chlorpromazine for controlling vomiting.

Enemas: Enemas are liquid preparations that are instilled in the colon.

These are of two types:

1. Evacuation enema meant for purgation.
2. Retention enema is meant for giving drugs for systemic as well as local use, e.g. cortisone in ulcerative colitis. Active drug is given in 100 ml of water.

Some drugs are well absorbed from rectal mucosa. Drugs absorbed from the upper rectal mucosa are carried to liver while those from the lower part of the rectum enter directly into systemic circulation, e.g. indomethacin is given by this route in patients of rheumatoid arthritis with peptic ulcers.

Advantages

1. This route is frequently used when nausea and vomiting are present.
2. Irritation of gastric mucosa is avoided.
3. Those drugs which are destroyed by gastric acidity can be administered through this route.
4. Those drugs which are destroyed during first pass through liver can also be given through this route.
5. This route is convenient in the terminally ill patients.

Precautions for retention enema

1. Avoid stimulation of peristalsis.
2. Small amount of the fluid at body temperature should be given.
3. It should be given slowly and at low pressure.
4. After removal of tubing put pressure on the anus for some time.

Avoid over distention or manipulation of anal and rectal tissues as it stimulates vagus nerves.

PARENTERAL ROUTES (INJECTIONS)

Routes of administration of drugs other than alimentary tract are called parenteral.

Advantages

1. These routes are useful in unconscious and uncooperative patients and for getting quick response.
2. In patients suffering from vomiting and diarrhea.
3. To avoid destruction of a drug in the alimentary canal, e.g. insulin.
4. Drugs which irritate stomach or intestine or are not absorbed from the gut are given by these routes, e.g. streptomycin.
5. Onset of action is very rapid and predictable therefore these routes are used during emergencies.

Disadvantages

1. It is an invasive technique not liked by the patients.
2. Self medication is not possible in most cases.
3. Trained personnel is required to give injections.
4. Drugs given once cannot be easily withdrawn.
5. Are less safe and expensive.
6. Asepsis must be maintained.

Various parenteral routes are:
   (i) Intradermal (into skin)
  (ii) Subcutaneous (under the skin)
 (iii) Intramuscular (into the muscle)
 (iv) Intravenous (into vein)
  (v) Intracardiac (into heart)
 (vi) Intra-arterial (into artery)
(vii) Intrathecal, intraperitoneal and intra-articular into the respective cavities.

Intradermal (Intracutaneous): This route is employed for giving vaccinations (BCG and Smallpox) and for detecting allergy. The forearm and upper back are the chosen sites.

Techniques: Wipe the area with alcohol and allow it to dry.

Fill the tuberculin syringe to a desired level and inject into skin forming a wheal.

Injection will fail if no wheal is formed or if on withdrawal there is bleeding.

Subcutaneous Injections: Insulin and heparin are given by this route.

Advantages

1. Absorption of drug is slow, sustained and uniform.
2. Drug implants are put which act as depot of the drug.

Disadvantages

1. Only small amounts (0.5–1.0 ml) of water soluble drugs can be given by this route.
2. Injection of irritant substances can produce abscess or sloughing.

This route is not useful in patients suffering from peripheral vascular diseases, oedema or circulatory shock.

Uses

1. Jet injections are used for mass innoculation programmes.
2. Saline is given by this route in children, hyaluronidase is added to it to improve absorption.

Techniques

1. Appropriate site should be selected.
2. Clean the area with alcohol.
3. Insert needle under the fold of skin quickly and straight.
4. Inject slowly.
5. Massage the area after removal of the needle.

Newer techniques

(a) **Dermojet:** Using a gun, drug solution is projected at high speed into skin area. Drug gets deposited in subcutaneous area.

   Advantages: It is painless and is used for mass vaccination.

(b) **Pellet implantation:** Small pellet containing drug is implanted in subcutaneous tissue. Drug is slowly released in a few weeks/month. **Testosterone, desoxycorticosterone acetate** are given by this route.

(c) **Sialastic implants:** Drug is packed in sialastic tube and implanted subcutaneously. Slow but constant release occurs into blood and action lasts for months. Empty tubes are removed later.

Intramuscular Injections:

Gluteus and deltoid muscles are used in adult and the aging while biceps and triceps are used occasionally in the adult.

Advantages

1. Fat soluble drugs can be given only by this route.
2. Irritants, colloids and suspensions can also be given by this route.
3. Absorption is good, rapid and uniform.
4. Onset of action is early.

Disadvantages

1. Injections produce local pain and if infected produce abscess.
2. Maximum of 10 ml can be given by this route.

3. Risk of injury to nerve is present.

4. If wrongly done drug can enter into blood.

Techniques

1. Muscle should be relaxed.

2. Avoid injecting into a vessel, hence put the needle into muscle and suck to detect blood. If blood is detected in your syringe, avoid injecting.

3. Z-track injections are made to prevent leakage of drug and discolouration of skin, e.g. iron salts.

Intravenous: This route is employed when immediate effect is required.

Advantages

1. It produces rapid action.

2. Desired blood concentration is achieved.

3. Dose is easy to monitor and adjusted.

4. Large quantities of fluids can be given by this route.

5. Drug is not destroyed either by intestine or liver.

Disadvantages

1. Only water soluble drugs can be given.

2. Drug given once cannot be withdrawn.

3. It is highly unsafe.

4. Generalised infection can be introduced if care is not exercised.

5. Trained personnel is required to give this injection.

6. Leakage of the drug outside the vein can produce severe irritation.

7. Venous irritation can lead to thrombosis.

Precautions

1. Maintain asepsis.

2. Make sure you are in vein. This is done by checking blood in syringe.

3. Injection should be given slowly.

4. Minimum dosage should be employed.

Intravenous route is employed either for bolus administration or continuous infusion.

Bolus — when large dose is given initially, e.g. heparin. IV injection is generally given slowly.

Intravenous Infusion: It is a slow but continuous administration of drug.

Advantages

1. It reduces risk of repeated intravenous injections and irritant effect as the drugs can be administered in diluted form.

2. It maintains a constant level of drug in the blood.

3. Effect lasts longer.

4. It is used when large volumes are required to be given.

Disadvantages

1. Chances of infection are increased.
2. Chances of local injury are more.
3. Patients usually do not like this technique.

Nursing care

1. Maintain sterile conditions.
2. To avoid air embolism air must be allowed to escape as tubing fills the fluid.
3. Do not overfill the drip chamber as this obscures flow of drops by which flow is monitored.
4. Do not contaminate needle by touching surface.
5. Attach tape on the needle so that dressing can be changed without disturbing tape or needle.
6. Adding more drugs to fluid entails interactions. These should be kept in mind.
7. Rate of flow of injection should be closely monitored.

Intra-arterial, intrathecal, intraperitoneal, intramedullary and intra-articular injections are made only by the physician.

Intra-arterial route is used to administer drugs for cancer treatment or for diagnostic purposes, e.g. coronary and other angiographies and peripheral and vascular diseases.

Intrathecal: This route is employed to give antibiotics with a view to treat meningitis. Extradural/ Epidural — morphine is given through this route to produce relief.

Intraperitoneal: In infants it is used for giving large volumes of fluids (saline and glucose). For treating peritonitis antibiotics are given through this route.

Intra-articular route is employed to give gold and hydrocortisone in rheumatoid arthritis.

Iontophoresis: It is a special technique for introducing drugs into skin for systemic effects. Galvanic current is used to bring about this effect.

Inunction: Certain drugs when rubbed on skin can get absorbed and produce systemic effects, e.g. nitroglycerin ointment in angina. Application of drugs through this route reduces adverse reactions.

Factors determining selection of the route

(a) Desired speed of action — if immediate effect is wanted administer IV.
(b) Parenteral routes are preferred in the unconscious. In chronic states in the unconscious patient drugs can be given orally through gastric tubing.
(c) Solubility of the drug — water soluble drugs alone can be given IV. Fat based drugs can be given either orally or IM.
(d) Oral route is best for chronic use.
(e) In case of vomiting or ulcers in upper part of GI, drugs can be given per-rectum.

Syringes: Two types of syringes are available:

1. Glass   2. Plastic

Glass Syringes

Advantages

1. Are resistant to punctures.
2. Are accurate in scale and fluid level.

3. Being transparent, fluid level is seen clearly.
4. These are not easily disrupted by serial connections.
5. They can easily be sterilised by boiling.

Disadvantages

1. They break and crack easily and need careful handling.
2. There is greater risk of air embolism and airborne contamination.

Plastic Syringes

Advantages

1. These are resistant to cracking and breaking.
2. These are collapsible and allow emptying without denting hence less chances of air embolism.
3. These are too transparent.
4. Are disposable.

Disadvantages

1. They are not so accurate in scale.
2. They are easily disrupted by serial connections.
3. They cannot be sterilised in domiciliary practice.

Tuberculing syringe is of 1 ml capacity with 0.01 ml markings and is useful in giving small volumes.

6

Pharmacokinetics

The study of absorption, distribution, metabolism (transformation) and excretion of drugs in the body is termed as **pharmacokinetics**.

MECHANISMS OF ABSORPTION

Drugs are either absorbed by passive or active processes.

Characteristics of Passive Absorption: This mechanism does not utilise energy, hence is called passive. Following are the characteristics of passive absorption:

(a) Drug molecules move from regions of high concentration to areas of relatively low concentration.

(b) Rate of absorption or transfer is proportional to concentration gradient between the two compartments. Flow of drug takes place from a higher to a lower concentration compartment.

(c) Degree of absorption is limited by the surface area of the absorptive membrane.

(d) After the steady state is reached movement of molecules is in both directions.

(e) Degree of absorption is determined by size of the molecule and polarity. Small size molecules and unionised drugs are better absorbed.

Characteristics of Active Absorption

(a) Absorption can occur against concentration gradient.

(b) A carrier is required.

(c) This process requires energy.

(d) The system is designed to transport only specific or similar chemical structure (s).

(e) Capacity of the system is limited by the number of carrier units.

(f) Rate of transfer is proportional to concentration of drug, until carrier is saturated.

(g) The motility of drug molecules is in one direction only.

Drug factors influencing absorption

1. Disintegration and dissolution time of tablets/capsules determine rate of absorption. Thus rate of absorption depends on drug formulation.

2. Lipid solubility — lipid soluble drugs are better absorbed.

3. pH and ionisation: ionised drugs are poorly absorbed. Most drugs are weak electrolytes and ionise depending on pH of the area of absorption site. Acidic drugs (aspirin and barbiturates) are better

absorbed in acidic pH of stomach while alkaline drugs (pethidine and ephedrine) are normally absorbed from gut.

4. Particle size: Small particles are better absorbed hence aspirin, grisiofulvin are available as microfined drugs.

Human Factors Influencing Absorption

1. Surface area and vascularity of that area–larger the area better the absorption, e.g. small intestine.
2. Presence of food delays gastric emptying, thus delays absorption. Food constituents may form complexes, with drug and make it unabsorbable, e.g. absorption of tetracyclines is reduced in presence of milk. Rifampicin, ampicillin and roxithromycin are better absorbed in empty stomach.
3. Intestinal motility—Increased motility reduces absorption and vice versa.
4. Metabolism—certain drugs like nitroglyecrin and insulin are metabolised in gut and cannot be given through this route some drugs undergo first pass metabolism in (propranolol, salbutamol) their dose has to be increased to achieve effect.

PASSAGE OF DRUGS ACROSS BODY BARRIERS

Drug Absorption through Skin

1. Skin is less permeable to drugs than other membranes.
2. Only lipid soluble substances are absorbed through intact skin.
3. Abraided skin absorbs drugs.

Drug Absorption by Mucous Membranes

1. Drug is absorbed directly into blood circulation when given by sublingual, buccal, nasal, conjunctival, vaginal and rectal routes.
2. Absorption is rapid.

These routes are used when it is not possible to use oral route or when the drug is likely to be destroyed by the digestive enzymes.

Laxatives, adsorbants, antidiarrhials and antacids are given for local effects. Ingested drugs must be resistant to degradation by digestive process.

Absorption from Intestine: **Carriers** for active absorption of **sodium, potassium, vitamins, amino acids, simple sugars, uracil, thymine, bile salts** are present in the intestine. Chemically similar drugs such as **5-fluorouracil, 5-bromouracil** are actively carried by these carriers and get absorbed.

Absorption of most drugs is dependent on passive diffusion. The rate of absorption is dependent on passive diffusion and is influenced by dissolution and ionization of the drug. Absorption of the drug depends upon particle size and chemical form of the drug and its solubility.

Absence of hydrochloric acid in stomach retards gastric absorption of acid drugs in stomach.

(a) Tablets and capsules disintegrate before absorption.
(b) Food delays absorption of most drugs.
(c) Mixtures are better absorbed than solids.
(d) Deficiencies of pancreatic and intestinal secretions may prevent dissolution of enteric coated tablets and capsules.
(e) Vomiting and diarrhoea reduce absorption.

Inhalation: Only gaseous form of drugs or those which can be given in fine mists can be given through this route.

Injectables are usually completely absorbed.

BIOAVAILABILITY

1. It is the amount of the drug that can be absorbed and transported by the body to its site of action. It is the amount of drug that reaches site of action that determines efficacy.
2. Particle size of the drug, its solubility, polarity and its crystalline structure influence the absorption of the drug.
3. Bioavailability is measured by determining the concentration of the drug in blood or tissues at a specified time following its administration.

DRUG DISTRIBUTION

This is influenced by (a) rate of circulation, (b) cardiac functioning and (c) the nature of the tissue barriers.

Exercise increases while cooling reduces drug distribution to the tissue. Tissues with less blood supply such as bone receive less drug.

Blood Brain Barrier (BBB)

1. Nature has provided this barrier to exclude certain chemicals from reaching the brain.
2. This barrier is constituted by glial cells and capillary endothelium in the brain.
3. Only lipid soluble, unionised drugs can cross this barrier.

All drugs acting on the central nervous system are lipophilic and cross BBB. BBB is missing from area of CTZ (vomiting centre).

Placental Barrier: Placenta behaves as a simple lipoidal membrane. Like blood brain barrier it selects out drugs. Carrier mechanism also operates at this level.

DRUG STORAGE

Plasma protein binding: On reaching blood most drugs get bound to plasma proteins free drug-unbound-produces effect and bound form of drug acts as store. Protein binding prolongs duration of action of drug. **Warfarin, tolbutamide, phenytoin, fursemide, salicylates and sulfonamides** are highly protein bound. The protein binding is influenced by presence of other drugs and one drug may compete with other for the binding site leading to drug interactions.

Certain diseases, e.g. liver and kidney failures cause reduction in albumen, leading to less binding. Dose of such drugs should be reduced in these patients.

Drugs may be stored in various tissues including bones and fat.

(i) Drugs which are stored in liver, e.g. chloroquine and mepacrine.
(ii) Thyroid concentrates iodine.
(iii) Drugs stored in fat-thiopentone sodium, DDT, benzodiazepines and estrogens.
(iv) Fluoride and tetracycline get concentrated in bone.
(v) Emetine is concentrated in muscles.
(vi) Chloroquine is stored in retina.

BIOTRANSFORMATION (METABOLISM) OF DRUGS

Drugs are subjected to chemical reactions. The metabolites so produced may be pharmacologically active or inactive. These actions are produced by enzymes. Generally metabolism makes drug biologically less active and more polar, thus easier to excrete through kidneys.

Chemical process involved in biotransformation

Phase I reactions

1. Oxidation
2. Reduction
3. Hydrolysis

Phase II reactions or synthesis

1. Alkylation
2. Methylation
3. Conjugation with glucuronic acid, sulfate, etc.

Examples of phase I reactions

Drugs undergoing oxidative metabolism—barbiturates, benzodiazepines, paracetamol, phenothiazines, phenytoin and steroids.

Drugs undergoing reductive metabolism—chloramphenicol and halothane.

Drugs undergoing hydrolysis—procaine, pethidine and choline esters

Examples of phase II reactions

Drugs undergoing glucuronide conjugation: aspirin, morphine and metronidazole.

Drugs undergoing acetylation: 1NH, sulphonamides and hydralazine.

Drugs undergoing methylation: adrenaline, histamine and nicotinic acid.

Drugs undergoing sulphation: sex steroids and chloramphenicol.

Drugs undergoing glutathione conjugation—paracetamol.

Examples of changes in pharmacological action produced by metabolism

(A) Active drug to	Active metabolite
1. Phenylbutazone	Oxyphenbutazone
2. Codeine	Morphine
3. Heroin	Morphine
4. Diazepam	Oxazepam
5. Chloral hydrate	Trichlorethanol
6. Propranolol	4-OH propranolol
7. Amitriptyline	Nortriptyline
8. Chloroquine	Hydroxychloroquine
(B) Inactive drug (prodrug)	Active metabolite
1. Benorylate	Aspirin and paracetamol
2. Cyclophosphamide	Alkylating metabolites

3. Telampicillin, becampicillin	Ampicillin
4. Levodopa	Dopamine
5. Prednisone	Prednisolone

(C) Active drug to   **Inactive metabolite**

1. Norepinephrine	Metanephrine (less active)
2. Cyanide	Thiocynate
3. Ethanol (alcohol)	Acetylaldehyde

(D) Active drug to   **Toxic metabolite**

1. Fluoroacetic acid	Flurocitric acid
2. Malathion	Maloxon
3. 1NH	Acetylhydrazine
4. Enflurane	Difluoromethoxy-difluoroacetic acid
5. Halothane	Trifluoroacetic acid

Factors influencing metabolism

(i) Genetic differences
- (a) Species
- (b) Familial

(ii) Physiological status
- (a) Age
- (b) Sex
- (c) Nutrition
- (d) Disease

(iii) Environmental status
- (a) Stress
- (b) Radiation
- (c) Effect of chemicals (enzyme inducers/inhibitors).

Genetic differences: The degree of availability of enzymes involved in metabolism determines the rate of metabolism of drug. The level of the enzyme is genetically determined. Hence, there are rapid metabolisers and slow metabolisers. Genetic influence on metabolism is seen in 1NH, alcohol, hydralazine, succinylcholine and tolbutamide.

Species: Enzyme systems involved in biotransformation in one species may be completely or partially absent in others.

Age: Infants do not have full capacity to metabolise chemicals. Their immature livers are not capable of handling either the range or total quantity of chemicals that adult systems can. Therefore less dosage is given in children and the elderly also have a limited capacity to handle drugs.

Sex: Rate of metabolism of benzodiazepines, estrogens and salicylate is more in males than females.

Hormones: Hypothyroidism increases half life of digoxin.

Nutrition and Drug Metabolism: Coffee or cola nuts increase oxidative metabolism of antipyrine. Low carbohydrate and high protein diet increases metabolic capacity.

Environmental factors: Cigarette smokers metabolise a few drugs more rapidly than non smokers. This is because smoke induces metabolising enzymes.

Enzyme induction: Microsomal enzymes in liver are responsible for metabolising drugs. Synthesis of these enzymes can be increased by certain pollutants in environment (cigarette smoke, DDT) and by a few drugs (rifampicin, phenobarbitone, griseofulvin, carbamazepine and alcohol). Enzyme induction reduces effects of other drugs, e.g. rifampicin causes failure of contraceptive pill and increases toxicity of paracetamol. **Tolerance to drugs may develop.**

Clinical uses of enzyme inducers
(a) Phenobarbitone is used to treat congenital non-hemolytic jaundice.
(b) Phenytoin reduces clinical manifestations of cushing syndrome.

Enzyme inhibitors: On the contrary certain drugs **inhibit the metabolising enzymes**, e.g. cimetidine, ketoconazole, erythromycin and ciprofloxacin. These tend to prolong the life of drugs co-administered with them, e.g. pheniprazine, iproniazid and chloramphenicol.

Disease: Diseases of liver limit biotransformation of drugs. Certain drugs that cause liver damages and are dependent totally on liver for elimination need to be avoided in patients with liver diseases. Half-lives of diazepam and chlordiazepoxide are increased in cirrhosis and viral hepatitis. Thus even in normal doses these drugs may severely depress brain. Cardiac diseases reduce blood flow to liver thus limiting drug metabolism.

By altering hormone levels and neural activity in the body **stress** affects metabolism.

DRUG EXCRETION

Drugs are excreted from the body as intact molecules (drug as such) or its metabolites. Pathways of elimination include respiration, urination, fecal excretion and exocrine secretion.

The rate of removal of drug from the body is termed as **clearance**.

Half life ($t_{1/2}$) is another term frequently used to estimate how fast a drug leaves the body. By definition, half life of a drug is the length of time necessary for the concentration of drug to decrease by half.

Lungs excrete paraldehyde, alcohol, volatile general anaesthetics.

Skin: Arsenic, mercury, sodium and potassium are excreted through skin.

Bile: Novobiocin and erythromycin are secreted in bile. Phenolphthalein is secreted in the bile and reabsorbed from intestine (enterohepatic circulation) which prolongs its life.

Drugs undergoing enterohepatic circulation — erythromycin, ampicillin, rifampicin, tetracycline phenolphthalein and oral contraceptives.

Intestine: Heavy metals, cascara sagrada and senna are secreted in intestine.

Milk: Penicillin, streptomycin, erythromycin, phenothiazines, diazepam, caffeine, alcohol, tolbutamide, quinidine, barbiturates, heroin and morphine are secreted in milk. Few of these drugs (antibiotics) may be of use to the infant but others are likely to produce adverse reactions in the breast fed baby. Drugs which are secreted in milk and are harmful to the child should be avoided by the mother. Mother should be advised not to breast feed the child while taking these drugs.

Saliva: Iodine, heavy metals, lithium, thiocyanates, rifampicin and metronidazole are excreted in saliva. Lead compounds get deposited on the gums.

Kidneys are far most important for excretion of drugs.

Urinary excretion is influenced by:
(a) the rate of glomerular filtration,
(b) changes in urinary pH and
(c) competetion for reabsorption.

Drugs which are removed unchanged by the kidneys-lithium gentamicin, methotrexate, ethambutol and cephalexin and furosemide.

Drugs which partly undergo metabolism in liver and are partly excreted through kidneys, e.g. penicillins, methyldopa, lincomycin, digitoxin and para-aminosalicylic acid.

By increasing volume of urine and allowing less time for reabsorption (**forced diuresis**) poisonous substances can be got rid off.

Barbiturates and salicylates are quickly excreted in alkaline urine.

Pethidine, mecamylamine, quinine and amphetamine are better excreted in acidic urine.

7

Factors Modifying Drug Action

Several factors influence drug response both qualitatively and quantitatively. These factors depend both on the drug and the biological nature of the patient.

1. Age: Children require lesser dose

(i) as their body weight is less

(ii) blood brain barrier is poorly formed and

(iii) the enzymes responsible for metabolism of drugs are not completely formed.

In the **elderly,** the rate of metabolism and excretion is reduced, therefore, they also require lesser dose.

Dose for child can be calculated by using Young's formula.

Young's formula

(a) $\dfrac{Age}{Age+12} \times$ adult dose = dose for child

2. Body Weight: Drug gets more diluted in the heavily built individual, consequently the effects are less.

$\dfrac{Weight\ in\ kg}{70} \times$ adult dose = calculated dose for the particular patient

Surface area is considered a better basis for calculation of the dose of toxic drugs, e.g. anticancer agents.

$\dfrac{Body\ surface\ area\ in\ sq.\ meters}{1.7} \times$ adult dose = dose for a specific patient with that surface area

3. Sex: Women generally require less dose because of smaller body weight. During menstruation, pregnancy and lactation the use of many drugs has to be restricted.

4. Individual Variation: Some individuals are naturally hypersusceptible to certain drugs.

5. Racial Species and Genetic Differences: Ephedrine produces mydriasis in caucsians but not in negroes.

Species variation: Atropine is ineffective in rabbits (due to presence of atropinesterase). Digitalis does not produce vomiting in rats.

Genetic differences: Synthesis of enzymes responsible for metabolism of the drug or its action is dependent upon genetic pattern of individual hence genetic differences in drug metabolism. Science dealing with genetically mediated variations in drug responses is called **Pharmacogenetics.**

(i) Rate of acetylation of drugs is genetically determined. There are slow and fast acetylators. The lifespan of 1NH, hydralazine, procainamide in body is determined by rate of acetylation.

(ii) Effect of succinylcholine (a skeletal muscle relaxant) normally lasts for 30 secs but in individuals deficient in pseudocholinesterase it is prolonged. This may result in apnea and death.

(iii) Primaquine, sulphones and quinolones produce haemolysis in G6PD deficient individuals.

6. Presence of Disease:
Disease of liver and kidney affects the elimination of drug. Half life of morphine is increased in liver disorders.

Gentamicin and tetracycline tend to produce greater toxicity if kidney functions are impaired.

Drugs are poorly absorbed in malabsorption syndrome and CHF.

Morphine is better tolerated during pain.

Prodrugs are less effective in a patient with liver disease.

Protein binding of drugs is reduced in liver diseases hence free drug concentration in blood is higher leading to its toxicity.

Permeability of BBB is increased in kidney failure hence smaller doses of CNS active drugs are required.

7. Time of Drug Administration:
Sleep producing drugs (hyponotics) act better when given at night. Corticosteroids produce less pituitary depression if given early morning.

8. Emotional Factors:
Personality of patient modifies drug effect, e.g. dose of tranquillisers required for agitated patient is more than for sober patients. Emotional state also affects the absorption of drug.

9. Physiological Variables:
Pregnant uterus is more sensitive to oxytocin than non pregnant uterus. Acidosis inhibits the diuretic activity of acetazolamide.

10. Tolerance:
On repeated administration of certain drugs response of the individual is reduced and to produce the same degree of effect a higher dose is required. Tolerance is seen with **alcohol, barbiturates** and griseofulvin, etc.

Cross tolerance: Tolerance to one drug of a particular chemical group results in tolerance to other drugs of chemically similar group, e.g. patients tolerant to pethidine are tolerant to morphine.

Tolerance can be natural or acquired.

Acquired tolerance can be due to:

(i) Enzyme induction.

(ii) Less absorption of the drug (pseudotolerance).

(iii) Change in sensitivity or release of neurotransmitter.

(iv) Change in homeostatic mechanism.

Small dose is less effective while higher dose produces toxicity. The degree of pharmacological action depends on dose.

11. Dose: Physiological dose of vitamin D promotes calcification while higher dose causes decalcification. Neostigmine causes increase in muscle tone but large dose causes paresis.

12. Route of Administration of Drug: This affects the quantitative as well as the qualitative responses of drug.

(a) **Quantitative:** Drug given by intravenous route produces higher degree of response than oral route.

(b) **Qualitative:** Magnesium sulphate when given orally produces diarrhoea and dehydration while when applied locally it reduces swelling. Given rectally it reduces intracranial tension and when given by injection it exerts anticonvulsant effect.

13. Frequency of Dose Administration and Cummulative Action: When the rate of administration of a drug is more than its rate of elimination it accumulates in the body, e.g. digoxin. Drugs which are strongly bound to plasma or tissue proteins also tend to accummulate in the body. They exert their effect for long time and produce long lasting toxicity.

Frequency of dose depends on its pharmacokinetic profile. Aim is to provide continuous optimum range of blood concentration.

14. Combined Effects of Drugs: When two drugs are given together, they are present in the body at the same time. Presence of one drug affects the function of the other.

Examples:

(a) **Synergism:** when the effect of one drug is additive to the other, combination is termed beneficial and is of synergistic nature, e.g. combination of ephedrine and aminophylline.

(b) **Potentiation:** Combined effect of two drugs is more than summation of their individual effects, e.g. physostigmine and acetylcholine or ammonium chloride and mercurial diuretics.

(c) **Antagonism:** When action produced by one drug is countered by the other drug, e.g. histamine produces bronchoconstriction and adrenaline produces bronchodilatation.

  (i) Chemical antagonism: Acids neutralising alkalies, e.g. antacids are given to treat hyperacidity in stomach.

  (ii) Physiological antagonism when two drugs with different physiological effects are combined, e.g. histamine and adrenaline.

  (iii) Antagonism at receptor level: Atropine blocks effect of acetylcholine by blocking cholinergic receptors. This type of antagonism may be reversible or irreversible. Reversible antagonism is seen between acetylcholine and atropine. Higher concentrations of acetylcholine can overcome blockage caused by atropine and d-tubocurare.

Irreversible antagonism is seen between adrenaline and phenoxybenzamine. Excess of adrenaline cannot overcome blockade.

Clinical uses of antagonism

1. To treat adverse effects of drugs, e.g. phenobarbitone is added to ephedrine.
2. To treat drug poisoning, e.g. naloxone counters morphine poisoning.
3. To avoid combinations which reduce efficacy, e.g. penicillin with tetracycline.

15. Drug Dependence: WHO has defiend drug dependence as 'A state, pshychi or physical which results from interaction between a living organism and a drug and condition is characterised by compulsion of drug intake'.

Examples of drugs which cause dependance.

1. Morphine its semisynthetic and synthetic preparations.

2. Alcohol

3. Barbiturates

4. Amphetamine

8

Pharmacodynamics

Pharmacodynamics is the study of effects of drugs on human body and their mechanisms of action.

When a drug given in therapeutic doses reaches its site of action it produces pharmacological actions which may be desirable (**therapeutic effects**) and undesirable effects (**unwanted side/adverse effects**). Doses higher than therapeutic dose produce **toxic effects**.

Efficacy is the effectiveness of the drug in terms of degree of therapeutic effect produced by it.

Safety and toxicity: No active chemical is free of toxicity. The incidence and severity of adverse reactions produced by a drug determines its safety. The difference between therapeutic and toxic dosages determines the margin of safety of a substance.

When considering use of drugs, its adverse reactions must be weighed against its benefits.

Potency is the concentration of active drug in the preparation. When the chemical nature of the active ingredients is unknown, potency is measured by testing in animals (**bioassay**). When the chemical nature of the active ingredient is know potency is measured by chemical assay.

MECHANISM OF DRUG EFFECTS

Drugs do not generate any new function they only modify or replace the existing function of the body.

Drug may either increase the activity of the cell (**stimulation**) or decrease its activity (**inhibition**) or it may act by replacing the deficiency of the substances in body. In addition drugs may act by irritation and killing of microbes (**anti-infective action**).

1. **Stimulation:** Selective increase in activity of specialised cells is termed stimulation, e.g. increased, salivary secretion by pilocarpine, increase in heart rate and its force of contraction by adrenaline.

2. **Inhibition or depression:** This is selective decrease in the activity of specialised cells, e.g. cocaine depresses conductivity in sensory nerves, barbiturates depress central nervous system, quinidine depresses junctional tissue of the heart.

3. **Dual actions:** Some drugs may stimulate one type of cells while depressing others, e.g. morphine stimulates CTZ center but depresses respiratory and cough centers.

4. **Irritation:** This term is used for non-specific tissues, e.g. epithelial, endothelial and connective tissues, e.g. irritant purgatives stimulate peristalsis, volatile oils act as carminatives.

   Counter irritant is a term applied when an irritant agent applied locally on skin relieves visceral pain. Examples are use of liniment turpentine, camphor, iodex, hot water bottle, etc. Irritants stimulate sensory nerves in the skin. The impulses so generated are relayed through cerebrospinal axis to brain. These interfere with the impulses coming from the viscera, which get gaited. In addition irritants stimulate vasomotor fibers to the internal organ which helps in removal of pain producing substances from the viscera.

5. **Replacement:** Use of hormones, vitamins, minerals, calcium, sodium and potassium, etc. in states of deficiency, e.g. insulin in diabetes mellitus, thyroxine in myxoedema, vitamin D in rickets, iron in microcytic anaemia, etc.

6. **Anti-infective action:** These kill or selectively reduce growth rate of microorganisms with little or no adverse effects on the host cell, e.g. streptomycin in tuberculosis and griseofulvin in fungal infections.

7. **Stimulating or inhibiting immune system:** Vaccines and sera act by improving immunity and steroids produce good effects by suppressing antigen-antibody reactions.

Site of drug action: The site where the drug acts and how the drug acts are two important aspects of pharmacology.

(a) Drug may act at the site of application, e.g. nystatin ointment and local anaesthetics–they produce their effect without getting absorbed.

(b) Drug may act during its transportation, e.g. osmotic diuretics like mannitol, glycerol and urea.

Drugs which act after absorption are said to produce systemic action.

(c) Drugs may act by getting concentrating in a particular tissue, e.g. anaesthetics get concentrated in brain and produce generalised effects or digitalis in heart.

Site of the drug can be anatomically and physiologically identified, e.g. in case of digitalis it is heart and in case of thiazides it is renal tubules. The site of action can be biochemically localised, e.g. organophosphorus compounds inhibit cholinesterase. It is also possible to localise the pharmacological site of action namely **receptor site**.

MECHANISMS OF DRUG ACTIONS

Drug can produce action in the following ways:

1. Physical means, e.g.
    (a) Chelation.
    (b) Osmotic action, e.g. osmotic diuretic or osmotic purgatives.
    (c) Adsorption, e.g. kaolin and activated charcoal act as anti-diarrheal as they adsorb toxins.
    (d) Demulcents and soothing agents — lozenges are used in pharyngitis.
    (e) Radioactive substances, e.g. ^{131}I ^{32}P in thyrotoxicosis and polycythemia vera respectively.
    (f) Radio-opaque substances are used in X-rays for diagnosis, e.g. barium sulphate for detection of lesions in gastrointestinal tract.

2. **Drugs may act through chemical reactions:** antacids (anti-acids) are alkaline in nature and are used to neutralise acidity of the stomach, e.g. sodium bicarbonate.
    Ammonium chloride is used in case of alkalosis.

3. **Drugs may produce their effect by initiating reflex,** e.g. turpentine oil relieves pain and acts as counter irritant (reflex action helps).

4. **Drugs acting on enzymes:**
    (i) Some drugs may inhibit enzymes to produce their effect, e.g. organophosphorus compounds inhibit cholinesterase. Allopurinol — a xanthine oxidase antagonist is used in treatment of gout.

Salicylates inhibit prostaglandin synthetase and act as anti-inflammatory agents.

(ii) Some enzymes may be used as drugs, e.g. papain, chymotrypsin, etc.

5. **Action through receptors:** Most of the drugs act by combining with their receptors.

Receptor is a locus (which may be present on the cell membrane or be intercellular) with which drug combines and produces pharmacological action. This combination takes place only if the receptor has affinity for the drug, which is determined by the chemical configuration of the receptor and the drug.

Drug receptor combination then brings about an action called **intrinsic activity**. If a drug has intrinsic activity it is called an **agonist**, e.g. acetylcholine and adrenaline. In certain conditions drug combines with the receptors but fails to bring about intrinsic activity, these drugs are called **antagonists**, e.g. atropine. **Partial agonist,** a drug which has affinity but low intrinsic activity, e.g. nalorphine.

Dose response relationship with increase in dose, there is an increase in response till maximum is reached. Further increase in the dose does not increase response (graded response).

Therapeutic index: It indicates safety margin of the drug.

9

Adverse Drug Reactions

Side effects are actions of drugs that are not specifically desired in a treatment and are exerted at therapeutic dose levels.

Side effects may be mild or severe. The less serious ones are often undiagnosed except in long-term therapy. Adverse reactions of drugs take variable time to develop and any tissue in the body can be affected.

Among common undesirable side effects are nausea, vomiting and skin rashes.

1. **Allergic reactions:** These reactions to drugs are the result of body's immunological response to a drug. These reactions may be produced by the drug or its metabolite or even by inert substances added to the active drug during manufacturing. Allergic reactions do not occur during first exposure to a drug. These reactions may manifest as:

   (i) **Skin reactions:** Itching, rash (urticaria).

   (ii) **Cardiovascular reactions:** Anaphylactic shock characterised by dyspnoea (difficulty in breathing), cyanosis, angioedema, hypotension and acute cardiovascular collapse. Type I reactions.

   (iii) **Respiratory reactions:** These may range from rhinitis to asthma.

   Allergic tendencies are familial and a family history of allergies should be elicited at the time of administration.

   Type II reactions: Antigen-antibody complexes cause lytic effect on RBC, WBC and platelets resulting in anaemia, agranulocytosis and thrombocytopenia. In severe cases aplastic anemia may be produced.

   Type III (Arthus reaction): Antigen-antibody complexes are deposited on walls of blood vessels resulting in fever, arthralgia, lymphadenopathy, serum sickness and Stevens-Johnson syndrome.

   Type IV: Delayed hypersensitivity: It is due to A/G + A/B acting on T cells and results in local reactions, e.g. contact dermitis.

2. **Idiosyncratic responses:** These are defined as genetically determined—unexpected responses to drug. Examples: Primaquine produces haemolysis in negroes and in G6PD deficient individuals.

TESTING FOR ALLERGIES

Skin Testing

Advantages

1. It is simple.
2. It allows many substances to be tested simultaneously.
3. It provides immediate results.

There are two techniques available for skin testing:

(a) Intradermal skin test   (b) Prick test

Intradermal skin test: The 0.02 ml solution of the agent is injected intradermally so as to make a wheel. It is declared positive if the flare (erythema) spreads to 21–30 mm area.

Precautions

1. Reading should be taken 15–20 minutes after injection.
2. If two or more substances have to be tested the injections should be at least 10 cm apart.

Prick Test: It is carried out by placing a drop of drug on the skin, then pricking the skin with a needle. After about a minute the extract is wiped off. Area is observed for flare after 15–20 minutes.

Anti-histaminics taken before the test interfere with its results.

Disadvantage: In both techniques false positive and negative are possible.

Other tests: These are highly specialised tests and carried out by only a few laboratories in India. Their utility in day-to-day nursing and medical care is limited.

1. Estimation of levels of immunoglobulins IgE in blood and serum can be done.
2. Isolation of allergens.
3. Estimation of antigen and antibody reaction.

Treatment of allergies includes:

1. Removal of the allergen
2. Use of antihistamines.
3. Use of beta-adrenergic drugs, aminophylline, corticosteroids — if bronchospasm is present.
4. Nasal decongestants (for allergy restricted to nasal mucosa).

Nursing care

1. Careful and accurate history is important.
2. Test for allergy.
3. Advice patient to discontinue antihistaminics and steroids for at least 4 days before this test.
4. Advise patient to avoid the known allergen.

Adverse reactions	Drug responsible for reactions
(i) Hepatotoxicity	Alcohol, paracetamol, INH, CPZ
(ii) Bone marrow suppression	Chloramphenicol, antineoplastic drugs
(iii) Fluid and electrolyte imbalance	Ethosuximide, diuretics, minerals, corticosteroids
(iv) Cushing's syndrome	Corticosteroids

(v) Nephrotoxicity	NSAIDs, sulfonamides, aminoglycosides and gold salts
(vi) Ototoxicity	Streptomycin, quinine, frusemide
(vii) Optic damage	Chloroquine, ethambutol, methyl alcohol
(viii) Joint pains	Rubella vaccine, sulfizoxazole, penicillin, diazepam, methylphenidate
(ix) Photosensitivity	Hydroxyzine, tetracycline, chloroquine, chlorpropamide, hexachlorophene.
(x) Acne	Androgens, corticosteroids
(xi) Gangrene of extremities	Propranolol and ergotamine
(xii) Cardiac arrhythmias	Digoxin
(xiii) Postural hypotension	Alpha blockers
(xiv) Hypertension	Steroids, contraceptive pill

Signs and Symptoms of Adverse Drug Reactions

1. *Bone marrow suppression*—anemia, leukopenia, thrombocytopenia, weakness, dysponea, unusual tiredness or weakness. Fever, chills, repeated infections like sorethroat. Unusual bleeding following trauma, haemorrhage.

2. *Arthralgia:* Joint pain.

3. *Allergy:* Skin rashes, bone marrow suppression, hepatitis and glomerulonephritis.

4. *Hepatotoxicity:* Anorexia, nausea, jaundice, hepatic tenderness, increase in SGOT, SGPT and alkaline phosphatase.

5. *Nephrotoxicity:* Oliguria (decrease in urine formation) oedema, weight gain, albuminuria and crystalluria, increase in blood urea.

6. *Ototoxicity:* Ringing in ears, increased sensitivity to noise initially but difficulty in understanding of speech.

7. *Gastrointestinal irritation:* Dysphagia, anorexia, nausea, vomiting, abdominal pain. Bloody or black tarry stools and diarrhoea.

8. *Central nervous system:* Forgetfulness, disorientation, anxiety, irritability and sleeplessness, etc.

Nursing care

1. Nausea and vomiting—serve attractive food preferred by the patient. In severe cases antiemetic can be given before the meals.

2. Postural hypotension — patient must be instructed to take large volumes of fluids. Change of posture by the patient should be very gradual. Before standing he must sit up—this provides time for adaptation.

3. Itching—instruct patient to apply pressure on the area and avoid scratching. If possible identify the allergen and avoid its use in medicine.

4. Constipation—Instruct patient to take fluids and food rich in fiber content.

5. Diarrhoea—Advise patient to avoid irritant foods. Tea acts as astringent.

6. Reassure patient: mental and emotional disturbances can be reduced.

7. Advise patient not to ever medicate himself.

Drug Interactions: When two or more drugs are given at the same time they may interact resulting in either increase or decrease in desired effect. These interactions may sometime result in harmful effects, e.g. severe bleeding may occur when aspirin is combined with warfarin (an anticoagulant).

Beneficial drug interactions

1. Naloxone is used for treating poisoning due to opioids.
2. In treatment of hypertension, diuretics are given along with other drugs to counter Na^+ retention. Beta blockers are added to counter increase in renin and reflex tachycardia.
3. In treatment of tuberculosis drugs are combined to improve efficacy and reduce development of resistance.
4. In cancer therapy drugs are combined to improve efficacy and reduce drug toxicity.

Harmful drug interactions

1. Absorption of tetracyclines is reduced if given with milk.
2. Salicylates increase anticoagulant activity of warfarin by displacing warfarin from plasma protein binding sites.
3. Alkalies reduce excretion of amphetamine and increase its toxicity.
4. Alcohol potentiate CNS effects of phenobarbitone.

10

Drug Treatment during Pregnancy and Lactation

Fate of the fetus is tied to its mother. Agents affecting the mother are likely to affect the fetus too. Chemicals taken by mother (ingested, inhaled, or through injections) by crossing placental barrier reach the fetus. All these agents can be injurious to fetus and therefore care needs to be exercised.

Pregnancy is a physiological state with following differences:

1. Drugs not harmful to the mother may be harmful to the fetus.
2. There is increase in maternal blood and plasma volumes hence the drug gets diluted.
3. Maternal serum protein is lower. This lowers the capacity of the protein to bind drugs and amount of free drug is more.

Following drugs cross the placenta within minutes of administration: Ampicillin, penicillin G, cephalosporin, kanamycin, tetracycline, sulfonamides, streptomycin, diazepam, phenytoin, barbiturates, alcohol, pethidine, salicylates, lidocaine and propranolol.

Factors influencing the effect of drugs on the fetus

Amount of the drug reaching fetus: this depends upon

(a) Dose of drug.
(b) The gestational age of the embryo or fetus at the time of drug administration—first trimester is most sensitive.
(c) The duration of the exposure to drugs.

Alcohol, Cigaratte Smoke and Caffeine: Fetal alcohol syndrome occurs in women who consume alcohol during pregnancy. Neurological, psychological or behavioral changes are noticed in infants born to these mothers. Women taking over 300 mg of caffeine per day appear to have higher incidence of abortions, stillbirths and premature births.

Children born to mothers who smoke during pregnancy are usually low weight, have smaller liver and suffer from hypoglycemia. Rate of abruptio and placenta previa is more in these women. Neurological symptoms are seen in these infants due to presence of excess carbon monoxide in smoke.

Principles to be remembered

1. Drugs given during the first 14–17 days of gestation interfere with cell division (may result in abortion).
2. Drugs given between 18th to 55th days of gestation interfere with organ differentiation (may result in malformations).
3. Drugs used near term interfere with uterine activity of the mother.

Certain diseases like hypertension, diabetes and congestive cardiac failure tend to worsen during pregnancy. For treatment of hypertension during pregnancy hydrallazine and methyldopa are preferred because,

(i) this combination gives maximum efficacy, and

(ii) produces fewer adverse effects.

To maintain control of blood glucose during pregnancy patient should be put on multiple injections of short or intermediate acting insulin. A continuous subcutaneous pump of insulin gives best results.

Propranolol, procainamide and disopyramide (antiarrhythmic drugs) all induce premature labour, these should be avoided.

Use of thiazides produces low birth weight infants. Their use should be restricted. Qunidine and digoxin can be safely used.

The severity of asthma is reduced during pregnancy. Administration of theophylline is considered safe during pregnancy.

Drugs can be given to mother to treat fetal conditions, e.g. Rho (D) immune globulin is given to mother to prevent Rh incompatibility (jaundice).

Glucocorticoids are given to mother to treat respiratory distress syndrome.

Penicillin, digoxin, thyroxine and biotin are given respectively to treat syphilis, heart failure, hypothyroidism and biotin deficiency of fetus.

Drug to mother	Effect on fetus
1. Anti convulsants (trimethadone and phenytoin)	Facial deformities, mental retardation
2. Alcohol	Growth retardation and mental retardation
3. Diethylstilbestrol	Vaginal adenosis and uterine anomalies
4. Androgens	Masculinization of female fetus
5. Folic acid antagonists	Multiple malformations
6. Oral contraceptives	Limb and cardiac effects
7. Diazepam	Facial clefts and cardiovascular defects

Drugs to be avoided or used with caution during pregnancy

1. Drastic purgatives as they stimulate uterine contractions.
2. Diuretics specially thiazides should not be used as they tend to produce thrombocytopenia in the newborn.
3. Diazoxide inhibits uterine activity during labour and produces diabetes in neonate.
4. Oral anticoagulants should be replaced with heparin.
5. Aminophylline produces irritability and apnea in the neonate.
6. Hypnotics depress neonatal respiration. They should be avoided near term.
7. Live vaccines given during first trimester induce congenital malformations.
8. Vitamin A during first and vitamin K during third trimester are injurious to foetus.
9. Fansidar, maloprin, and quinine all have teratogenic potential.
10. Aminoglycosides and tetracyclines should not be administered during 2nd and 3rd trimester while trimethoprim should be avoided during first trimester.

11

Drugs in Renal Failure

In renal failure drugs may produce:
- (a) Further damage to kidneys.
- (b) May accumulate in the body as they cannot be fully excreted therefore normal doses of these drugs lead to toxicity.
- (c) Certain drugs (thiazides) are rendered ineffective in renal failure.

Therefore care is excercised in prescribing drugs during renal failure.

(A) Drugs that can damage kidneys should be avoided, e.g.

1. Heavy metals, aminoglycosides, sulphonamides, amphotericin.
2. Drugs producing hypercalcaemia or uricosuric effect produce injury to renal tubules as calcium and uric acid tend to get deposited in kidneys.
3. Certain drugs (penicillins, hydrallazine, rifampicin and isoniazid) produce immunological injury to kidneys.

(B) Dosage schedule

(i) Drugs dependent entirely upon kidneys for their elimination are prescribed in lower doses, e.g. lithium, gentamycin, methotrexate and ethambutol.

(ii) Drugs which are partly eliminated by kidneys and are partly metabolised in liver (e.g. ampicillin, penicillins, methyldopa digoxin) are given in smaller quantities. Dose of these drugs depends upon the creatinine clearance.

(iii) Sodium and potassium salts of the drugs should be avoided as they tend to accumulate and precipitate oedema.

(iv) Drugs which are eliminated through metabolism should replace those which are eliminated through kidney excretion, e.g. digitoxin should be preferred over digoxin.

(v) Thiazides become ineffective and should be avoided as diuretics. Frusemide continues to act and should be preferred.

(vi) Urinary tract infections are very difficult to treat as antibiotics do not reach site of action.

12

Nursing Care of Patients with Terminal Illness

Nurse must ensure three things
1. Patient should be made as comfortable as possible.
2. Should remain in a state of consciousness.
3. Should remain free of pain.

In domiciliary practice

(a) Reassure the family
(b) Reassure the patient
(c) Attend to his emotional problems as far as possible and make the family understand his needs.

In hospital practice

1. Nurse must give time to her patient and listen to his complaints. This comforts the patient.
2. Environment must be made free of tension and noise.

Analgesics: Aspirin and paracetamol if given regularly are a great help.

Naproxen, flurbiprofen and indomethacin can be given rectally.

Morphine is most useful and is a strong analgesic. It should be given in the smallest effective dose. Subsequently the dose can be increased. Sustained release oral preparations of morphine may be useful or morphine patches/epidural morphine can be given.

Antiemetic (prochlorperazine) can be given to prevent nausea and vomiting associated with morphine.

Headache due to increased intracranial tension responds to glucocorticosteroids.

Persistent cough in these patients responds to dimorphine.

For treating cardiac dyspnea morphine can be administered.

Bed sores should be prevented by rubbing alcohol.

Superinfections should be treated by appropriate antibiotics.

Mouth washes prevent the occurrence of stomatitis.

Anorexia may be helped by the use of prednisolone given in the dose of 15 to 30 mg daily.

Laxatives should be given to prevent constipation.

Autonomic Nervous system (ANS)

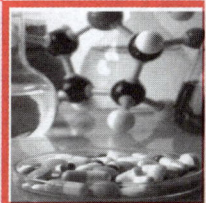

13

Autonomic Nervous System (ANS)

This system differs from the somatic system in following aspects.

(a) There is no voluntary control over this system hence the name **autonomic**. It functions below the level of consciousness. ANS controls visceral functions.

(b) On removal of the nervous connection the organs innervated by this system (heart, intestine, etc.) continue to show contractile activity while denervation of the skeletal muscle produces paralysis.

(c) Tissues innervated by ANS exhibit rhythmic movements.

ANS is composed of afferent as well as efferent nerves. The controlling centers are in medulla oblongata and the highest integration of ANS takes place in the hypothalamus.

Ganglion lies between pre-and postganglionic nerve on the efferent side.

The ANS consists of two divisions:

1. Sympathetic nervous system.
2. Parasympathetic nervous system.

Generally both sympathetic and parasympathetic nerves innervate an organ. Some organs, however, are supplied by only one system, e.g. parasympathetic nerves alone supply ciliary muscles of the eye, glands of stomach and pancreas.

Splenic blood vessels, hair follicles and sweat glands are supplied by only sympathetic system.

Parasympathetic nerves are of craniosacral origin (III, VII, IX and X cranial nerves carry parasympathetic fibers) while sympathetic nerves come from thoracolumbar region. **Adrenal gland is a sympathetic gland.**

The functions of the sympathetic system is to prepare the body for emergency. **Effects of stimulation of sympathetic nervous system are widespread while they are localised on the parasympathetic side.**

Transmission of the impulse across a synapse of neuroeffector junction is mediated through a chemical substance called **neurotransmitter**.

Noradrenaline and dopamine are transmitters on the sympathetic side. While acetylcholine is transmitter on parasympathetic side.

14

Parasympathomimetic or Cholinomimetic Agents

Acetylcholine is a neurotransmitter on the parasympathetic side. It is synthesised by cholinergic neurons. It is stored in vesicles from where it is released.

Acetylcholine is released at the following sites:

1. The preganglionic nerve endings of sympathetic and parasympathetic system.
2. At the postganglionic nerve endings of the parasympathetic nerves.
3. At the neuromuscular junction of the skeletal muscles.
4. At the postganglionic sympathetic nerves of sweat glands.
5. Nerve endings supplying adrenal medulla.
6. In certain regions of brain.

Sensory nerves in this system perform following functions:

(a) Mediate sensations from viscera (sensation of pain is not mediated through these nerves) to brain. Sensations from respiratory and cardiovascular system are relayed to brain.

(b) Rise in blood pressure or change in pH stimulates carotid sinus, carotid body and aortic arch. Impulses are carried by glossopharyngeal and vagus nerves and hypotension is produced reflexly.

Motor or efferent nerves of the parasympathetic system are contained in III, VII, IX and X cranial nerves and second, third and fourth sacral segments of spinal cord.

Cranial nerves supply: Eye (III nerve), lacrimal, submaxillary and sublingual salivary glands (VII and IX nerves) and visceral organs (X nerve).

Lower one-third of the gastrointestinal tract however is supplied by the sacral nerves. Rectum and sexual organs are also supplied by sacral nerves.

There are two types of cholinergic receptors:

(a) **Muscarine receptors:** M_1, M_2 and M_3
(b) **Nicotinic receptors:** N_m and N_n

Distribution of receptors

Nicotinic receptors are found in:

(a) Neuromuscular junctions of skeletal muscles N_m
(b) Ganglia of both sympathetic and parasympathetic systems N_n
(c) Certain areas of brain (N_n)

Muscarinic receptors are located in following regions:

1. In certain areas of brain (M_1)
2. In heart (M_2)
3. In abdominal viscera (stomach, intestine, ureters, urinary bladder, uterus) (M_3-muscles, sphincters and glands, M_1-motility)
4. In blood vessels (M_3 in muscle) — cholinergic blood nerves are missing.
5. Sweat glands
6. In eye-iris as well as ciliary muscles (M_3)
7. In bronchial musculature (M_3)
8. Salivary and lacrimal glands (M_3)
9. At presynaptic nerves endings — M_1 causes inhibition of ACh release while N_m increases release of ACh.

M_2 and M_1 are involved in regulation of sympathetic control.

Acetylcholine acts on both muscarinic as well as nicotinic receptors.

Stimulation of **muscarinic receptors** of parasympathetic system leads to following effects:

1. Eye: Pupilis get constricted and intraocular tension is reduced.
2. Heart: There is reduction in heart rate (bradycardia) and conduction of impulses in conducting tissue. The contractile strength of heart is also reduced. This leads to reduction in cardiac output and fall in blood pressure.
3. Exocrine glands: All secretions are increased.
4. Smooth muscles

   (a) Smooth muscles of the bronchi get contracted. A condition like asthma develops. In an already asthmatic patient these drugs may produce serious consequences.
   (b) Smooth muscles of the intestine are stimulated. In small concentrations there is increase in motility as well as tone, but in higher concentrations tone markedly increases and the motility is subsequently reduced. These drugs, therefore, can produce colicky pain.
   (c) Increase in secretions in the gut.
   (d) Stimulation of parasympathetic system produces contraction of ureter and urinary bladder resulting in micturition.
   (e) Central nervous system is initially stimulated and later depressed.

Stimulation of nicotinic receptors

(a) Skeletal muscles: Stimulation of nicotinic receptors (N_m) in skeletal muscles produces muscle contraction and twitchings.

(b) Ganglion: Stimulation N_n in ganglion leads to rise in blood pressure.

Acetylcholinesterase is an enzyme that destroys acetylcholine and shortens its lifespan.

Acetylcholine cannot be used therapeutically because:

(a) It has to be given intravenously to produce effects.
(b) It is short acting: actions last for 10–30 seconds.
(c) It produces stimulation of both muscarinic and nicotinic receptors.

CHOLINOMIMETIC DRUGS

Drugs that stimulate parasympathetic system are classified as follows:

Directly acting

(a) Esters of choline—carbachol, methacholine and urecholine

(b) Alkaloids—pilocarpine, muscarine and arecoline

Indirectly acting cholinomimetics or cholinesterase inhibitors or anticholinesterases

(a) Reversible type: Carbomates—physostigmine, neostigmine, pyridostigmine, demecarium and ambenonium.

(b) Irreversible type: Organophosphorus compounds—insecticides and war gases, oxotremorine, suman, sarin, parathion, malathion, ecothiophate.

Carbachol

Advantages

1. Carbachol is not destroyed by cholinesterase and is stable in the gut therefore it has long duration of action and can be given orally.
2. Its actions are more pronounced on intestine and urinary bladder.
3. It can be used in eye for causing pupillary constriction.
4. Does not cross BBB.

Disadvantages

1. It is very potent and very toxic. It should **never** be given intravenously.
2. It stimulates muscarinic as well as nicotinic receptors, therefore, has too many adverse reactions.

Adverse reactions

1. Sweating
2. Salivation and defecation.

Dose

1–4 mg orally
0.25–0.5 mg subcutaneously
0.75–3.0% solution for eye.

Uses

1. Atony of bladder.
2. Paralytic ileus.
3. Glaucoma–0.75–3.0% solution.

Bethanechol (Urecholine)

Advantages

1. It has predominant effects on gastrointestinal and urinary tracts.
2. It does not stimulate nicotinic receptors.
3. It is not destroyed by cholinesterases.

Uses

1. Treatment of acute postoperative and postpartum urinary retention.
2. Treatment of postoperative distension and postvagotomy gastric retention.

Dose: 10–30 mg orally.
2.5 to 5 mg subcutaneously.

Methacholine

Advantages

1. It is destroyed only by true cholinesterase and that too at a slower rate. Therefore, it has longer duration of action (but less than that of carbachol).
2. It acts mainly on muscarinic receptors, therefore, adverse reactions are less.
3. It can be given orally as well as subcutaneously.

Actions on cardiovascular system are more marked. Therefore, cardiac arrhythmia or even cardiac arrest may occur.

Uses: It was sued to control supraventricular paroxysmal tachycardia. Not clinically used for this purpose as better drugs are available.

All these agents should not be used in following conditions:

1. Hyperthyroidism
2. Bronchial asthma
3. Peptic ulcer
4. Myocardial infarction (to avoid development of hypotension and arrhythmias).

ALKALOIDS

Pilocarpine: This is an alkaloid derived from plants (pilocarpus microphyllus or pilocarpus jabarandi):

1. It has predominant effects on eye, sweat and salivary glands.
   (a) In the eye it produces constriction of pupils and lowers intraoccular tension.
   (b) It increases sweating and increases heat loss.
   (c) Salivary secretions are markedly increased.
2. It stimulates ganglion and unlike other cholinomimetic agents, it produces rise in blood pressure.
   It is very toxic and not given systematically.

Uses: Locally applied in eyes

   (i) to treat glaucoma — 0.5–5% aqueous solution is used.
   (ii) to treat toxicity of atropine and its substitutes
   (iii) to break adhesions between the lens and the iris
   (iv) Alzheimer's disease

Muscarine and arecoline are important only from **toxicological point**. Symptoms of toxicity due to muscarine (*Amanita muscaria*) resemble cholera. There is vomiting, diarrhoea and vasomotor collapse. In addition jaundice appears. Arecoline is an alkaloid obtained from betel nut. It serves no therapeutic purpose.

Poisoning due to muscarine is treated by:

(a) Correcting fluid and electrolyte imbalance.

(b) Atropine injection reverses all its ill effects.

ANTICHOLINESTERASES

Anticholinesterases inhibit the enzymes (cholinesterases) which destroy acetylcholine in the body. Through this mechanism they preserve acetylcholine which shows its effects.

Cholinesterases are of two types:

(a) acetylcholinesterase (true), and

(b) butarylcholinesterase (pseudo).

True cholinesterase is present in cholinergic neurons and synapses and at neuromuscular junctions. It causes rapid destruction of acetylcholine and is more active against physostigmine but less active against organophosphorus compounds.

Pseudocholinesterase is found in serum and is more active against organophosphorus compounds.

Inhibition of these enzymes can be reversible or irreversible.

Reversible type of inhibition of cholinesterase is produced by **neostigmine, physostigmine, edrophonium** and **ambenonium**.

Physostigmine: It is an alkaloid obtained from plant called *Physostigma venenosum*.

1. It effectively crosses the conjunctival barrier and produces miosis and reduction in intraocular tension.

2. It increases skeletal muscle tone so is used in myasthenia gravis.

3. It counters toxicity of atropine and atropine substitutes and is used to treat poisoning due to these drugs.

4. It is used to treat toxicity of antidepressant drugs.

Precaution: Aqueous solution of physostigmine should be freshly prepared as it deteriorates on standing.

Neostigmine

1. It resembles physostigmine but has predominant direct effect on skeletal muscles (N_m receptors). It increases tone of skeletal muscles by preserving acetylcholine and also by a direct action of muscle. **It is the drug of choice in myasthenia gravis.**

2. Effects on cardiovascular system and gastrointestinal system are same as with other cholinomimetic agents.

It does not affect central nervous system.

Uses

1. Myasthenia gravis — 15–30 mg three or four times daily (orally) or 0.5 to 20 mg subcutaneously.

2. For treatment of glaucoma 0.1–1.0 of % aqueous solution.

3. It is used as an antidote for reversal of curare induced skeletal paralysis.

Pyridostigmine: Has effects like neostigmine but has slower onset and longer duration of action and is used for treating myasthenia gravis.

Edrophonium: It resembles neostigmine in pharmacological actions, but has very short duration of action.

Uses

1. For diagnosis of myasthenia gravis.
2. For differentiation between cholinergic and myasthenic crisis.
3. For evaluation of response to drug regimens for myasthenia gravis.

Benzpyrinium: It is used to treat postoperative paralytic ileus and urinary retention.

Demecarium: Used as long acting miotic (which cause pupillary constriction) in treatment of glaucoma and convergent strabismus.

Disadvantages

1. Intense contraction of ciliary muscles produces headache.
2. Moment to moment control of intraocular tension is not possible. There are peaks and valleys in intraocular tension which are not desired.
3. Tends to produce cataract.

Irreversible inhibitors of cholinesterase —Ecothiophate, isoflourophate and organophosphorus compounds

Ecothiophate is non-lipid soluble.
It is used as long acting miotic.

Organophosphorus Compounds: Parathion, malathion, mipafox, masidox, sumithion (TIK–20) and dyflos are used as **insecticides**. These drugs (diazone) exist in inactive form and are activated in the body through metabolism. Insects with higher rate of metabolism are more sensitive to their effect than man.

Soman, tabu, sarin are also used as **war gases** (chemical war fare).

Poisoning by organophosphorus compounds is quite common in agriculture persons involved in spraying of insecticides. These drugs are often consumed for suicidal purposes (baygon, flit, etc.).

Symptoms of poisoning: Patient develops nausea, anorexia and mental confusion.

Vomiting, colicky pain in abdomen, sweating and excess salivation follow later. Pupils are constricted. There is twitching of skeletal muscles and convulsions. Breathing becomes difficult (asthma type). Respiratory depression, cardiovascular collapse and coma develop subsequently.

ENZYME REACTIVATORS

There are certain drugs (**oximes**) which can reactivate cholinesterases. These drugs have been developed to counter toxicity of cholinesterase inhibitors (organophosphorus compounds).

Limitations of these drugs

1. These agents are **effective only if given in the early stages** of poisoning.
2. These agents can counter skeletal muscle paralysis but not muscarinic effects of organophosphorus compounds. Therefore, atropine must be given along with these agents.

Few oximes that are available for clinical use are—pralidoxime and MINA, DAM and obedoxime.

ADRs: Tachycardia and hypotension, drowsiness.

Treatment of organophosphorus poisoning and nursing care

1. Patient should be removed from the contaminated atmosphere and given bath with sodium bicarbonate solution.
2. Nurse patient in prone position and clear respiratory passages and intubate.
3. Perform gastric lavage (if drug has been taken orally).
4. Artificial respiration should be started.
5. Atropine (2.0 mg) is given intramuscularly or intravenously at once and repeated every 15 minutes till the patient recovers or has dilatation of pupils and absence of rales.
6. Cholinesterase reactivator: Pralidoxime (1–2 g) is given intravenously and repeated depending upon the condition of the patient. In severe cases initial dose is 2.0 gm.
   DAM—1 gm IV slowly (20 mg of minute) can be repeated after 20 minutes.
   Obedoxime: It is more potent then pralidoxime—3–6 mg/kg is given IV and repeated every 20 mins.
7. Diazepam is given to control convulsions.
8. Fluids are given if the patient is dehydrated.
9. Treat shock and give prophylactic antibiotics.
10. Patient to be monitored for 2–4 weeks as delayed toxicity can manifest.

15

Clinical Situations where Cholinomimetics are used

TREATMENT OF MYASTHENIA GRAVIS

Myasthenia gravis is characterised by weakness of the skeletal muscles. The muscle tone as well as power of contraction are reduced.

1. Neostigmine is the drug of choice. It acts by increasing acetylcholine at the neuromuscular junction and also by directly stimulating the muscle (15 mg every 6 hours).
2. Pyridostigmine, physostigmine are also useful.
3. Ephedrine and potassium chloride are used as adjuvants.
4. Germine diacetate has been tried. It is veratrum alkaloid but does not produce hypotension or vomiting.
5. Prednisolone (10 mg/kg/day) is given if the above fail.
6. Immunosuppressants (azathioprine, cyclosporine) plasmaphoresis as adjunct have also been tried and found effective in a few patients.

Nursing care of myasthenia patient

1. Parasympathomimetics should be given before meals.
2. Watch patients for respiratory distress. Prompt action needs to be taken in the case of respiratory tract obstruction.
3. Administer these drugs at regular intervals (2–4 hours). Sustained releasing preparations can be given less frequently. Patient should be woken up at night and the drugs administered.
4. Inform patients about the adverse reactions of these drugs. Educate them about handling these reactions.
5. These patients should be advised not to take drugs that relax muscles such as amikacin, gentamycin, kanamycin, neomycin, streptomycin, tobramycin and pancuronium.

DRUGS USED IN GLAUCOMA

Glaucoma is a condition associated with increased intraocular tension. It may also be congenital. It can be of the following types:

(a) Primary
(b) Secondary

Primary glaucoma can be of two types:

(a) Narrow angle (acute congestive glaucoma)

(b) Wide angle (chronic simple glaucoma).

Treatment of the secondary glaucoma needs treating the cause.

Drugs used in Acute Glaucoma: Pilocarpine nitrate (4%) with physostigmine (0.5%) every 10 minutes can be combined with mannitol (20%) or glycerol (10%) IV infusion.

Acetazolamide (0.5 gm) orally reduces tension. Surgery needs to be done.

Drugs used in Chronic Simple Glaucoma: Drugs increasing outflow of aqueous humor.

(a) 1% physostigmine and 4% pilocarpine — these are instilled into the eye every 10 minutes for one hour. Demecarium (0.125–0.25%), ecothiophate (0.03–0.25%) can also be used.

(b) Prostaglandin analogues — latanoprost (0.005%).

Drugs reducing production of aqueous humor:

(a) Nonselective beta-adrenergic blocker–timolol (0.5%).

(b) Selective β-blockers–betaxolol (0.5% twice daily).

(c) Adrenaline (0.1–2.0%).

(d) Selective α_2 agonists.

  (i) Apraclonidine.

  (ii) Brumonidine 0.2%.

(e) Thymoxamine is given.

Combination of anticholinesterase with sympathomimetic agent is most effective.

Long-term use of long acting anticholinesterases produce lenticular opacities.

Timolol a non-selective beta blocker without membrane stabilising activity, is long acting. It reduces intraocular tension by reducing formation of aqueous humor. It does not affect pupillary size, tone of ciliary muscles or outflow of humor.

Propranolol is not used as it predisposes to corneal damage.

16

Parasympatholytics or Cholinergic Blocking Drugs

The parasympathetic blocking agents comprise atropine and hyoscine and their synthetic and semisynthetic substitutes.

Atropine an alkaloid is derived from plant Atropa belladona.

Hyoscine (scopolamine) is obtained from Hyoscymus niger and Datura stramonium.

These drugs block muscarinic receptors and classified as follows:

1. Natural alkaloids — atropine and hyoscine

2. Semisynthetic and synthetic derivatives which are used for application in the eye (for refraction)
   - (a) Homatropine
   - (b) Eucatropine
   - (c) Tropicamide
   - (d) Cyclopentolate

3. Synthetic and semisynthetic preparations used for relieving smooth muscle spasm.
   - (a) Atropine methonitrate
   - (b) Methscopolamine bromide
   - (c) Methantheline
   - (d) Propantheline
   - (e) Oxyphenonium
   - (f) Adephenine hydrochloride

4. Used in treating Parkinsonism
   - (a) Benzhexol
   - (b) Cyrcimine hydrochloride
   - (c) Procyclidine hydrochloride
   - (d) Biperiden hydrochloride
   - (e) Benztropine mesylate

Atropine (as prototype)

It blocks muscarinic receptors at therapeutic doses. At very high doses it can block nicotinic receptors.

Pharmacological Actions

1. Smooth muscles of the intestinal tract and the bronchi are relaxed.

2. Reduces secretions of exocrine glands, e.g. tears, salivary, bronchial, intestinal and sweat.
   Does not have profound effect on the pancreatic secretions. Secretion of milk is not affected.

3. Heart rate may be initially reduced but later increased with atropine and other drugs of this group.

4. Central nervous system as well as respiratory center are stimulated by small doses of atropine but larger doses depress it. Hyoscine depresses CNS in all doses.

5. Pupils are dilated and the eye is focused for far vision. **Intraocular tension is raised**. Produce loss of light reflex.

Uses of Atropine

1. To relieve colicky pain of the biliary, urinary and intestinal tracts—it is given along with pethidine or morphine. Atropine is preferred in very acute state but tincture belladona is also effective.
2. In eye it is used:
   (a) To produce mydriasis for fundoscopy and refraction studies.
   (b) Alternatively given with miotic for breaking adhesions between the lens and the iris.
   (c) For treating acute iritis, iridocyclitis and keratitis.
3. Few patients of dysmenorrhoea benefit from atropine
4. In treatment of organophosphorus and carbamate poisoning atropine is given to counter muscarinic activity
5. For treating Parkinsonism.
6. AV block due to excessive vagal activity.

Adverse Reactions

1. Dryness of mouth and constipation.
2. Blurred visions with mydriasis.
3. Hyperpyrexia associated with dry skin.
4. Excitement or delirium both are possible.
5. Retention of urine.
6. Precipitation of glaucoma.

Treatment of Poisoning due to Atropine: It is treated by giving physostigmine (1–4 mg intravenously) and diazepam (for controlling convulsions and excitement).

HYOSCINE

This alkaloid has two prominent effects
1. Secretions of exocrine glands are markedly reduced.
2. It produces sedation and inhibits vomiting due to motion sickness.

It was used as preanaesthetic medication and as lie detector.

Nursing care

Atropine is highly potent and toxic substance
1. Press the tear duct while instilling atropine eye drops.
2. Any behavioural change following atropine instillation should be treated as atropine toxicity.
3. Patient should be informed about blurring of vision and photophobia following atropine. Change of glasses does not necessarily eliminate this problem.
4. Inform patient about adverse reactions namely constipation and difficulty in passing urine. He can avoid these two symptoms by taking laxatives and excess fluids respectively.

Atropine administration should be avoided in patients
(a) over 40 years of age   (b) of acute asthma
(c) with enlarged prostate

PARASYMPATHOLYTICS USED IN EYE

Homatropine: It produces both cycloplegia and pupillary dilatation.

The effect is short lasting hence preferred.
2–5% solution is used.
Onset 45–60 min; duration 3–6 hours.

Cyclopentolate — onset 30–60 mins duration–24 hours, is useful in children.

Tropicamide — onset 20–40 mins, duration 3–6 hours — it is quickest acting with shortest duration, it causes both mydriasis and cycloplegics.

Atropine: It is potent mydriatic and cycloplegic (loss of accommodation) but has slow onset of action (30 min–1 hr) and very long duration of action (7–10 days). 1% ointment is used. It is mydriatic of choice in children. Causes increase in intraocular pressure therefore avoided in elderly.

DRUGS USED AS SPASMOLYTICS

Atropine Methonitrate: It can be given orally (dose–0.2 to 0.4 mg/4–6 times daily).

Uses: To treat congenital hypertropic pyloric stenosis.

Methscopolamine: It does not produce adverse reactions associated with central nervous system.
Uses

1. To treat renal colic.
2. To treat frequency of micturition associated with cystitis.
3. In treating peptic ulcer.

Dose: 2.5 mg orally three times a day.

Methantheline (Banthine)

1. It has higher selectivity, greater effect on gastrointestinal tract than on other systems.
2. Its duration of action is longer than that of atropine.

Adverse reactions: It may produce urinary retention, postural hypotension, impotency and acute psychosis.

Dose: 50–100 mg orally or 15–25 mg intramuscularly.

Propantheline (Probanthine): It resembles methantheline in its actions but is more potent.

Uses

1. To treat diarrhea associated with irritable bowel syndrome.
2. To treat pain due to diverticulitis and peptic ulcer.

Adiphenine: This drug is a powerful smooth muscle relaxant.

Uses

1. Spastic colon
2. Biliary colic
3. Dysmenorrhoea

Ipratropium bromide is used in chronic obstructive pulmonary disease (asthma) with accumulation of secretions. It is given by inhaler.

17

Clinical Situations where Parasympatholytics are used

Parasympatholytics used in treating:

1. **GIT diseases:** Peptic ulcer—pirenzepine (M1 blocker).
   Hypermotility syndrome for symptomatic—relief belladona tincture.

2. **Cholinergic poisoning**—atropine.

3. **For respiratory disorders**
   (a) As preanaesthetic medication—to dry up secretions—atropine and glycopyrolate.
   (b) In chronic obstructive pulmonary disease and asthma—ipatropium bromide inhalation.

4. **Cardiovascular disorders**
   (a) Reflex bradycardia after M1 (inferior block).
   (b) Hyperactive carotid sinus reflexes.
   (c) Idiopathic dilated cardiomyopathy.

DRUGS USED IN TREATMENT OF PARKINSONISM

Parkinsonism is characterised by tremors of the hands, rigidity of muscles and mask like face. These patients lose facial expressions because the muscles of the face become too rigid. In advanced state of the disease there is rigidity in walking. These patients have suffling gait and they have increased salivation.

Parkinsonism is a disease of basal ganglion, here there are two systems which balance each other, cholinergic system is stimulatory while dopaminergic system is inhibitory. Parkinsonism can result due to over activity of cholinergic system or under activity of dopaminergic system. **Treatment therefore lies in either giving anticholinergic agents or/and dopaminergic agonists.**

Treatment with drugs is aimed at reducing rigidity of the muscles and muscle tremors. It is unwise to start treatment until it is absolutely necessary as:

(i) Some patients do well even without drugs.
(ii) Drugs used in this condition have many serious adverse reactions.
(iii) Patients become refractory to treatment after some time.

I. DOPAMINE ENHANCING DRUGS

Levodopa: Levodopa is a precursor of dopamine and in the body it is converted to dopamine. **Akinesia, rigidity and tremors all are reduced** by this agent. Most of the patients (66%) respond to this drug.

Disadvantages

1. It has cardiac toxicity (arrhythmias).
2. It is ineffective in drug induced Parkinsonism.
3. It takes 4–8 weeks to produce effect.

Adverse reactions

1. Nausea, vomiting and anorexia.
2. Hypotension and cardiac irregularities.
3. Involuntary movements of limbs are produced.
4. Late toxicity
   (a) Behavioural toxicity—confusion and depression suicidal tendencies are produced.
   (b) Blood urea nitrogen and SGOT increase.
5. Tolerance develops to good effects.

Addition of decarboxylase inhibitors **carbidopa and benzerazide** to levodopa helps:

(a) In increasing efficacy.
(b) In better control of symptoms.
(c) Required dose of levodopa is reduced by 75%.
(d) Reducing adverse reactions (cardiac effects are prevented).

Precautions

1. This drug should not be given to patients already suffering from cardiac diseases or use with caution.
2. Reserpine, phenothiazines and vitamin B_6 should not be given along with this drug as these reduce its efficacy.

Tolcapone: It inhibits COMT and preserves levodopa thereby increasing its duration of action. It is given in combination with levodopa.

Bromoergocriptine: It is effective in parkinsonism. Its actions are similar to levodopa but is slower acting.

Ropinirole: It is well absorbed when given orally its actions are similar to bromocriptine but acts faster and causes less nausea. However, some patients develop sleep disorders.

Pramipaxole: Same effects like ropinirole.

Pergolide is also used to treat Parkinsonism. It is more potent than bromocriptine.

Adverse drug reactions

- Orthostatic hypotension
- Hallucinations
- Pleuropulmonary and retroperitoneal fibrosis
- Nausea, vomiting and hypotension

Selegiline (Deprenyl): It is MAO-B inhibitor. It inhibits metabolism of dopamine and increases dopamine. It is used in combination with levodopa. It reduces end off dose-wearing effect.

Apomorphine: Not used commonly as it causes renal damage.

Amantadine: This is an anti-viral agent. It is now used as an adjunct in Parkinoson's disease.

Dose: 100 mg once or twice daily.

It is less effective than levodopa.

II. ANTICHOLINERGIC DRUGS

These agents oppose the action of acetylcholine. They reduce tremors, salivation and to lesser extent reduce rigidity.

Atropine: This is given orally, often patients develop tolerance to this drug and there is a need to increase its dose frequently. Blurring of vision, photophobia and urinary retention often disturb the patient.

Dose: 0.5 mg twice or thrice daily.

Benzhexol Hydrochloride (Pacitane): This drug controls all symptoms (muscular rigidity, tremors, sialorrhoea and seborrhoea). In addition it induces euphoria in these patients. It has atropine like effects. It does not improve bradykinesia and loss of postural reflexes.

Advantages

1. It is free of serious adverse reactions.
2. It is well absorbed and rapidly disappears from tissues.
3. It can be used even in presence of hypertension and cardiac diseases.
4. It is useful in drug induced and postencephaletic Parkinsonism.

Adverse reactions: Like atropine it produces blurred vision, nausea, dizziness and restlessness. It precipitates urinary retention.

Dose: Initial dose is 1–2 mg/day. This can be increased to 10–30 mg/day.

Benztropine, procyclidine, orphenadrine and ethopropazine are other drugs used in Parkinsonism. These drugs have actions similar to benzhexol hydrochloride.

Drugs likely to produce Parkinsonism like syndrome.

Certain drugs Phenothiazines, butyrophenones, thioxanthines, reserpine, methyldopa can precipitate/produce Parkinsonism.

These drugs should be avoided in therapeutics or their use should be minimised.

Drugs used in treatment of bladder spasm—oxybutynin (H_3 blocker).

Drugs used in urinary incontinence—oxybutynin, totterodine and imipramine.

18

Sympathomimetic Agents

The actions produced by these drugs resemble the actions produced by stimulation of sympathetic (adrenergic) system.

Noradrenaline is the main neurotransmitter of this system. Adrenaline is a **neurohormone**. Tyrosine and dopamine are the other important neurotransmitters of this system. These neurotransmitters are catechol derivatives and are called **chatecholamines**.

There are two types of adrenergic receptors namely alpha and beta. Each of these receptors has sub types: α_1, and α_2, β_1, β_2 and β_3.

Alpha receptors are predominantly present in the smooth muscles of the blood vessels (arterioles) and are of three types α_{1a}, α_{1b}, α_{1c}, α_1 receptors are post junctional while α_2 are prejunctional on nerve endings, postjunctional in brain, pancreas and heart.

β_1 receptors are present in heart, β_2 in bronchi, blood vessels and uterus. β_3 are present in adipose tissues.

Synthesis of dopamine, adrenaline (epinephrine) and noradrenaline (norepinephrine)

$$Phenylalanine \rightarrow Tyrosine \rightarrow Dopamine \rightarrow Adrenaline \rightarrow Noradrenaline$$

Adrenaline is formed only in adrenal medulla. Adrenaline (epinephrine) is a methylated noradrenaline. It is the main hormone of the adrenal medulla. It is released from the medulla into the blood steam and acts on tissues away from the site of its release hence, it is called neuro hormone.

Noradrenaline (norepinephrine) is the main transmitter at the postganglionic sympathetic nerve endings. Small amount of this agent is also released from adrenal medulla. Dopamine is a precursor of noradrenaline.

Important sympathomimetic drugs which do not occur naturally in the human body are isoprenaline (isoproterenol), ephedrine, phenylephrine, amphetamine, salbutamol, terbutaline and isoxsuprine.

Pharmacological actions of catecholamines (dopamine, adrenaline and noradrenaline):

Adrenaline acts on both alpha and beta receptors

Noradrenaline acts on alpha receptors all over the body and β_1 receptors of the heart.

Dopamine acts on presynaptic β receptors and causes release of noradrenaline. In addition it acts on D_1, D_2, D_3 and D_4 receptors.

1. **Heart:** Intravenous administration of these drugs produces increase in heart rate, increase in excitability, conductivity and contractility. In small concentrations these drugs produce increase in cardiac output and systolic blood pressure.

   There is tendency to produce arrhythmia including ventricular tachycardia and fibrillation.

   These drugs increase oxygen demand by the myocardium, therefore, they may precipitate angina and myocardial ischaemia.

2. **Blood pressure**

   (a) Systolic blood pressure is raised by both adrenaline and noradrenaline.

   (b) Adrenaline produces a fall in diastolic blood pressure while noradrenaline raises it. Therefore, **adrenaline cannot be used to raise diastolic pressure.**

   (c) Blood vessels in skeletal muscles are dialated by adrenaline but constricted by noradrenaline.

   (d) Blood vessels of skin and abdominal viscera are constricted by both these drugs.

   (e) Dopamine increases systolic pressure and pulse pressure. Diastolic pressure remains unchanged or is slightly increased, cardiac output is increased. **Blood flow to kidneys glomerular filtrate and sodium excretion are increased** while both adrenaline and noradrenaline reduce tissue perfusion.

3. **Smooth muscles** of the intestine and urinary bladder are relaxed by adrenaline as well as noradrenaline. **Bronchial smooth muscles are relaxed by adrenaline but not by noradrenaline.** Detrusor muscle is relaxed but sphincter is constricted. This helps in increasing holding capacity of bladder.

4. Adrenaline (noradrenaline) increases the break down of glycogen to glucose but noradrenaline has no such effect.

Uses

1. **Adrenaline** is useful in asthma and anaphylactic shock and for cardiac resuscitation. Noradrenaline is used to raise blood pressure.

2. Both are used along with local anaesthetics and are applied on skin and mucus membranes to control bleeding from arterioles and capillaries.

3. Adrenaline is also used (as 2% solution) in open angle glaucoma.

4. Adrenaline used in cardiac arrest.

Adverse reactions

1. Ventricular arrhythmias.

2. Subarachnoid haemorrhage.

3. Pulmonary oedema.

4. Blood sugar is increased.

5. CNS stimulation (anxiety, tremors and subjective feelings of fearfulness is produced).

Dose

(i) For local application: Adrenaline is used in concentrations of 1:20,000 to 1:10,000.

(ii) 2% solution of adrenaline is used for glaucoma.

(iii) For asthma 0.2 to 0.5 ml of 1:1000 solution of adrenaline can be given subcutaneously. 1% solution is given by inhalation.

(iv) For cardiac resuscitation 0.2 to 0.3 ml of 1:1000 solution of adrenaline is given. Injection is made directly into the heart.

(v) For anaphylactic reaction: Please refer **Anaphylaxis**

(vi) Noradrenaline when used for raising blood pressure is given inravenously as infusion. Usual dose range is 2–4 ug/minute.

Precautions and nursing care during administration of adrenaline and noradrenaline

1. Adrenaline tends to get oxidised and turns pink. Any solution of adrenaline that is pink should not be administrated.
2. Before injecting adrenaline subcutaneously in asthmatic patient you must be certain that the needle of the syringe is not in vein.
3. If these drugs are being given intravenously (as in anaphylactic reaction, etc.) patient should never be left unattended.
4. The site of infusion should be changed every 12 hours.
5. Check for any extravasation of these drugs as they are liable to cause necrosis.
6. These drugs should be avoided in patients who have received isoproterenol or certain anaesthetics (halothane, trichlorethylene, etc.).
7. Blood pressure should be checked every 15 minutes.
8. Infusion of these drugs should not be stopped abruptly as severe hypotension is precipitated.
9. Patient with myocardial infarction, thyrotoxicosis and hypertension show greater sensitivity to these drugs.
10. Repeated use of adrenaline in asthma produces resistance.
11. Subcutaneous injection of adrenaline in asthma should be made very slowly.
12. Hypovolemia and acidosis cause refractoriness to the hypertensive effect of these drugs. These conditions should be corrected before the drugs are declared ineffective.

Dopamine: It acts on alpha, beta as well as dopamine receptors (D_1, D_2, D_3 and D_4). In low to moderate doses:

1. It increases contraction of the heart but has little effect on the heart rate and therefore is less likely to produce arrhythmia.
2. It does not reduce blood supply to kidneys and the abdominal viscera as it dilates renal blood vessels and **improves renal** functioning. It can therefore, be used in shock.
3. It does not reach brain in large amounts.

It is ineffective by oral route.

Higher doses act on α receptors and cause increase in BP, these should be avoided.

Adverse reactions

1. Nausea and vomiting
2. Anginal pain in the susceptible individuals
3. Leakage of this drug outside veins causes sloughing.

Use: It is the drug of choice in management of shock.

Dose: Infusion of dopamine should go at the rate 0.5 to 1.0 mg/kg/minute.

Precautions

1. Solution of dopamine is unstable in alkaline medium. It should therefore **be given in saline or dextrose**. Even in these solutions, it lasts for 24 hours only.

2. Leakage of this drug in the subcutaneous tissue should be avoided as it causes necrosis and gangrene.

Dobutamine: This drug resembles dopamine. It has positive inotropic effect.

Does not change peripheral resistance.

Does not act on D_1 receptors.

Acts on β receptors.

Does not cause release of noradrenaline.

It is found to be **useful in low output cardiac failure and acute heart failure not associated with hypertension.**

Dose: 2.5–10 mcg/kg/min IV infusion

Isopropyl-noradrenaline (Isoprenaline): It is the most potent stimulator of beta receptors. Its main effects are on heart, and bronchial smooth muscles ($\beta_1 + \beta_2$). It can be given sublingually and also by inhalation (in asthma) which helps in reducing toxicity. It has been replaced by selective β_2 agonists (salbutamol).

Ephedrine: It is an alkaloid derived from plant Ephedra. It causes awakening and relaxes urinary bladder and bronchial smooth muscles. It can be given orally and effects are long lasting.

Uses

1. As nasal drops in nasal congestion.
2. It is given to prevent asthmatic attack and treat mild attack. Hence, was given in between the acute attacks.
3. It is given to children at night to prevent bed wetting.
4. It is also useful in myasthenia gravis and is given along with other drugs.
5. It is used to treat narcolepsy.

Dose: 30–60 mg/three times a day.

Precautions: Last dose should not be given after 5 p.m.

Adverse reactions

1. Insomnia (sleeplessness).
2. Tremors and psychotic symptoms.
3. Difficulty in micturition.
4. Tachycardia.

Amphetamine (Benzedrine): It has predominant effects on the central nervous system.

(a) Produces euphoria (feeling of happiness).

(b) Causes postponement of sleep—it is abused by medical and paramedical students for this effect.

(c) Suppresses appetite—this effect is short lasting.

(d) Reduces the feeling of fatigue. It is for this effect that it is taken by athletes.

(e) Possesses weak anticonvulsant activity.

Uses

1. Narcolepsy.
2. It is added to barbiturates in the treatment of epilepsy (it counters the sleep produced by barbiturates but does not counter its antiepileptic effect.)
3. It is used in treating hyperkinetic syndrome in children.

Cautions

1. This drug should not be used as better drugs are available and as it tends to produce habituation.
2. It should not be used to induce wakefulness as it hampers with judgement and intellectual work.

Phenylephrine: It acts only on alpha receptors.

It resembles noradrenaline in actions but has longer duration of action.

Uses

1. It is used to dilate pupils.
2. It reduces intraocular tension and is used in glaucoma.
3. It is used as nasal decongestant.

CLINICAL SITUATIONS WHERE SYMPATHOMIMETICS ARE USED

1. **Pressor agents:** Noradrenaline, adrenaline, dopamine, mephenteramine.
2. **Cardiac stimulants:** Adrenaline, isoprenaline, ephedrine, dobutamine.
3. **Nasal decongestants:** Ephedrine, pseudoephedrine, xylometazoline, oxymetazoline and naphazoline.
4. **Bronchodilators:** Salbutamol, terbutaline, salmetrol, retodrine and isoetharine.
5. **Anorectics:** Fenfluramine, dexfenfluramine, mazindol.
6. **CNS stimulants:** Ephedrine, amphetamine, methamphetamine.
7. **Uterine relaxants and vasodilators:** Isoxsuprine, salbutamol, terbutaline.

NASAL DECONGESTANTS

Congestion of the nose occurs due to dilatation of vessels in the nasal mucosa. Drugs on instillation cause α_1 receptor stimulation leading to vasoconstriction which relieves nasal congestion.

Drugs in this group are **xylometazoline, oxymetazoline, nafazoline and ephedrine.**

Advantages

1. Small children (infants) cannot suck milk if their nose is blocked. These drugs are helpful in relieving this problem.
2. The action is restricted to nose.

Disadvantages

1. Overuse of these drugs may cause damage to nasal mucosa.
2. If care is not exercised then few of these drugs may get absorbed from nasal mucosa producing central effects.

Ephedrine is the best drug for nasal decongestion because it:

(i) is highly effective

(ii) is cheap and

(iii) stimulates central nervous system.

Nursing care

Press medial canthus to stop the drug from entering into nose.

DRUGS USED IN ASTHMA

Salbutamol, terbutaline, salmetrol and fenoterol. All these drugs are specific β_2 stimulants and cause bronchodilation.

Advantages

1. All these drugs have greater effect on β_2 receptors in lungs than β_1 receptors in the heart. Thus, these drugs produce bronchodilation without causing tachycardia. Due to this selectivity of action the adverse effects associated with heart are reduced.

2. These drugs have longer lasting action. Repeated dosing is not required.

3. Most of these drugs can be given by various routes to suit the convenience of the patient.

Salbutamol: Can be given orally as well as through inhaler. Dose is 2 mg three times daily.

Terbutaline: 4–5 mg three times a day.

Salmetrol: It is longer acting (effect lasts for 12 hours) other long acting drugs are—formetrol, fenoterol pirbuterol and reprotelol.

Uses

1. For prevention and treatment of asthma

2. To prevent premature labour.

Drugs used to suppress appetite: Amphetamine, phenylpropanolamine and fenfluramine.

These drugs suppress appetite but are linked with serious adverse events, e.g. phenylpropanolamine produces severe hypertension and increased risk of strokes.

Fenfluramine causes suicidal tendencies.

Amphetamine is habit forming.

DRUGS USED IN PERIPHERAL VASCULAR DISEASES AND PREVENTION OF PREMATURE LABOUR

Nylidrine and isoxsuprine hydrochloride have predominant effect on the β_2 receptors. These drugs are used to dilate blood vessels in peripheral vascular diseases and to prevent premature labour.

Isoxsuprine (Duvidilan): Causes uterine relaxation and is used in treatment of dysmenorrhoea, threatened abortion, premature labour and peripheral vascular diseases.

Adverse reactions: Nausea and vomiting, palipitation, nervousness and trembling.

Drugs elevating mood: Methylphenidate, amphetamine and pemoline.

All these drugs are habit forming and have abuse potential.

SELECTIVE α₂ AGONISTS

Clonidine, apraclonidine, alpha methyldopa and guanfecine. These drugs inhibit release of catecholamines and are used to treat hypertension and increased intracranial pressure.

Clonidine: Stimulates α_2 receptors in brain and causes fall in cardiac output and BP hence is given to treat hypertension. It produces sedation and hypothermia.

Uses

1. For treatment of moderate hypertension
2. For prophylaxis of migraine
3. In the treatment of withdrawal symptoms of alcohol, opioids and barbiturates.

Adverse reactions

1. CNS: drowsiness, depression, and headache
2. Dry mouth, nasal stuffiness and constipation
3. Rebound hypertension is produced if stopped suddenly.

Apraclonidine is used to lower intraocular tension.

Alpha Methyldopa: After entering brain it is converted to its active metabolites namely alpha methyl dopamine and alpha methyl noradrenaline which stimulate α_2 receptors in the brain and produce effects like clonidine.

Adverse effects

1. CNS: drowsiness, depression and headache.
2. Dry mouth, nasal stuffiness and constipation.
3. Thrombocytopenia.

Use: To treat hypertension.

19

Sympathetic Blocking Drugs

These drugs block the responses of sympathetic stimulation. There are three types of these drugs:
1. Alpha receptor blocking agents.
2. Beta receptor blocking agents.
3. Alpha and beta receptor blocking agents.

ALPHA RECEPTOR BLOCKERS

Following are alpha receptor blocking agents:
(a) Phenoxybenzamine (dibenzyline).
(b) Ergot alkaloids.
(c) Tolazoline and phentolamine.
(d) Yohimbine, piperoxen and azeptine.

α_1 selective blockers: Prazosin, terazosin, dexozosin and alfluzesin and urapidal.

α_2 selective blockers: Yohimbine, prostadil.

Phenoxybenzamine (Dibenzyline)

This drug produces irreversible blockage of all alpha receptors.
1. Produces fall in blood pressure.
2. Prevents cardiac arrhythmias produced by adrenaline and similar drugs.

Advantages

1. It is highly effective.
2. The action is long lasting therefore used in chronic cases not responding to other drugs.

Disadvantages

1. Onset of action is delayed.
2. Accumulates in the body.

Adverse reactions

1. Lethargy or fatigue.
2. Nausea and vomiting.
3. Nasal stuffiness and failure of ejaculation (impotency) are produced.

Ergot Alkaloids: These alkaloids are obtained from fungus. These are not used for their alpha blocking effects, but are used for treatment of migraine and for producing contraction of uterus after delivery.

Priscoline and Phentolamine: These drugs produce

(a) Arteriolar dilatation with resultant fall in blood pressure
(b) Increase in force of contraction of the heart and tachycardia (reflex actions)
(c) Increase in secretions of stomach and salivary glands.

Adverse reactions

1. Diarrhea
2. Postural hypotension
3. Excessive sweating
4. May aggrevate peptic ulcer
5. Failure of ejaculation and nasal stuffiness.

Uses: These drugs are used in peripheral vascular diseases and in the diagnosis of pheochromocytoma.

Dose: Tolazoline: 50 mg 2 to 4 times a day and phentolamine—5 mg lM.

Azeptine: It produces dilatation of blood vessels by blocking alpha receptors and also causes direct relaxation of vessels.

Adverse reactions

1. Nasal congestion.
2. Precipitation of peptic ulcer.

Prazosin: It blocks α_1 receptors selectively and dilates arteries and veins. Produce severe hypotension when given for the first time (first dose effect). It reduces tone of internal sphincter of bladder and is used to improve urinary outflow in benign prostatic enlargement. It does not **cause tachycardia.**

Doxazosin, Afluzosin, Terazosin: Actions same as prazosin but effects lasts longer:

Tamulosin acts specifically on prostatic α_{1c} adrenergic receptors.

BETA RECEPTOR BLOCKING AGENTS

(A) **Nonselective ($\beta_1 + \alpha_2$) blockers:**
(a) Beta blockers with intrinsic activity—propranolol.
(b) Without intrinsic sympathomimetic activity: nadolol, timolol.
(c) With intrinsic sympathomimetic activity: (partial activity)—pendolol, oxprenolol and alprenolol.

(B) **Selective β_1 blockers:** Metoprolol, atenolol, acebutalol, besoprolol, esmolol, betaxolol.

(C) **Selective β_2 blocker:** Butoxamine.

Drugs which are commonly used from this group are:
Propranolol, metoprolol, atenolol, acebutolol and timolol.

Propranolol: It blocks both β_1 and β_2 receptors. In addition it **possesses local anaesthetic activity**. This latter activity is exerted only in high doses and contributes to certain effects on the heart.

All the therapeutic effects are attributed to its β_1 blocking effect.

By blocking β_2 receptors it tends to precipitate asthma.

To overcome this problem few drugs have been developed which block only the β_1 receptors and are called cardioselective beta blockers, e.g. acebutalol. These drugs do not produce asthma.

Pharmacological Actions

1. Cardiovascular system:
   (a) On heart and blood vessels—heart rate and contractile activity of heart are reduced which causes reduction in cardiac output. Oxygen demand is reduced, therefore these drugs are used in angina pectoris.
   (b) Release of renin is reduced. Blood pressure is lowered by these drugs.
   (c) These drugs reduce the flow of blood to extremities that remain cold.

2. Central nervous system:
   (a) Propranolol inhibits skeletal tremors
   (b) It is effective in migraine
   (c) It has anxiolytic activity

3. Break down of glycogen to glucose is reduced. In addition symptoms due to hypoglycemia (sweating and palpitation) are also blocked.
4. Intraocular pressure is reduced.
5. **Increase serum triglycerides.**

Adverse reactions of beta blockers

1. On heart
   (i) These drugs produce severe bradycardia and cardiac stand still may occur.
   (ii) Heart block is produced which can lead to arrhythmias.
   (iii) All these drugs can precipitate congestive cardiac failure.
   Due to its membrane stabilising activity, propranolol produces greater amount of reduction in cardiac contraction.

2. Asthma is precipitated or aggrevated
3. Hypoglycemic responses of the drugs are potentiated
4. Mental depression is produced
5. Allergic reactions are manifested by a few individuals.

Timolol is used to Treat Glaucoma

1. It does not irritate the eye when instilled.
2. It is highly effective.
3. It does not produce local anaesthesia.

Partial beta agonists: Certain beta blockers alprenolol, oxprenolol and pindolol possess intrinsic activity—that is—in addition to beta blockade these are capable of stimulating beta receptor activity to a small **extent.**

Advantages of partial agonists
1. These drugs are less likely to produce cardiac failure.
2. Bronchospasm is less marked.
3. AV block is not produced.

Labetalol, celiprolol and carvedilol block both alpha and beta receptors. Are highly effective in the treatment of hypertension.

Uses of beta blockers

  (i) Cardiac arrhythmias not associated with heart block

 (ii) Angina pectoris

(iii) Treatment of hypertropic obstructive cardiomyopathy

 (iv) Hypertension (specially the one associated with increased renin activity in the blood)

  (v) Pheochromocytoma

 (vi) Chronic open angle glaucoma

(vii) In anxiety states propranolol is given to reduce symptoms

(viii) Thyrotoxicosis and thyroid crisis (before antithyroid drugs take effects)

 (ix) Migraine.

Precautions

1. Sudden withdrawal of beta blockers produces serious cardiac arrhythmias. These drugs should therefore be gradually withdrawn.
2. These drugs should not be used in patients
   (a) of complete heart block,
   (b) with impending cardiac failure.
3. Propranolol should be used with caution in patients receiving:
   (a) Insulin.
   (b) Other sympathoplegic drugs such as guanethidine and reserpine.
   (c) MAO inhibitors.

20

Drugs Acting on Autonomic Ganglion

Ganglion is synaptic site between pre-and postganglionic nerves in sympathetic as well as parasympathetic system. Acetylcholine is the main neurotransmitter in the ganglion. Nicotinic receptors predominate in the ganglion while muscarinic and adrenergic receptors are also present.

1. **Ganglionic stimulants:** Large doses of acetylcholine, nicotine and lobeline.
2. **Ganglionic blockers:** Trimethaphan, hexamethonium, mecamylamine and pentolinium tartrate.

GANGLIONIC STIMULANTS

Nicotine: It is the chief alkaloid of tobacco (Nicotina tobacum). Tobacco smoke contains nicotine and carbon monoxide along with various other carcinogenic chemicals.

Actions

1. In small doses it stimulates central nervous system, causes vomiting, increase in respiration and exerts antidiuretic effect (inhibition of urine formation).
2. Produces tachycardia and rise in blood pressure.
3. Increases motility of the gut.

Heavy smoking increases risk of lung cancer, angina pectoris, myocardial infarction, peptic ulcer, chronic bronchitis and atherosclerosis.

GANGLIONIC BLOCKING AGENTS

These drugs block the passage of impulses across sympathetic as well as parasympathetic ganglia.

These drugs produce following actions:
1. On cardiovascular system
   (a) bradycardia, postural hypotension,
   (b) cardiac output is reduced, and
   (c) blood flow to kidneys and other organs is also reduced.
2. On gut — constipation, flatulence and dryness of mouth
3. On eye — mydriasis and cycloplegia are produced
4. On reproduction — impotence and failure of ejaculation are produced which are undesirable effects.

These drugs are not popular in clinical practice because of the above mentioned effects.

Uses

1. These drugs are used only in severe type of hypertension where the disease is not responding to other drugs. To control hypertensive crisis.
2. These drugs are used to achieve controlled hypotension during surgery.

Adverse reactions

1. Visual disturbances.
2. Dryness of mouth, constipation.
3. Urinary retention.
4. Postural hypotension.
5. Pulmonary oedema is produced by hexamethonium.
6. Allergic reactions are common with trimethophan.

Nursing care of patients receiving ganglion blocking agents

1. Reassure patient regarding his disease and adverse drug reactions.
2. Blood pressure should be reduced gradually.
3. Rate of infusion of these drugs should be carefully controlled if these drugs are being administered intravenously.
4. Warn patient against postural hypotension. Patient should be advised to shift slowly during change of posture.
5. Warn patient against sudden stoppage of these drugs.
6. Equipment should be ready to maintain vital functions if cardiovascular problems develop.

Section III

Central Nervous System

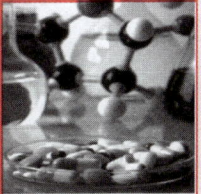

21

Central Nervous System

GENERAL ANAESTHETICS (GAs) AND PRE-ANAESTHETIC MEDICATION

General anaesthesia is a reversible progressive irregular descending paralysis of central nervous system.

Purpose of anaesthesia is to:

1. Make the patient unconsious.
2. Provide analgesia — relief from pain during surgery which may extend to postoperative period as well and cause amnesia (loss of memory).
3. Relax skeletal muscles.

General anaesthesia is usually given during major surgery. General anaesthetics are of two types:

(a) Those which are intravenously administered.

   (i) Ultrashort acting barbiturates, e.g. thiopental sodium, methohexitone.

   (ii) Non-barbiturates: Propanidid, ketamine, althesin, diazepam (IV) and fentanyl.

(b) Inhalational, e.g.

   (i) Gases: Nitrous oxide, cyclopropane.

   (ii) Volatile liquids: Ether, halothane, trichloroethylene, methoxyflurane, enflurane and isoflurane.

ULTRASHORT ACTING BARBITURATES

Thiopentone

Advantages

1. Can be easily administered.
2. Action starts immediately (unconsciousness in 11 seconds).
3. Induction of anaesthesia is smooth.
4. Does not sensitise the myocardium to catecholamines.
5. Produces less complications postoperatively.
6. Recovery from anaesthesia is fast (10–20 minutes).

Disadvantages

1. Degree of analgesia produced is very poor, therefore painful procedures should not be done.
2. Death may occur due to respiratory failure.

3. Necrosis and gangrene can occur if leakage occurs.

4. Residual depression of respiration can last up to 12 hours.

Uses

1. For induction of general anaesthesia.

2. For surgical procedures to be carried out in short time, e.g. dental extraction.

3. To control convulsions which are not responding to other treatments.

Precautions: Patients should not be discharged from hospital for 15 hours.

Adverse reactions

1. Laryngospasm (is prevented with atropine premedication).

2. Shivering and delerium.

3. Can precipitate intermittent porphyria.

4. In shock, sepsis and hypovolemia — can cause cardiovascular collapse.

Propanidid: Anaesthesia with this drug lasts for 20–30 minutes. It produces greater degree of analgesia than thiobarbiturate.

Adverse reactions

1. Twitching and tremors.
2. Fall in blood pressure.
3. Haemolysis.

Due to presence of cremophor which causes anaphylactoid reaction its use is limited.

Ketamine: It is given IM, causes unconsciousness in 3 minutes that is maintained for 15 minutes.

Advantages

1. It produces strong analgesia even in very small doses. The analgesic effect lasts even during postoperative period.

2. It increases blood pressure and can even be used during shock.

3. Respiration is not affected.

4. **Causes bronchodilation,** therefore is safe in asthmatics and is good for patients with hypovolemia.

Disadvantages

1. It cannot be used in hypertensive individuals.

2. It produces hallucinations.

3. Reflexes in the pharynx and larynx are not abolished.

Use: It is used in children under going cardiac catheterisation and bronchoscopy.

Etomidate
Advantages

1. Has greater safety margin as dose that produces anaesthesia does not depress respiration or CNS.
2. Does not cause prolonged hangover.

Disadvantages

1. Causes involuntary movements
2. Postoperative — nausea and vomiting.

NEUROLEPTANALGESIA

It is produced by combining **neuroleptic drug** with an **analgesic** (droperidol and fentanyl). The patient is mentally detached from his surroundings.

Advantages

1. Onset of anaesthesia is smooth and rapid.
2. Recovery from anaesthesia is smooth.
3. Vomiting and coughing are suppressed and do not interfere with surgery.
4. These agents do not produce changes in blood pressure.

Disadvantage: Muscle relaxation is absent.

Adverse reactions

1. Hallucinations and respiratory depression.
2. Mental depression.
3. Parkinsonism like condition can be produced as these block D_2 receptors. It is used as supplement to GA.

PREANAESTHETIC MEDICATION

It is given to patient before anaesthesia. It is done to achieve the following:

(a) Sedation of the patient—this is done to reduce anxiety due to surgery as presence of anxiety is bad during anesthesia.

(b) To prevent pre as- well as postoperative pain.

(c) To counter certain adverse reactions of anaesthetic agents, e.g. ether (anaesthetic) increases bronchial secretions—atropine is given as preanesthetic agent to reduce them.

(d) To inhibit bronchial secretions.

Narcotic analgesics: Morphine (15 mg IM) or pethidine (100 mg IM) to produce analgesia.

Advantage: Produces good degree of analgesia.

Disadvantages

1. Both interfere with pupillary size.
2. Respiratory center is depressed.
3. Both produce fall in BP that adds to fall in BP produced by general anaesthetic agents.
4. Morphine produces vomiting.
5. These agents produce bronchoconstriction.

Presently, diazepam and atropine are used as preanaesthetic medications.

Diazepam: This is used to reduce anxiety.

Advantages

1. It sedates the patient.
2. It is safer than barbiturates or morphine.
3. It can be given orally.
4. If produces less degree of respiratory depression.
5. It produces skeletal muscle relaxation.

Barbiturates were used earlier but they have been replaced by diazepam.

Atropine

Advantages

1. It produces some amount of stimulation of respiration.
2. It dries up secretions in the respiratory tract.
3. Protects against bradycardia and hypotension.

Glycopyrolate: As compared to atropine it is longer acting, is better in reducing secretions and is less likely to cause significant tachycardia.

Antiemetics: Metoclopromide, domperidone (domstal) or ondansetron (emeset) may be used. Antihistaminics with antiemetic properties may also be used.

INHALATIONAL ANAESTHETIC AGENTS

These drugs are administered in the following ways:

1. **Open method:** Anaesthetic agent (liquid) is put on the sheets of gauze which is kept on the nose of the patient. Patient while breathing inhales anaesthetic agent. No special apparatus is required. It can be carried out easily outside the hospital.

2. **Semi open method:** It requires a mask. Liquid anaesthetic agent is put on this mask. Less amount of anaesthetic is lost to air as compared to open method.

Disadvantage

It encourages accumulation of carbon dioxide in the patient.

3. **Closed method:** General anaesthetic agent is administered through a special machine. Patient inhales and exhales through this machine. Soda lime is put on the side of expiration that removes carbon dioxide and the exhaled air (minus carbon dioxide) is re-breathed by the patient and loss of anaesthetic agent is further reduced.

Chloroform: Chloroform is no more used as it is **hepato and cardiotoxic.**

Ether: It is one of the oldest anaesthetic agents in use.

Advantages

1. It is potent and safest anaesthetic agent. It can be used even by a nurse.
2. It produces **good analgesia**.
3. It produces **skeletal muscle relaxation**.
4. It produces less inhibition of respiratory center than other anaesthetic agents.
5. It does not affect heart.

6. It does not interfere with liver or kidney functions.
7. It can be given by all techniques.
8. It can raise blood pressure.

Disadvantages

1. It catches fire.
2. Induction of anaesthesia as well as recovery are slow.
3. Vomiting is likely to occur postoperatively.
4. Generalised convulsions are produced specially in children.

Halothane: It is the only inhalational anaesthetic that is metabolise in liver. When given with nitrous oxide delivery of halothane to lungs is increased.

Advantages

1. It does not catch fire.
2. Tracheal intubation is easier.
3. It provides bloodless field during surgery.
4. It produces good skeletal muscle relaxation.

Disadvantages

1. Special apparatus is required for its induction.
2. Sensitises the heart to adrenaline and noradrenaline.
3. Produces marked fall in BP.
4. Produces inhibition of respiration.
5. **Does not produce analgesia**.

Uses

1. as anesthetic agent.
2. to measure cerebral and coronary blood flow.
3. to control convulsions.

Ethylene
Advantages

1. It produces good analgesia.
2. It is safe as it does not adversely affect heart, lungs, kidneys or liver.

Disadvantages

1. When this gas is combined with oxygen it is liable to catch fire.
2. Deeper planes of anesthesia are not produced.

Trichloroethylene
Advanatages

1. It is potent analgesic, analgesia extends to postoperative period.
2. It is non-irritant to respiratory airways.
3. It is non-inflammable.

Disadvantages

1. Induction of anaesthesia and recovery from it are slow.
2. Skeletal muscle relaxation is not adequate.
3. It causes nausea and vomiting in the postoperative period.

Enflurane, Isoflurane, Methoxyflurane, Sevoflurane and Desflurane

Enflurane: Enflurane depresses cardiac functioning. It precipitates epilepsy.

Advantages

1. Induction and recovery from anaesthesia are rapid.
2. Produce good analgesia and skeletal muscle relaxation.
3. Do not sensitise heart to catecholamines.
4. It is non-irritant.
5. Does not cause renal damage (unlike methoxyflurane).

Disadvantage: Respiratory depression is more marked than with most other drugs.

Isoflurane: Causes stimulation of beta receptors.

Sevoflurane: It is latest fluorinated anaesthetic with good patient acceptability. It is not pungent but is not recommended for closed circuit administration because it is degraded by soda lime.

Desflurane

Advantages

1. Postoperative cognitive impairment is short lived.
2. Patient can be discharged earlier than with halothane.

Nitrous Oxide: It is not considered complete anaesthetic therefore not be used alone as general anaesthetic.

Advantages

1. It is non-inflammable.
2. Non-irritant.
3. It is non-toxic to liver, kidney and brain.
4. It has good analgesic activity (equivalent to morphine) onset of action is quick and smooth. Recovery is rapid.
5. Nausea in post anaesthesia period is not much.

Disadvantages

(a) Low potency.
(b) Unconsciousness cannot be produced in therapeutic doses without hypoxia.
(c) It is poor muscle relaxant.
(d) Prolonged administration can cause leukopenia and megaloblastic anaemia.

It is given as 70% nitrous oxide with 30% oxygen.

Use: Used for obstetric and dental analgesia.

Cyclopropane Gas
Advantages
1. It has potent anaesthetic activity.
2. Induction of anaesthesia and recovery from anaesthesia are smooth and rapid.
3. It does not irritate respiratory passages.
4. It only slightly affects blood pressure or cardiac functions.
5. It produces good amount of skeletal muscle relaxation.
6. It is used for major cardiac and abdominal operations.

Disadvantages
1. Interferes with eye signs of anaesthesia.
2. Sensitises the heart muscle to catecholamines and arrhythmias are produced if adrenaline or noradrenaline are given to a patient receiving cycloprapane.
3. Depresses respiratory center.

BASAL ANAESTHESIA
It is useful for alcoholics, psychotics and extremely apprehensive candidates requiring surgery.

Paraldehyde: It is given per rectum. It possesses sedative and anticonvulsant properties.

Disadvantages: Absorption of this drug varies from individual to individual. It becomes difficult to regulate anaesthesia.

Other drugs that are given during anaesthesia
1. Skeletal muscle relaxants.
2. Short acting ganglion blockers (trimethophan), if surgeon wishes to produce controlled hypotension.
3. Oxygen is added to inhalational agents to prevent hypoxia.

Following drugs are kept ready to meet any challenge during surgery/anaesthesia:

(i) **Vasopressors** — phenylephrine, methoxamine or angiotensin, (ii) steroids, (iii) antibiotics for instillation into pleural cavities.

Sequence of events before anaesthesia:
1. A hypnotic is given a night before surgery.
2. Premedication (morphine sulphate or pethidine, atropine sulphate and diazepam) is given two hours before surgery.
3. For induction of anesthesia intravenous thiopental is given.
4. Short acting skeletal muscle relaxant (succinylcholine) is given intravenously before intubation.
5. Mixture of general anaesthetics is given.
6. Skeletal muscle relaxant (d-tubocurarine) is given if relaxation is required, e.g. in abdominal surgery.
7. Additional analgesic is given when the anaesthetic agent employed does not produce sufficient degree of analgesia.

Nursing care

(A) In preoperative period

1. Alloy anxiety by reassuring the patient and by administering diazepam at night.
2. Pre-medication should not be delayed as:
   (i) It increases toxicity of the anaesthetic drugs.
   (ii) Recovery from anesthesia will be difficult.

(B) During surgery

1. Patient should be placed in posture as required by the surgeon, but patient should be made comfortable in this posture.
2. Needle for intravenous administration should be placed correctly.
3. Hearing is the last function to be lost. Nurse must make all efforts to avoid noise.
4. Patient must be protected from injury. Watching vital signs of the patient is a responsibility of the anesthetist.
5. Most of the anaesthetic drugs used are inflammable. Nurse must exercise all care to prevent fire in theater.

(C) Postoperative care

1. Patient must be encouraged to breathe deeply. This helps in removal of the anaesthetic drug from the body.
2. Patient should be monitored for complications of anesthesia, e.g. urinary retention, abdominal distension, respiratory depression and liver or kidney impairment.
3. Early ambulation minimises complications of anesthesia.
4. Nurse must protect herself against exhaled anaesthetic gases.

22

Skeletal Muscle Relaxants

Drugs that relax skeletal muscles are needed

(i) During surgery.

(ii) For treatment of sprains.

(iii) For setting fractured bones.

(iv) In spastic disorders such as hemiplegia, tetanus, status epileptics and chorea.

Classification

1. **Central acting:** Diazepam, mephenesin, meprobamate and chlormezanone.

2. **Neuromuscular blocking agents:**

   (A) Non-depolarising competitive blockers

   (a) Long acting-d-tubocurarine, pancuronium, doxacuronium and pepecuronium.

   (b) *Intermediate acting*: Atracurium, vecuronium, rapcuronium, cisastracurium.

   (c) *Short acting*: Mivacurium

   (B) Depolarising agents: Succinylcholine (suxamethonium), decamethonium.

3. **Directly acting:** Dantrolene sodium.

CENTRALLY ACTING MUSCLE RELAXANTS

Mephenesin: It acts on the central nervous system. In addition it produces sedation

Adverse reactions

1. Anorexia, nausea and vomiting.

2. Nystagmus and diplopia.

3. Lowering of blood pressure.

Uses

1. In spastic conditions such as tetanus and status epilepticus.

2. For resetting of fractured bones.

Carisoprodol

1. It relaxes skeletal muscles.
2. It is sedative.
3. It has weak analgesic, antipyretic and anticholinergic effects.

Use: In treatment of decerebrate rigidity.

Side effects

1. Drowsiness
2. Nausea and constipation
3. Rashes.

Methocarbamol: It is longer acting skeletal muscle relaxant than mephenesin. It blocks polysynaptic spinal reflexes.

Advantages

1. It has fewer side effects.
2. Does not cause sedation.
3. Incidence of hemolysis and thrombophlebitis is low.

Side Effects: Drowsiness, allergic rash, blurred vision and headache.

Orphenadrine: In addition to relaxation of skeletal muscles it causes analgesia.

Chlorzoxazone: It has same properties like mephenesin. Causes relaxation by acting at spinal cord level.

It is given in combination with analgesic (diclofenac) to relieve pain due to muscle spasms.

Diazepam: It is employed for treatment of status epilepticus and in conditions like myositis and spasms associated with arthritis.

Baclofen

It inhibits polysynaptive impulses in spinal cord. It is as effective as diazepam but produces less sedation.

It is well absorbed when given orally.

Uses

1. In spasms due to hemiplegia and paraplegia.
2. Trigeminal neuralgia.

Adverse reactions: Drowsiness and precipitates and worsens epilepsy.

Uses of centrally acting muscle relaxants

1. To relieve muscle spasms like sprain, tearing of ligaments, fibrositis and dislocation
2. Torticolis
3. Lumbago

4. Spastic neurological diseases, e.g. hemiplegia, paraplegia, spinal injury, multiple sclerosis, cerebral palsy and amyotropic lateral sclerosis

5. Tetanus (mainly diazepam is used)

6. Orthopedic manipulations

NEUROMUSCULAR BLOCKERS

Non-depolarising Agents

D-tubocurarine: This is an alkaloid derived from plant called Chondrodendron tomentosum.

Actions

1. Skeletal muscles are relaxed.
2. Blocks autonomic ganglion and produces fall in the blood pressure
3. Releases histamine which is responsible for fall in blood pressure, bronchoconstriction and allergic reactions.

Onset of action—4–6 min. Duration of action—80–120 minutes.

Adverse reactions

1. Hypoxia and respiratory paralysis.
2. Hypotension.
3. Allergic reactions.

Drug interactions

1. Halothane, ether and aminoglycosides increase its effects. These drugs should not be used with d-tubocurarine or the dose of d-tubocurarine should be reduced.
2. Higher doses of d-tubocurarine is required during respiratory alkalosis.
3. Lower doses of this drug are needed in respiratory acidosis, during fever and in infants.

Dose: 6–10 mg is given intravenously.

Gallamine (Flaxedil): This drug produces relaxation of the skeletal muscles and tachycardia. It does not release histamine.

Adverse reactions: In addition to adverse reactions of tubocurarine it produces cardiac arrhythmias.

Initial dose is 1 mg/kg intravenously.

Atcuronium and **pancuronium** have actions similar to d-tubocurarine. Pancuronium is 5 times more potent than d-tubocurarine, vecuronium is shorter acting.

Persistant Depolarising Agents

Succinylcholine

1. Before relaxing muscles it produces muscle twitching. Action lasts for very short duration.
2. Initially it produces bradycardia and hypotension followed by hypertension and tachycardia.

Adverse reactions

1. Cardiac arrhythmias.
2. Respiratory arrest may occur in few patients specially who have atypical cholinesterase.
3. Pain or fatigue of muscles.

Factors influencing the effect of succinylcholine

1. Infants and patients with liver disease, and those with atypical pseudocholinesterase are highly sensitive to this drug.
2. Procaine increases its efficacy and duration.

It is given in the dose of 0.1 to 0.5 mg/kg slowly by intravenous route.

Uses

1. As muscle relaxant for intubation.
2. As adjuvant to GA for short surgeries.
3. For surgical diagnostic procedures such as bronchoscopy/laryngoscopy.
4. In treatment of convulsions due to tetanus and status epilepticus.
5. During electroconvulsive therapy.

Decamethonium

It resembles succinylcholine in its actions.

It is five times more potent than d-tubocurarine.

It releases histamine and causes fall in blood pressure.

Adverse reactions

1. Respiratory paralysis.
2. Iodide containing salt of this drug produces allergic reactions.

Dose: 10–60 microgram per kilogram body weight given intravenously.

DIRECT ACTING MUSCLE RELAXANTS

Dantrolene: It reduces the contraction and relaxes the muscles through a direct inhibitory effect on the release of Ca^{++}.

Uses

1. It is specially useful in treating **malignant hyperthermia** in susceptible individuals.
2. Multiple sclerosis.
3. Skeletal nuscle spasms due to spinal injuries.

Adverse reactions

1. Liver damage.
2. In early stages fatigue is reported.

Nursing care

All these drugs are employed either in operation theater or in casualty.

(a) Nurse must ensure that correct muscle relaxant is handed to the anesthetist.
(b) Positive pressure artificial respiration with oxygen should be ready before administering these drugs.
(c) Antagonist to these drugs should be kept ready in the tray to meet emergency.
(d) Neostigmine and atropine are needed for treating tubocurarine poisoning.

23

Alcohols

Ethyl and methyl alcohol are important from medical point the former for uses and addiction while latter is famous for causing deaths amongst poor drinkers.

ETHYL ALCOHOL

Ethyl alcohol is available as liquors, wines, spirits and for medical purposes as:

Absolute alcohol—90% w/w dehydrated alcohol.

Rectified spirit—90% w/w ethyl alcohol with methyl alcohol.

Local Actions

Local application of alcohol produces:

1. Maximum bactericidal effect at 70% concentration.
2. It has mild rubefacient and counter irritant effect.
3. It produces cooling of skin.
4. On injection it produces pain, inflammation and necrosis followed by nerve damage. Due to this action it is used to treat neuralgias.

Systemic Effects

CNS: It depresses CNS and the individual becomes less inhibited and more talkative. In higher quantities individual loses self-control and gait becomes unsteady. There is drowsiness, **impairment** of vision and muscular co-ordination—driving becomes difficult.

Still higher doses produce paralysis of respiration and cardiovascular centers and death occurs.

Cardiovascular system: It produces dilation of cutaneous and gastric blood vessels leading to feeling of warmth. Loss of heat is increased and the body temperature is reduced.

Moderate doses increase heart rate. Alcohol is usually employed as a home remedy for syncope. Coronary arteries of the heart get dilated but the workload of heart is increased. Small quantities of alcohol are not harmful but large quantities of alcohol should be discouraged in cardiac patients as it produces depression of myocardium and vasomotor center.

Liver: Long use of high doses of alcohol destroys liver. Initially fatty liver is produced which is followed by cirrhosis. Moderate doses do not damage liver provided there is no nutritional deficiency.

Kidney: It reduces the release of anti-diuretic hormone and exerts diuretic effect. Alcohol cannot be used as diuretic in clinical practice.

GIT: It increases acidity in stomach. Higher quantities reduce acid secretion.

Other effects: There are wrong notions about alcohol that has encouraged its use. One of them being its aphrodisiac (increase of sexual activity) property.

If taken during pregnancy it **damages fetus**.

Uses

1. It is applied locally for
   (a) Treating hyperthermia
   (b) For antiseptic activity
   (c) Injected into nerve to relieve pain of trigeminal neuralgia
   (d) For prevention and treatment of bed sores.
2. Systemic uses: In moderate quantities it increases HDL and reduces LDL.
3. It is given in debilitated patients to improve appetite.

Adverse reactions

1. Acute behavioural changes
   (a) Euphoria and minor motor disturbances occur with 2 oz of whisky.
   (b) Nystagmus and errors in simple tests are produced.
   (c) Impaired driving ability occurs with doses of 3 oz.
   (d) Motor incoordination.
   (e) Amnesia (forgetfulness).
   (f) Coma occurs when blood levels are over 300 mg/100 ml blood.
2. Hangover
3. *Alcoholic coma:* Withdrawal syndrome—delirium tremens—anxiety, sweating, nausea, vomiting, tachycardia and convulsions characterize this condition.

   It is treated by:

   (a) Giving IV fluids.

   (b) Creating a congenial atmosphere.

   (c) Tranquillisers like chlorpromazine are given.

   (d) Convulsions are treated with diazepam.
4. Nutritional deficiencies of folic acid, iron, nicotinamide and thiamine are common. Haematinics and vitamins should be supplemented.
5. *Hepatic damage:* Cirrhosis is a common complication of alcoholics.
6. Chronic alcoholism is increasing in our country. **Crime rate is directly proportional to addiction rate.**
7. Addiction due to alcohol should be treated.

ISOPROPYL ALCOHOL

It is used as antiseptic. It is more toxic. This alcohol is added to ethyl alcohol rendering it unfit for internal use (denatured alcohol).

DISULFIRAM

It is given to produce aversion to alcohol.

This drug is given and the patient is asked to take his choicest drink after it. Patient then experiences warmth, throbbing headache, nausea and vomiting and a hangover. Aversion develops to drinks. Similar reaction is produced by metronidazole and griseofulvin therefore patients taking these drugs should be advised against taking alcohol.

Precautions: This drug should not be given in patients of cardiovascular disease, epilepsy and cirrhosis.

Nursing care

1. Advise patient to take alcoholic beverages with food. This prevents gastric irritation and delays its absorption.
2. In patients suffering from acute alcohol toxicity support vital functions.
3. When taking drug history specially ask for alcohol as it interacts with many drugs and influences their actions.
4. While treating chronic alcoholism, monitor the patient for withdrawal symptoms.
5. Encourage patients of alcoholism to seek medical help.

TOXIC ALCOHOLS

Methyl alcohol or methanol is encountered as adulterant in illegal liquour. Alcoholics ingest it mistakenly or in desperation. Methanol is metabolised to formic acid and its effects last longer.

Unlike ethanol, methanol is not a strong CNS depressant but it produces severe acidosis. Human optic nerve is especially vulnerable to this acidosis.

Treatment

1. Treatment must be initiated early. Patient be kept in dark room.
2. Simultaneous administration of **ethanol** reduces the conversion of methanol to formic acid. 50% alcoholic equivalent of beverage is given orally followed by 0.5 ml/kg every 2 hours for 4 days.
3. Acidosis is neutralised by sodium bicarbonate given orally (if the patient is conscious and not vomiting) or intravenously. Urine is made alkaline by potassium chloride.
4. **Fomepizole** (4-methyl pyrazole) is specific inhibitor of alcohol dehydrogenase and retards metabolism of methyl alcohol.
5. Folate therapy: Lowers formic acid by increasing its metabolism.
6. Haemodialysis can save the patient.

24

Hypnotics and Sedatives

Sleep is not a passive but an active phenomenon. Hypnotics are drugs that induce sleep while sedative reduces excitement. In higher dose sedative too can induce sleep.

Anxiety, pain, dyspnoea or discomfort of any kind can give the patient sleepless nights. In domiciliary practice hypnotics are more often misused than used. In some patients difficulty in sleeping may be the first sign of depression, treatment lies in giving antidepressants rather than hypnotics.

The most commonly used hypnotic agents are barbiturates, benzodiazepines, chloral hydrate, ethyl alcohol, glutethimide and paraldehyde.

All hypnotics and sedatives cross placental barrier during pregnancy and are also detectable in breast milk.

Barbiturates

Actions

1. These are powerful cerebral depressants.
   (a) In smaller doses they produce sedative and in higher doses hypnotic action. **REM sleep is depressed**, this produces hangover and increases dreaming and nightmares on withdrawal.
   (b) Specific **anticonvulsant effect is exerted by phenobarbitone**.
2. In hypnotic doses the blood pressure is reduced marginally but in larger doses fall in BP is appreciable.
3. In hypnotic doses barbiturates do not exert much effect on kidneys, heart, liver and intestine.
4. Chronic use of barbiturates results in induction of liver enzymes (P450) responsible for drug metabolism. This action is responsible for number of drug interactions.

Disadvantages

1. These agents **do not relieve pain**, in fact these agents increase the feeling of pain. This point is of clinical importance as these drugs cannot induce sleep in presence of pain. No amount of barbiturates will put the patient to sleep if he is experiencing pain. Pain must be relieved before barbiturates can induce sleep.
2. These drugs interact with too many drugs.

Uses

1. For sedating the patient. These drugs have been used to relieve anxiety and tension during treatment of hypertension, peptic ulcer and hyperthyroidism.
2. Short acting barbiturates (secobarb, etc.) are employed to induce sleep. Intermediate acting barbiturates are used in patients who have tendency to wake up in middle of the night.
3. Phenobarbitone may be used in grandmal epilepsy. It also controls severe types of convulsions such as status epilepticus and eclamptic fits.
4. It was used as preanesthetic medication.
5. It is given in premature children to treat kernicterus.

Adverse reactions

1. Tolerance develops. Once the patient becomes tolerant there is need to step up the dose.
2. Drug dependence develops — barbiturates cannot be suddenly withdrawn as abstinence syndrome is precipitated. Convulsions are the main features of this withdrawal.
3. If administered along with chlordiazepoxide or diazepam or alcohol these drugs produce severe CNS depression (coma).

Nursing care

1. Ideally barbiturates should not be given to the patient who complains of insomnia (sleeplessness) without investigating the cause.
2. Elderly patients should not be given barbiturates. These drugs occasionally induce confusion and disorientation and during phase of forgetfulness, these individuals consume many tablets leading to toxicity.
3. These drugs are metabolised in the liver and excreted in urine — these agents should be given cautiously in patients with renal and hepatic disorders.
4. Barbiturates should not be combined with other drugs — especially CNS depressants.
5. Patients must be warned against taking alcoholic drink along with barbiturates.

Poisoning with barbiturates: Severe poisoning with barbiturate is still not uncommon. Patient is brought in an unconscious state with weak and thready pulse. Respiration is shallow Chyne stokes rhythm may be seen. Pupils are constricted but later get dilated.

Treatment

(a) Gastric lavage with saline — provided patient has been brought in within 2 hours of taking barbiturate tablets.
(b) Endotracheal intubation is done to maintain patent airways. Artificial respiration is continued till patient recovers.
(c) IV fluids are given. Mannitol or lasix is given along with sodium bicarbonate. This hastens the excretion of barbiturates through kidney.
(d) Haemodialysis is done if the barbiturate levels in the blood are more then 6 mg%.

Chloral Hydrate: This is safe mild hypnotic of special value in children and young infants. Increases anticoagulant effect of warfarin.

Advantages

1. It induces sleep but does not suppress REM sleep.
2. It does not affect respiration and blood pressure.
3. It is cheap.
4. Tolerance does not develop.

Disadvantages

1. It has bad smell and bad taste.
2. It does not maintain good sleep.
3. Does not have anticonvulsant effect.

Adverse reactions

1. Nausea and vomiting.
2. It produces pin point pupils.
3. In large doses it produces depression of respiration.

Dose: 0.5–2.0/g at night.

Precautions

1. Should not be given to patients suffering from liver or kidney damage.
2. Not to be given to patients of gastritis and peptic ulcers.

Paraldehyde

(a) It is extremely effective hypnotic.
(b) It is also valuable in the treatment of status epilepticus.
(c) It can be given orally, intramuscularly as well as per rectally.

Disadvantages

1. It is foul smelling.
2. Air around patient smells of paraldehyde as the patient excretes it through lungs.

Adverse reactions

1. Irritates gastric as well as rectal mucosa.
2. Produces excitement in the presence of pain.
3. It is rarely used as hypnotic nowadays.

Uses

1. As an anticonvulsant in status epilepticus.
2. To control convulsions of tetanus and eclampsia.
3. It is rarely used as hypnotic.

Nursing care and precautions to be taken

1. Paraldehyde dissolves plastic syringes and should be injected with glass ones only.
2. This drug decomposes to acetic acid and acetaldehyde. Death can occur syringes if the decomposed drug is used.

3. Patient should not take alcohol or alcohol containing medicaments with this drug.

4. This drug should be avoided in patients of liver and lung disease.

To avoid these dangers

(a) Paraldehyde must be stored in a cool and dark place.

(b) Paraldehyde kept for more than 6 months should be discarded.

Benzodiazepines: **Diazepam, flurazepam and nitrazepam** are used as hypnotics.

These drugs produce following actions:

(a) **Sedation or calming:** Aggressiveness is reduced. Because of this effect these agents are used in anxious neurotic patients.

(b) **Hypnosis:** Sleep resembling normal sleep is produced. Unlike barbiturates benzodiazepines do not interfere with REM sleep.

(c) **Anticonvulsant activity:** They possess strong anticonvulsant activity. These agents are used in status epilepticus.

(d) They **relax skeletal muscles** and are used in treatment of spastic disorders.

(e) Benzodiazepines **lower blood** pressure and are usually prescribed for hypertension.

(f) Exert antigrade amnesia.

Advantages over barbiturates

1. Sleep produced by these drugs is near normal, as they do not suppress REM sleep. There is no hangover and no rebound.

2. Safety margin is more (dose which produces sleep is too small as compared to one which is toxic).

3. Drug interactions are less.

4. Even high doses do not suppress CVS and respiration.

Adverse reactions

Tolerance and physical dependence both develop.

High dose and chronic treatment alone produce dependance.

Uses

1. These agents are used as sedatives (in anxiety and neurotic patients).

2. As hypnotic.

3. In treatment of status epilepticus (diazepam).

4. As pre anaesthetic medication.

5. During withdrawal in alcoholic addicts.

6. As muscle relaxants.

Dose

Diazepam	5–10 mg
Flurazepam	15–30 mg
Nitrazepam	5–10 mg
Alprazolam	0.25–0.5 mg

Precautions

1. Patient should be warned not to take other CNS depressant drugs along with these agents.
2. In the elderly patients these agents tend to produce ataxia (unsteadiness of gait) hence should be avoided.
3. Flurazepam is long acting and if repeated it accumulates in body. Administration of this drug should be well spaced.

ANTAGONIST OF BENZODIAZEPINES

Flumazenil

Actions

1. Blocks CNS effects of benzodiazepines only.
2. It is used to treat toxicity due to benzodiazepines.
3. It has short half life. It is given IV.

Adverse reactions

1. Convulsions and cardiac arrhythmia
2. Agitation and confusion.

Antihistaminic drugs also produce sedation as well as hypnosis. The CNS depression produced by these drugs adds to the effect of other agents. Hypnotics should not be given along with antihistamines.

Bromide: This drug is not used in advanced hospitals, but in Primary Health Center and less developed regions of this country it is still in use.

Adverse reactions on chronic administration
1. Dermatitis
2. Anorexia
3. Gastric irritation
4. Slurred speech.

Nursing care of insomnic patient

1. Patients in wards often complain of sleeplessness. It is the duty of the nurse to reassure the patient. This reduces anxiety and induces sleep. Nurse must create an atmosphere congenital to sleep. Lights must be put off and noise terminated.
2. Drugs which reduce sleep (ephedrine, amphetamine, etc.) should not be given later than 4.0 p.m.
3. In domiciliary practice patient should be advised to take heavy dinner. This in itself helps the patient to sleep. Milk products induce sleep.
4. Occasional loss of sleep does not need treatment. **Avoid repeating sleeping pill**. Try to diagnose the cause of sleeplessness and treat it.
5. It is important to remember that **sleeping pill should not be given in pain**. Pain be relieved by analgesic first and hypnotic to be given later.
6. If everything fails, diazepam can be given to the patient provided he is not on drugs which interact with it.

NEWER AGENTS

Buspirone, ipsapirone and gepirone: These drugs produce sedation lack hypnotic, anticonvulsant and muscle relaxant effects.

Zolpidem: Actions similar to benzodiazepine but lacks muscle relaxant and anticonvulsant effects.

Zopulone: It is BZI receptor agonist. Has rapid onset and shorter duration. Tolerance and dependence not reported.

25

Non-narcotic Analgesics

These drugs are also referred to as **non-steroidal anti-inflammatory agents** (NSAIDS) or analgesic antipyretic agents.

These drugs differ from narcotic analgesics in the following ways:

	Non-narcotics	*Narcotics*
Examples	**Aspirin**	**Morphine**
1. Addiction liability	NIL	++++
2. Site of action	Peripheral	Central
3. Changed reaction to pain	Absent	Present
4. Efficacy	In somatic pain associated with inflammatory conditions	In visceral pain
5. Sleep	Not induced	Induce sleep

CLASSIFICATION

I. Non-selective (Block both COX-1 and COX-2)

Salicylates: Aspirin, diflunisal.

Paraminophenol derivatives: Paracetamol.

Pyrazolone derivatives: Phenylbutazone and oxyphenbutazone.

Indole derivatives: Indomethacin.

Propionic acid: Ibuprofen (safest), naproxan, ketoprofen and flurbiprofen.

Anthralic acid derivatives: Mefenamic acid and enfenamic acid.

Aryl-acetic acid derivatives: Diclofenac sodium, acceclofenac sodium.

Oxicam derivatives: Piroxicam and tenoxicam.

Pyrolo-pyrole derivatives: Ketolac.

Pyrazolone derivatives: Metamizol (novalgin), prophenazone (saridon).

Benzoxazocin: Nefopam.

II. Preferential COX-2 Blockers

Nimesulide, meloxicam, etodolac, sulindac and nabumetone.

III. Selective COX-2 Inhibitors

Celecoxib, rofecoxib, etoricoxib, paracoxib.

IV. Block Prostaglandins and Leukotriene Pathways

Locafelone (no risk of peptic ulcer).

NSAIDS

Salicylates: **Aspirin** is chemically acetyl salicylic acid. This simple substance has complex actions.

1. **Analgesic activity:** Aspirin produces marked degree of analgesia. Unlike narcotic analgesics it does not induce sleep. It is more effective in relieving dull aching pain of low intensity. Visceral pain responds to these agents to a lesser extent.

   Unlike narcotics these agents do not change the reaction of the individual to pain.

2. **Antipyretic action:** Have excellent antipyretic activity. In fever these agents bring down the body temperature to normal **but never below normal**. That is these drugs **are not hypothermic agents.**

3. **Anti-inflammatory and antirheumatic effect:** Inflammation is a response of the body to injury. There are three components of inflammation — redness, heat and oedema. All the three components of inflammation are inhibited by these drugs. Pain is due to inflammation and when inflammation is reduced, pain is reduced and process of healing sets in. Salicylates are the best anti-inflammatory agents.

4. **Blood:** These drugs
   (a) decrease ESR
   (b) decrease fibrinogen
   (c) reduce platelet aggregation. Aspirin is longest acting anti-platelet agent as **irreversibly inhibits** cyclooxygenase in platelet.

5. Respiration is slightly stimulated.

6. **Gastrointestinal tract:** Epigastric distress, nausea and vomiting are produced. They erode the gastric mucosa leading to gastric bleeding.

7. In higher doses these drugs increase the excretion of uric acid through kidneys. **In normal doses increase serum uric acid.**

In normal doses hepatic and renal functions are not affected.

Adverse reactions

These may be divided into two:

1. Those which occur at therapeutic dose level.
2. Those which are produced only in large doses.

I. Those occurring in therapeutic dosage

(a) Nausea, vomiting and dyspepsia
(b) Haematemesis and melena
(c) Precipitation of asthma

(d) These drugs increase bleeding tendencies by lowering prothrombin and vitamin K dependent factors.

(e) Chronic use produces fatty infiltration of liver and destroy kidneys.

Aspirin and related drugs exert a local irritant effect on the gastric mucosa thereby nausea and vomiting may be produced. Some patients experience abdominal pain after taking aspirin tablets. All these symptoms are more prone to occur in patients predisposed to gastric ulcers. These reactions are reduced by giving these drugs after meals or giving antacids along with them or using enteric coated tablets.

Some asthmatic patients are particularly sensitive to aspirin in that the drug may induce a severe and occasionally fatal attack of asthma.

II. Salicylism is produced only in large doses

Salicylism is a syndrome characterised by headache, dizziness, vertigo, tennitus, mental confusion. Respiratory alkalosis may be present. Hyperglycemia, dehydration, hyperpyrexia and gastrointestinal bleeding are seen in cases of acute poisoning.

Uses

1. To relieve pain in neuralgias, myalgia, toothache, headache and dysmenorrhoea.
2. Treatment of fever including rheumatic fever.
3. For the treatment of rheumatoid arthritis.
4. Large doses can be used in gout but are not tolerated.
5. After myocardial infarction it is given to prevent platelet aggregation.
6. In diarrheas.

Contraindications

1. In patients with peptic ulcer or those at risk.
2. Not used in children.
3. Needs to be stopped one week before elective surgery.
4. Not given before labour.
5. Not given to pregnant women or lactating women.

PARA-AMINOPHENOL DERIVATIVES

Phenacetin and Paracetamol: **Phenacetin** is added to aspirin and caffeine (APC). Phenacetin is not preferred these days because:

1. Analgesic activity is weak.
2. It has poor anti-inflammatory activity.

Adverse reactions

1. Renal damage occurs with phenacetin.
2. Methemoglobinaemia is produced.
3. May sometimes produce anaemia.

Tolerance and habituation develops with phenacetin.

Paracetamol: It has antipyretic and analgesic activities but lacks anti-inflammatory activity.

Advantage: It does not cause gastric irritation.

Disadvantage: It does not produce suppression of inflammation. **It is hepatotoxic** and 10 gm of this drug can cause death.

Uses

(a) This can be used as antipyretic in children
(b) As analgesic and antipyretic in patients of gastric ulcers.

Dose: Paracetamol 300–600 mg/4 times a day.

Toxicity of paracetamol is treated by acetylcysteine

PYRAZOLONE DERIVATIVES

Drugs in this group are phenylbutazone, oxyphenbutazone, aminopyrine and antipyrine — the last two being toxic are not used.

Phenylbutazone: It has potent anti-inflammatory activity.

Adverse effects

1. It suppresses bone marrow. It may even produce agranulocytosis.
2. It causes retention of Na^+ and water leading to oedema formation.
3. It interferes with thyroid functions. The use of this drug should be restricted.

Uses

1. Gout
2. Ankylosing spondylitis
3. Rheumatoid arthritis and osteoarthritis
4. It should not be given for treating minor ailments.

Drug Interaction

1. It increases efficacy of tolbutamide and acetohexamide.
2. It increases toxicity of oral anticoagulants.

Oxyphenbutazone: It is a metabolite of phenylbutazone. It differs from its parent compound (phenylbutazone) as it causes less gastric irritation. It has same uses and adverse reactions.

Indomethacin: It has antipyretic, analgesic and anti-inflammatory activity.

Advantages

1. It is more effective than aspirin.
2. It can be administered per rectum.
3. It has longer duration of action.
4. It is highly effective anti-inflammatory agent.

Uses

1. Acute gouty attacks. Presently, it is drug of choice as it is preferred over colchicine.
2. Rheumatoid arthritis.
3. To relieve pain in pericarditis and pleurisy.
4. Ankylosing spondylitis.

Adverse reactions

1. Headache
2. Mental confusion
3. Blurring of vision.

Precautions

(a) It should be taken with meals or antacids. Chronic use of this drug should be avoided.
(b) Except for treatment of patent ductus arteriosus it should not be given in children.

Ibuprofen: It has good anti-inflammatory and analgesic activities but gastric irritation is less. Safest non-selective NSAID.

Uses

1. Rheumatoid arthritis and osteoarthritis.
2. In soft tissue injury.

Caution: Concomitant use of this drug with aspirin reduces anti-inflammatory activity.

Ketoprofen: It inhibits lipoxygenase and cyclooxygenase. It stabilises liposomes.

It is as effective as aspirin but produces adverse effects on CNS.

Mefenamic Acid: It has analgesic activity but is less effective than aspirin as anti-inflammatory agent. It has lesser antipyretic activity, causes diarrhoea.

Analgin: It has analgesic as well as anti-inflammatory activity. It does not increase excretion of uric acid therefore it is not used in gout. Toxic effects are like phenylbutazone.

Naproxen: It has anti-inflammatory, analgesic and antipyretic activities.

Uses

1. In treatment of rheumatoid arthritis
2. In treating osteoarthritis
3. In ankylosing spondylitis
4. It has also been used in dysmenorrhoea.

Adverse drug reactions

1. Abdominal pain
2. Drowsiness, headache and dizziness
3. Gastric pain and gastric bleeding
4. Individuals sensitive to acetylsalicylic acid are also sensitive to this drug.

Dose: 250–500 mg twice a day.

Meclofenamate: It has effects like salicylates but is not superior. It is used to treat chronic rheumatoid arthritis and osteoarthritis.

Adverse reactions

1. Gastrointestinal disturbances as with any other anti-inflammatory agent.
2. Diarrhea.
3. Not to be given to pregnant ladies and children.

Diclofenac: It has analgesic, antipyretic and anti-inflammatory activities **It gets concentrated in synovial fluid hence is effective in relieving joint pains. It is effective when applied locally.** Aceclofenac is safer than diclofenac sodium.

Piroxicam: Has anti-inflammatory, analgesic and antipyretic activities.

Half life is long, hence is given once a day. It is well tolerated.

Adverse drug reactions

1. Peptic ulcer.
2. Allergic reactions.
3. Toxic to kidneys.

Tolmetin

1. It is anti-inflammatory, analgesic and antipyretic agent. It is as effective as salicylates but is better tolerated.
2. It is completely and rapidly absorbed from the gut.
3. It is used in rheumatoid arthritis.
4. It has to be given 4 times a day.

Caution: Patients who are sensitive to acetylsalicylic acid are sensitive to tolmetin also.

Nimesulide: It inhibits Cox-2 more than Cox-1.

It is more effective antipyretic than indomethacin, diclofenac, piroxicam and ibuprofen.

Analgesic activity is equal to aspirin and anti-inflammatory activity equal to indomethacin. In addition to inhibition of synthesis of prostaglandins it acts through other mechanisms to inhibit inflammation.

Uses

1. To relieve pain.
2. To control inflammation in osteoarthritis.

Advantages

1. It is well tolerated, causes less gastric irritation.
2. It has fewer side effects.

Contraindications

1. Peptic ulcer.
2. **Moderate-to-severe hepatic dysfunction.**

Sulindac: It is prodrug.

1. It has anti-inflammatory, analgesic and antipyretic properties.
2. It is less potent than indomethacin.
3. Does not interfere with renal PGS and is safe in patients with hypertension.

Uses

(i) Ankylosing spondylitis.
(ii) Rheumatoid arthritis and osteoarthritis.

Caution: Patients sensitive to acetylsalicylic acid are sensitive to this drug also.

Ketorolac: Acts on opiod as well as non-opioid receptors. It is used for dental extraction. Not suitable for more than 3 days.

Nursing care of patients with pain

1. Try and find the cause of pain and treat this cause, e.g. amyl nitrite in angina, antacids in peptic ulcer, miotics in glaucoma and muscle relaxants in sprains.
2. Dull aching pain is relieved by non-narcotic analgesics. These should be tried in full dosages and at the earliest.
3. Elicit history of allergy to these drugs.
4. If patient has peptic ulcer treating physician should be informed about it.
5. Combination of drugs should be discouraged specially those which contain narcotic analgesics of low potency. These drugs do not give any benefit to the individual but makes him liable to abuse the drug.

   In anxious patients with severe pain codeine may be combined in full dosage.
6. In conditions of chronic pain the selection of the drug must be made with care depending upon the health of his kidneys, liver and heart.
7. Counter irritants and hot water bottle go a long way in relieving pain and potentiating the effect of these drugs.
8. Making the atmosphere of the patient physically and emotionally comfortable adds to effects of these drugs.

Patient is advised to take these drugs after meals and certainly not on an empty stomach. Disprin is better than most of the other drugs because it is effective, cheap and causes less gastric irritation.

Nursing care of the patients receiving anti-inflammatory agents

1. Elicit information regarding sensitivity of the patient to these drugs specially acetylsalicylic acid (aspirin).
2. Elicit history of peptic ulcer in these patients as all these drugs have tendency to aggrevate this problem.
3. Have a clear understanding about other drugs consumed by this patient (so as to avoid interactions).
4. Instruct patient to take the drug immediately after meals.
5. Teach the patient or his relative to watch for adverse reactions.

Nursing care of the patient receiving non-narcotic agents

1. Patients receiving these drugs feel better than their condition demands as the symptoms get suppressed and it becomes difficult to evaluate the disease process. The patient, therefore, be watched carefully.

2. Patient should be instructed not to discontinue the drug prematurely.

3. Nurse must warn the patient against increasing the dose of analgesic antipyretic drugs above the recommended levels as toxicity develops.

4. If the patient is not responding to usual doses, physician should be consulted.

Selection of the drug is determined by the functional condition of liver, kidney and gastric mucosa of the patient.

26

Pharmacology of Gout

Gout is characterised by over production of uric acid and its deposition in joints (tophi) resulting in degenerative changes, acute attacks of pain and swelling of joints (one or more small joints may be involved such as those of toes and fingers).

Principals of treatment of gout

1. To give immediate relief in acute pain — indomethacin, colchicine, corticosteroids are given for this purpose.
2. To increase excretion of uric acid by uricosuric agents, e.g. phenylbutazone, sulphinpyrazone and probenecid.
3. To reduce production of uric acid, e.g. allopurinol.

PAIN RELIEVERS IN GOUT

Colchicine: It is an alkaloid toxic to mitotic spindle and does not allow leucocytic migration and phagocytosis.

(a) It is specific for acute gout as it relieves pain of gouty joints only.
(b) It is highly toxic.
(c) **Does not decrease serum uric acid.**
(d) **It has no analgesic activity.**

Adverse reactions

1. Gastrointestinal upset and diarrhea.
2. Leucopenia.

Dose

1.0 mg is given orally followed by 0.5 mg every two hours until pain is relieved, or diarrhea is produced or maximum of 3 mg is reached. It **should not be repeated within 7 days.**

Indomethacin: This drug has strong anti-inflammatory as well as analgesic activity. It has long duration of action and is required to be given only twice daily.

Glucocorticoids: These drugs are not used routinely because of their adverse reactions. The anti-inflammatory activity of these agents is responsible for giving relief in gout.

Dose: Prednisolone is given in the dose of 30–40 mg initially followed by 5–10 mg everyday.

URICOSURIC AGENTS

Drugs increasing the excretion of uric acid are called uricosuric agents. Uric acid is excreted as well as partly reabsorbed in the renal tubule. Uricosuric drugs act by inhibiting reabsorption of uric acid in the renal tubule. This helps in removal of uric acid from tophaceous deposits in the joints leading to relief from pain.

Since these drugs increase uric acid in the urine there is tendency to develop uric acid stones in the kidneys. This can be prevented by advising the patient to drink large volumes of fluid and to keep the urine on the alkaline side.

These drugs should not be given during acute attack of gout.

Probenecid: It has biphasic action. Smaller doses of this drug decrease tubular secretion of uric acid while larger doses (therapeutic doses) decrease its reabsorption producing net loss of uric acid in the urine.

It does not produce adverse reactions though there are interactions.

Interactions: It increases level of penicillin, indomethacin, heparin and dapsone in blood.

Sulphinpyrazone: It is a metabolite of phenylbutazone. It has slight anti-inflammatory but more marked uricosuric activity which is equivalent to that of probenecid.

Dose: 100–200 mg three times daily.

This drug is effective only if the kidneys are functioning properly.

Adverse reactions

1. It precipitates and aggravates peptic ulcer.
2. Bone marrow is depressed.
3. Inhibits platelet aggregation.

Benzbromarone: It reversibly inhibits urate-anion exchanger in the proximal tubule resulting in the inhibition of reabsorption of uric acid in renal tubule thereby lowering serum levels of uric acid. It has strong anti-inflammatory and analgesic activity.

Interactions: Aspirin and sulfinpyrazone inhibit uricosuric effect of this drug.

Dose: 25–50 mg/four hourly. In patients with peptic ulcer it can be administered as 100 mg suppository.

Uses: It is given in mild-to-moderate attack of gout after colchicine has controlled initial pain of severe gouty arthritis.

Salicylates also possess uricosuric activity but for this effect they are required to be given in high doses (3–5 g/day).

DRUGS INHIBITING SYNTHESIS OF URIC ACID

Allopurinol: By inhibiting the xanthine oxidase enzyme allopurinol inhibits conversion of hypoxanthine to xanthine and its conversion to uric acid. This drug also increases the excretion of hypoxanthine and xanthine which are more water soluble than uric acid.

Adverse Reactions: Incidence of side effects is low. Allergy, nausea and vomiting may sometimes be reported.

Uses

1. In patients of gout during chronic stage.
3. It is useful in patients with gouty tophi or uric acid stones in kidney.
4. It is given along with cytotoxic agents that produce excess of uric acid.

Nursing care of patients with gout

1. Fluid intake of these patients should not be less than two litres a day.
2. pH of the urine should be maintained on the alkaline side by giving sodium bicarbonate.

Patient should be instructed to avoid diets and drugs which can precipitate gout, e.g. thiazides, cytotoxic agents, alcohol and meat.

27

Drugs used in Rheumatoid Arthritis

Drugs are needed to relieve pain and reduce muscle stiffness and inflammation. Treatment of this condition if started at an early stage shows better results. In addition to drugs rest and physiotherapy are helpful.

1. NSAIDS and chloroquine.
2. Disease modifying agents: Penicillamine, sulphasalazine, gold and TNF blocking drugs.
3. Immunosuppressants: Methotrexate, azathioprine, cyclophosphamide.
4. Adjuvants: Glucocorticoids.

Indomethacin

This drug has strong anti-inflammatory as well as analgesic activity.

Advantages

1. It has long duration of action. It is required to be given only twice daily.
2. Given at bed time it controls the early morning stiffness.
3. In cases of peptic ulcer this drug can be given in the form of suppository.

Diclofenac

Acts by nimesulide prostaglandin synthesis. It is long acting NSAID.

Adverse reactions

1. GI bleeding
2. Allergic reactions
3. Fluid retention and oedema.

Tolmetin, nimesulide and nabumetone reportedly cause less GI bleed.

Piroxicam

20 mg b.d. for two days for owed by 20 mg o.d.

Disadvantage

All NSAIDS relieve pain but **progression of disease is not halted**.

DISEASE MODIFYING AGENTS

Chloroquine: It is a popular antimalarial which in addition has anti-inflammatory activity exerted through inhibition of phospholipase A.

Advantage: This agent is less toxic than gold, penicillamine and azathioprine.

Disadvantages

1. It takes about 4–12 weeks for this drug to produce its response in rheumatoid arthritis.
2. Only 50% patients respond to this drug.
3. It causes retinal damage.

Hydroxychloroquine causes less ocular toxicity.

Adverse reactions

1. Nausea and vomiting.
2. Corneal opacity and retinal damage (it takes about a year to produce this effect).
3. Vertigo, malaise and depression.
4. If given during pregnancy it produces foetal damage.

Precautions

1. Repeated eye check ups should be done.
2. It accumulates in the body. Repeated administration for long duration should be avoided. It is advisable to give this drug for 4–6 months. A gap of 3 months is given and the drug can be restarted.

Penicillamine: It is a chelating agent and helps in removal of copper. In addition it is beneficial in rheumatoid arthritis.

Advantages

1. It is effective when other therapies including gold have failed.
2. Use of corticosteroids can be avoided.

Disadvantages

1. Onset of action is late. It takes 2–3 months for the drug to become effective.
2. It produces anorexia, nausea and taste loss.
3. Long-term use can damage the kidney leading to marked nephrotic syndrome.

Precautions

1. As it can damage the kidneys urine should be repeatedly checked.
2. It causes thrombocytopenia or neutropenia, therefore blood should be routinely checked and the drug withdrawn at the appropriate time.
3. It interferes with the functioning of taste buds, therefore, the compliance rate is poor. Nurse must question the patient regarding intake of this drug whenever patient complains of loss of taste.

Gold: It is the most effective agent against rheumatoid arthritis. If taken at an early stage it prevents the progression of arthritis. It act by inhibiting cell mediated immunity. This stops progression of disease and normalises C factor.

Dose: 250 mg/day is increased gradually to 500 or 1000 mg/day.

Disadvantage: It is highly toxic.

Adverse reactions

1. It causes renal damage — glomerulonephritis.
2. Pruritis, glossitis, diarrhea and stomatitis are the usual features of early stages of its toxicity.
3. Liver damage is produced — cholestatic jaundice.
4. Peripheral neuritis.
5. Encephalopathy can also be produced.
6. Aplastic anemia.
7. Pulmonary fibrosis.
8. Postural hypotension.

Contraindications

1. Renal and hepatic dysfunctions
2. Haematological disorders.

Levamisole: It is an immunostimulant drug which is found to be effective in rheumatoid arthritis. It is not favoured as it produces rash, fever, myalgia and agranulocytosis.

Sulfasalazine: It has been in use for treating ulcerative colitis but lately has shown good effects in rheumatoid arthritis.

50–100 mg given 6 hourly has been found to be effective.

IMMUNOSUPPRESSIVE DRUGS

Corticosteroids: These drugs exert anti-inflammatory and immunosuppressive activities.

Prednisolone

Advantages

1. Highly effective.
2. Prednisolone (5 mg) at bed time effectively relieves pain of joints at night and the early morning stiffness.

Disadvantages

1. These agents have many adverse reactions.
2. **Disease may progress without manifesting symptoms.** Injection of hydrocortisone can be given in the joint. This reduces the systemic adverse reactions.

Uses: These agents are employed only in patients who fail to respond to salicylates, penicillamine, gold or azathioprine.

Azathioprine: It suppresses immune responses in the body.

Advantages

1. It is as effective as gold or penicillamine.
2. Can prevent or delay the use of steroids.

Disadvantages

1. It has carcinogenic activity.
2. In pregnant ladies it produces deformities of the foetus (teratogenic effect).

Precautions

Repeated blood counts should be done.

If patient complains of sore throat or fever he is advised to seek immediate medical help and this drug is withdrawn.

Uses: It is given only if the patient is not responding to less toxic agents.

Methotrexate is also used.

Cyclosporine is effective but causes kidney damage.

28

Narcotic Analgesics

Pain is one of the major sufferings of mankind.

An analgesic is a drug that results in the abolition of sensation of pain and is different from an anaesthetic agent. An anaesthetic agent causes abolition of all modalities of sensation. For example, morphine which is an analgesic drug makes the patient unable to appreciate the sensation of pain although he can still appreciate the sensation of touch or of heat.

Local anaesthetic (e.g. procaine) when injected near the nerve causes loss of all sensations — but only in a localised area. Since pain, touch, heat and all other sensations are lost therefore it is wrong to name it local analgesic.

Pain can be relieved by:
(a) Treating the cause, e.g. antacid to relieve acidity and antispasmodics in colicky pain.
(b) Interrupting conduction of pain, e.g. local anesthetics.
(c) Centrally acting drugs which increase threshold of pain perception, e.g. non-narcotic and narcotic analgesics.

A narcotic induces drowsiness, sleep, stupor or insensibility in a patient. It produces drug dependence. **Many of these drugs produce euphoria** therefore are addicting**.**

These drugs differ from hypnotics as these produce sleep as well as analgesia.

Narcotic drugs are divided into three groups:
1. Natural: Opium and its alkaloids (morphine, codeine).
2. Semisynthetic derivatives of morphine and codeine, e.g. pholcodeine, oxycodone, diacetyl morphine (heroin).
3. Synthetic derivatives: Pethidine, methadone, pentazocine, etc.

Endogenous opioid peptide receptors: Opioid peptides—endorphins, encephalins, dynorphins and beta endorphins — are present in brain, pituitary, spinal cord and the gut and the opioid receptors (μ, k, δ) are also present. Opium alkaloids act through these receptors.

Stimulation of mu (μ) receptor produces supraspinal analgesia, respiratory depression, reduction in gut motility, increase in tone of smooth muscles, sedation, euphoria and physical dependence. **Morphine exerts its effect primarily by stimulating m receptors.**

Stimulation of K (kappa) receptors leads to spinal analgesia, dysphoria and sedation. **Pentazocine** stimulates these receptors. **Nalbuphine and butorphanol** also act on kappa receptors and cause significant greater analgesia in women.

Delta receptor stimulation is associated with analgesia and changes in emotional behaviour.

Morphine

This drug occurs naturally and was known to the Indians for over five thousand years. The juice squeezed from the unripe seed capsule of poppy (Papaver somniferum in Latin means sleep bringing) is rich in opium. The main active ingredient of opium is morphine, which is obtained along with other alkaloids codeine, thebaine, noscapine and papavarine—the **last three lack analgesic activity**.

Actions of morphine

(A) On CNS

1. Morphine produces
   (a) Analgesia, euphoria and sedation. It relieves pain (analgesic activity) by increasing threshold to pain perception and altering emotional reactions to pain.

2. Morphine depresses
   (a) **Respiratory center**—which can cause death.
   (b) **Vasomotor center**—which results in fall in BP.
   (c) **Cough center**—therefore has antitussive activity.
   (d) **Thermoregulatory center**—in hypothalamus causes fall in body temperature.
   (e) **Cortical areas**—thereby produces sleep. It has sedative effect.

3. It stimulates
   (a) Chemoreceptor trigger zone and therefore induces vomiting.
   (b) Vomiting center.
   (c) Vagal center in brain and produces bradycardia.
   (d) Oculomotor center therefore causes constriction of pupils. **Morphine addiction and its toxicity can be diagnosed from this feature.**
   (e) Truncal rigidity.

4. Increases intracranial pressure.

(B) Extra CNS effects

(a) It causes contraction of smooth muscles of bronchi, gut and sphincters. Through this action it produces constipation, retention of urine and precipitation of asthma.

(b) It releases histamine in the body producing bronchoconstriction and fall in BP.

(c) Biliary tract—constricts bile duct resulting in biliary colic.

Special Features about its Effects

Sedative effects of morphine

Patients who are in extreme pain and are apprehensive due to disease such as myocardial infarction or injury need this drug. It relieves pain and by producing sedation it reduces their anxiety. These patients shortly after morphine injection drop off quietly into sound sleep.

Analgesic action of morphine

The dose of morphine required to produce analgesia varies from individual to individual. Although the dose normally given is 15 mg, the right dose of morphine is that which relieves patient's appreciation of pain.

Stimulation of the vomiting center

Vomiting is controlled by a center in the medulla. If the activity of this center is stimulated vomiting is produced. The therapeutic dose of morphine may produce vomiting in one-third of the patients while in others nausea alone may be produced.

This is highly undesirable effect of morphine because:
(i) Patients do not appreciate it.
(ii) It is hazardous in serious conditions such as myocardial infarction.

To overcome this difficulty morphine is sometimes given with an antihistaminic (promethazine) which blocks this effect.

Depression of respiratory center

Morphine directly depresses the activity of the respiratory center. Rate of respiration as well as tidal volume are reduced. There is depressed response to carbon dioxide in patients suffering from chronic respiratory diseases (who have reduced respiratory reserve), morphine can produce serious problems in these patients. Often patients of chronic bronchitis and emphysema pass into respiratory failure, coma and death after receiving morphine.

It precipitates bronchial asthma. Often doctors have difficulty in differentiating bronchial from cardiac asthma. Morphine is the drug of choice in cardiac asthma. Whenever, there is difficulty in differentiating (cardiac from bronchial asthma) the use of morphine should be avoided. **Aminophylline** can be administered in such situation till final diagnosis is made.

Morphine and the gut

By stimulation of mu (μ) receptors morphine causes spasmodic contraction of the smooth muscles of the gut. It also contracts the sphincters. Propulsion of food in the intestine is slowed. The reflexes of defecation are not appreciated and patient develops constipation. It can therefore be given in diarrhea.

Muscles of the bladder and the sphincter are contracted. In older patients **acute retention of urine** is likely to occur because many men in addition have enlarged prostate gland. Nurse should always be on the look out for this complication of morphine.

If morphine is given to a patient suffering from biliary or renal colic, it relieves his pain but **disease is intensified**. It is because the drug produces spasm of the sphincter of Oddi and ureters respectively. A rise in pressure may occur and cause the patient further pain. **In these conditions it should be given along with atropine**.

Morphine should not be given in undiagnosed abdominal pain till patient is hospitalised.

Routes of administration
1. Rectal — morphine hydromorphine.
2. Transdermal — fentanyl.
3. Intranasal — butorphanol.
4. Buccal transmuscosal — fentanyl citrate lozenges.

Uses of morphine
1. To relieve pain of the severe variety not likely to respond to non-narcotic analgesics.
2. In cardiac asthma (left ventricular failure).
3. For treatment of patients suffering from acute hemorrhagic shock.

4. As preoperative medication.

5. Intractable profuse diarrhea. Tincture opium is given orally.

Morphine is the drug of choice in left ventricular failure. Morphine helps these patients by reducing the sensitivity of the respiratory center to the messages from lungs. Morphine thus reduces the number of impulses to which it responds and reduces the rate of respiration thereby increasing the efficiency of respiration.

Adverse effects

1. It induces nausea and vomiting.
2. Produces constipation.
3. Precipitates bronchial asthma.
4. Produces acute retention of urine.
5. Depresses respiration.
6. Rarely allergic reactions may also be seen.
7. Increases intracranial pressure. **It should be avoided in head injury.**

Treatment of morphine toxicity

Toxicity of morphine results from accidental over dosing. Patient becomes stuperous, has shallow respiration. Heart rate and blood pressure both are reduced. Pupils are constricted initially, but near death they tend to dilate.

(a) Airways are kept patent and artificial respiration is given.

(b) Gastric lavage is done and the material preserved for legal purposes.

(c) Fluids are administered intravenously to raise blood pressure. Vasopressor (noradrenaline or dopamine) is added to the fluid.

(d) Specific antagonist of morphine **(naloxone)** is injected. If naloxone is not available nalorphine is injected.

Conditions in which morphine **should not be given:**

1. Head injury
2. Prostatic hypertrophy
3. Bronchial asthma and emphysema
4. Undiagnosed acute abdominal pain.

Tolerance means that the patient is capable of tolerating large doses of the drug. For example, if 60 mg of morphine can kill a normal man, a patient tolerant to morphine may not show any adverse effects to this dose. Some morphine addicts are able to inject themselves with doses of 100 mg or more without danger. They are said to have developed tolerance to this drug.

An individual with pain tolerates morphine better than the one without.

Drug dependence or drug addiction

All narcotic analgesics are drugs of addiction and are legally classified as dangerous drugs. An addict exhibits three features:

1. It is tolerant to drug
2. It is habituated to this drug
3. Shows withdrawal symptoms if his drug is stopped.

Habituation means that the addict is mentally dependent on the drug and shows mental irritability if he does not get his dose. This phenomenon is seen in cigaratte smokers.

Withdrawal symptoms show that the addict depends on his drug not only mentally but also physically. When this drug is withheld from the addict he develops symptoms such as tremors, dryness of mouth, photophobia (due to dilated pupils) and diarrhea. Withdrawal symptoms are nearly the opposite of pharmacological actions of the drug.

Morphine addiction is spreading like wild fire in this country. It is quite common among doctors and nurses. Two to three injections of morphine are sufficient to start the patient on path of addiction.

Codeine: It is chemically—methyl morphine. In the body it is partly converted to morphine. It differs from morphine in the following ways:

1. It is a less potent analgesic.
2. Can be given orally as it is well absorbed when given orally.
3. It has longer duration of action.
4. It is an excellent antitussive (supresses cough) agent. This effect is selective and is exerted at sub-analgesic doses.

Uses

1. It is used as antitussive agent. It is a common ingredient of most of the cough mixtures.
2. It is used for controlling diarrhoea.
3. It is used as analgesic in combination with NSAIDS.

Heroin: It is diacetylmorphine. It is 6 times more potent than morphine hence smaller dose is required to produce morphine like effects.

Dihydrocodeine is used as an analgesic.

Pholcodeine and dextromethorphan are better antitussive agents. They have fewer side effects. The addictive potential of these drugs is low.

Omnopon is a mixture of morphine and alkaloids of opium. It is administered parenterally. It is not considered superior to morphine. Not used now.

Pethidine: This is synthetic opiate that is commonly used in clinical practice. The analgesic activity of pethidine is as good as morphine but the dose required is more.

If differs from morphine in the following respects:

(a) It is less potent.
(b) It has quick onset but shorter duration of action.
(c) It **does not suppress cough.**
(d) It can be given orally.
(e) **It has atropine like activity and produces mydriasis.**
(f) **It produces tachycardia** along with hypotension.
(g) Nausea and vomiting are less marked effects.
(h) It is less constipating.

This drug is preferred in most of the clinical situations including labour as it produces less respiratory depression. It is used as preanaesthetic medication.

Warning and nursing care

In equianalgesic doses pethidine produces as much respiratory depression as morphine.

Respiratory rate is not much reduced but the tidal volume is reduced by pethidine. **Counting of respiratory rate alone therefore, may be misleading**.

Uses

1. Used as analgesic in conditions where morphine is used.
   (i) Where short time surgical intervention is required, e.g. gastroscopy, cystoscopy or pyelography.
   (ii) Where the pain needs to be controlled effectively and the associated anxiety needs to be suppressed, e.g. myocardial infarction, burns of major degree.
2. As preanaesthetic medication.
3. During labour for relieving pain. It is preferred over morphine as it does not interfere with uterine contractions.

Methadone: It acts on mµ (µ) receptors.

Advantages

1. It is effective when given orally. It causes less nausea and vomiting.
2. It has long duration of action therefore is useful in treating opioid addiction.
3. Degree of euphoria produced by this drug is less.
4. Withdrawal symptoms are mild and slow to appear.
5. Addiction liability is less.

Disadvantages

1. Injection of methadone produces local irritation.
2. Tolerance develops.
3. Withdrawal symptoms are mild but persist for longer time.

Adverse reactions

1. Mental clouding and dryness of mouth.
2. Nausea and vomiting are less frequent.

Propoxyphene: It has mild-to-moderate degree of analgesic activity. **It does not suppress cough.**

Warning

It has strong addiction liability. It is usually given in combination with non-narcotic analgesics. The use of this combination should not be encouraged.

PARTIAL OPIOID AGONISTS

Pentazocine: It is partial agonist of mµ (µ) receptors and agonist at kappa (κ) and receptors.

Advantages

1. It has analgesic activity.
2. It is less likely to produce addiction.

3. Less respiratory depression.

4. It can be given orally, subcutaneously and even through rectum.

Disadvantages

1. Withdrawal symptoms are not easily recognised.

2. It may produce psychotomimetic changes in some patients.

3. It has sympathomimetic effect hence is cardiac toxic, causes increase in BP and heart rate.

4. Partial agonist at mu receptors also acts on kappa receptors. It is good analgesic because it causes dysphoria.

5. **If given in narcotic addict it precipitates withdrawal symptoms.**

Adverse reactions

1. Chronic use produces subcutaneous and muscular fibrosis.

2. It increases systemic as well as pulmonary vascular pressure, therefore should be used with caution in patients of acute MI.

Buprenorphine: It is partial mμ (μ) agonist. **It is 25–50 times more potent than morphine and has long duration of action and can be given sublingually. It is therefore used for relieving acute severe pain.**

The actions of this drug are not reversed by naloxone.

Nalbuphine: It stimulates kappa receptors but blocks mu receptors. It needs to be injected. Degree of respiratory depression is less than with morphine. However, when respiration is depressed **it is not reversed by naloxone**.

Butorphenol: It has low addiction liability. Like pentazocine it strains heart and therefore is not recommended for treating pain associated with myocardial infarction.

Tramadol Hydrochloride: It is codeine analouage. It has antitussive activity. Tolerance and drug dependence are absent. It has good analgesic activity. It **does not produce respiratory depression, addiction and tolerance**. It is given to relieve severe acute or severe chronic pains. **Effects partially antagonised by naloxone.**

Dezocine is partial agonist at mu receptors. It is similar to morphine but effects are less marked.

Fentanyl, sufentanil, and remifenetanil are derivatives of pethidine.

Fentanyl

Advantages of fentanyl

1. It is ten times more analgesic than morphine.

2. Mild effect on CVS. It is safer than other opiods.

3. Does not increase intracranial tension.

4. Does not liberate histamine and can be given in asthmatics. Patches are available.

Adverse reactions

Nausea, vomiting, sweating and stupor.

Precautions to be taken while administering pethidine, morphine or any opioid

1. Morphine should be administered with care in patients of **emphysema, bronchiectasis** and **kyphosis** as morphine precipitates respiratory failure in these individuals.
2. Morphine should not be given to patients of **bronchial asthma** as it worsens asthma and causes respiratory depression.
3. **Myxeodematus** patiens are highly sensitive to morphine. Same is true about patients of **Addison's disease**.
4. Morphine should not be combined with tricyclic antidepressants and phenothiazines.
5. It worsens hypovolemic shock. Therefore, it should be avoided. If at all it is necessary it can be given after the fluid correction.
6. Elderly patients and young children need lower dose of these drugs.
7. It **raises intracranial pressure,** it should be avoided in patients of head injury as it interferes with the guiding signs (pupillary size, etc.).
8. Morphine tends to accumulate in patients with liver and renal failure. Dose must be constantly monitored in such patients.
9. Three to four injections of this drug produce addiction liability. It should be withdrawn at the earliest and substituted by a non-narcotic analgesic.
10. Morphine and pethidine are highly abused by the medical and para medical staff. There is need to keep these drugs under lock.

NARCOTIC ANTAGONISTS

These drugs oppose or antagonise the effects of narcotic agents by displacing them from their receptors.

There are two types of these agents:

1. Pure antagonist, e.g. naloxone and naltrexone.
2. Partial agonists, e.g. nalorphine and less important drugs such as propiram and profadol.

Nalorphine: It is partial agonist

1. Produces analgesia.
2. Produces drowsiness wih dysphoria or visual hallucinations.
3. Produces constriction of smooth muscles of the intestine, sphincters and bronchi.
4. In high doses it produces respiratory depression.

It abolishes euphoria, miosis and respiratory depression produced by morphine.

Effect of morphine on gastrointestinal tract and sphincters is also abolished.

Nalorphine is used

(a) For treating acute morphine poisoning if naloxone is not available.

(b) For diagnosis of opioid addiction.

Naloxone: It is a pure antagonist.

1. It antagonises the respiratory depressant effect of morphine.
2. It does not produce respiratory depression of its own.
3. Tolerance does not develop.

Disadvantages: Cannot be given orally. It has short duration of action, needs to be repeated.

Uses

1. For diagnosing addiction: Administration of this drug in narcotic addict precipitates withdrawal symptoms (diagnostic use).
2. For the treatment of poisoning due to narcotic agents: It reverses the respiratory depressant effect of most opioids.

   Dose: 0.1–0.4 mg IV

Naltrexone: Well absorbed orally but undergoes high first pass metabolism. Used to treat addiction.

Nalmefine: Only IV administration reverses effects of morphine in 1–3 minutes, normalizes respiration, level of consciousness, pupil size and bowel activity.

There is no tolerance to antagonistic effects of these agents.

Nursing care of patient of morphine poisoning

1. Give respiratory support.
2. Maintain BP.
3. Perform gastric lavage with potassium permanganate to remove morphine from stomach.
4. Naloxone 0.4–0.8 mg IV and repeat every 10–15 minutes.

29

Drugs used in Convulsive Disorders

Anti-convulsant drugs are used basically to treat epilepsy but are also effective in controlling convulsions due to other causes, e.g. convulsions produced by intracranial tumor or uremia.

Epilepsy is due to hyperexcitability of the neurons. It is sporadic in nature and is self limiting. Epilepsy is of various types:

1. Generalised convulsions are seen in:
    (i) Grandmal epilepsy (tonic-clonic epilepsy).
    (ii) Petitmal epilepsy (absence seizures) and its variance.
    (iii) Tonic seizures.
    (iv) Myoclonic seizures.

2. Partial convulsions (focal convulsions) are seen in:
    (i) Simple partial seizures.
    (ii) Complex partial seizures.
    (iii) Partial with secondary generalised tonic-clonic seizures.

Antiepileptic drugs are classified as follows

1. Long acting barbiturates: Phenobarbitone, mephobarbitone, methabarbitone and primidone.

2. Hydantoin derivatives: Diphenylhydantoin, mephenytoin and ethotoin.

3. Oxazolidindiones: Trimethadione and paramethadione.

4. Succinimides: Methsuximide, ethosuximide, phensuximide.

5. Phenalacetylureas: Phenacemide.

6. Valproic acid: Sodium valproate.

7. Iminostilbines: Carbamazepine.

8. Miscellaneous: Phenacemide, dexamphetamine, lidocaine, bromide and acetazolamide.

BARBITURATES

Phenobarbitone and other drugs belonging to this category (mephobarbitone and methabarbitone) are highly effective in grandmal epilepsy.

Phenobarbitone

Advantages

1. It is effective in controlling most of the convulsions (except absence seizures).
2. Cost is low.

3. Adverse reactions are few.

4. In children growth rate is not affected.

5. Can be combined with phenytoin.

6. Learning is not impaired in children.

Disadvantages

1. Not effective in petitmal epilepsy—may even aggravate this condition.

2. Not much effective in psychomotor type epilepsy.

3. May produce behavioural changes in children and older patients.

Adverse reactions: Drowsiness and lethargy. Both tend to disappear after few days.

Uses

To treat:
  (a) Grandmal epilepsy.
  (b) Cortical focal epilepsy.
  (c) Febrile convulsions.

Mephobarbitone: In liver it is converted to phenobarbitone and the anti-epileptic effect is due to this metabolite. It has no advantage over phenobarbitone. **Methobarbitone** is not better than phenobarbitone.

Primidone: In the body it is converted to phenobarbitone and phenylethylmalonamide.The parent compound as well its metabolites are anticonvulsants.

Advantages

1. It is broad spectrum antiepileptic agent. It is effective in grandmal, psychomotor and myoclonic epilepsies. Few cases of petitmal also respond to this drug.

2. It can also be combined with hydantoin derivatives.

Disadvantages

1. At the beginning of the treatment dizziness and drowsiness are sometimes severe.

2. It produces vertigo, ataxia, diplopia and dysarthria in some patients.

3. Rarely aplastic anaemia may also be produced.

Adverse reactions

1. Depression of central nervous system including respiratory depression.

2. Allergic reactions.

3. Neuralgias and myalgias.

Drug interactions: It can be safely combined with phenytoin.

HYDANTOINS

Phenytoin: It is effective in treatment of all types of epilepsy except absence seizures. Sensory aura associated with epilepsy is not much affected. It stabilises the membranes and inhibits fits. It can be given in combination with phenobarbiturates.

Uses

1. It is used in treatment of grandmal epilepsy, symptomatic convulsion and psychomotor epilepsy.
2. Trigeminal neuralgias.
3. Cardiac arrhythmias.

Adverse reactions

1. Nausea and vomiting.
2. Severe ataxia.
3. Allergic reactions.
4. Abdominal pain resembling appendicitis.
5. Hyperplasia of the gums — constant brushing of teeth reduces this problem.
6. Because of anti-folate effect it produces megaloblastic anaemia.
7. Vitamin D deficiency.
8. It is teratogenic.

Dose: 100 mg/three times a day orally. Intravenous injection of 50 mg/ml is also available. Dose should not exceed 50 mg per minute.

Warning: It should not be given intramuscularly.

Nursing care

1. Patients should be asked to brush their teeth frequently (3–4 times a day).
2. This drug should not be injected intramuscularly.
3. Supplements of folic acid should be given along with this drug. Over dosing with folic acid should be avoided as it counters the good effects of phenytoin.
4. Vitamin D and calcium can be supplemented.
5. If patient develops megaloblastic anaemia and does not respond to folic acid supplements, phenytoin should be gradually withdrawn and phenobarbitone started in such a patient.
6. Patients must be started on the second drug before the first is withdrawn.

OXAZOLIDINDIONES

Trimethadione (Troxidone): This drug is used to treat petitmal epilepsy.

Advantages

1. Most of the patients respond to this drug.
2. It takes 3–4 days to control petitmal epilepsy.
3. Acute toxicity is low.

Disadvantages

1. It aggravates grandmal epilepsy.
2. On chronic use it produces serious adverse reactions—agranulocytosis and renal damage.

Precautions

1. Family members of the patients should be asked to look for and report signs of serious toxicity.

2. Urine examination should be done frequently for presence of albumin.

3. Blood counts should be done at weekly intervals.

Paramethadione has effects like trimethadione but is not preferred as it produces drowsiness. It is used only in cases which fail to respond to trimethadione and ethosuximide.

SUCCINIMIDES

Ethosuximide: It is the drug of choice for petitmal epilepsy and is also effective in myoclonic spasms and akinetic epilepsy.

Adverse reactions

1. Anorexia and vomiting are produced due to gastric irritation.
2. Rarely allergic symptoms are seen.
3. Blood dyscrasias may be occasionally reported.
4. Parkinson like symptoms and photophobia.

Phensuximide and methsuximide do not aggrevate grandmal epilepsy. All other actions are like ethosuximide. Phensuximide is less effective and methsuximide more toxic than ethosuximide in petitmal epilepsy.

BENZODIAZEPINES

Diazepam, clonazepam, lorazepam are useful in treating petitmal and myoclonic epilepsies. Diazepam and clonazepam have short duration of action. Tolerance develops to these drugs hence utilised in severe acute epilepsy, e.g. status epilepticus.

They are effective against:
(a) Petitmal epilepsy.
(b) Myoclonic seizures.
(c) Status epilepticus.

GABAPENTIN

Used to treat refractory petitmal cases.

Adverse drug reactions

1. Sedation and ataxia
2. Dizziness and fatigue

On continuation of medicine adverse drug reactions tend to disappear.

SODIUM VALPROATE

It is broad spectrum antiepileptic.

It produces minimal sedation. It acts through GABA ergic system. It has following advantages:

1. It does not produce sedation.
2. Adverse effects are uncommon.
3. It is broad spectrum antiepileptic agent and is effective against petitmal, grandmal, myoclonic and temporal lobe epilepsies.

Dose: 600–1600 mg/day

Adverse reactions

1. GIT — anorexia, nausea and vomiting.
2. CNS — ataxia and tremors.
3. Hepatotoxicity, alopecia, increase in NH_3 in blood.

ACETAZOLAMIDE (DIAMOX)

It is useful in petitmal epilepsy. For details please refer DIURETICS.

SULTHIAME

It is effective in temporal lobe epilepsy. Grandmal and myoclonic epilepsies may also respond to this drug. It is not used because of its toxicity.

Adverse reactions

1. It may precipitate status epilepticus.
2. It produces psychotic reactions, kidney damage and blurring of vision.

Dose: 100–600 mg/day.

IMINOSTILBINES

Carbamazepine: It is effective in all epilepsies except petitmal including temporal lobe epilepsy. In addition it brings about a positive change in the personality of epileptic patient.

Uses

1. Temporal and grandmal epilepsies specially those refractory to other drugs.
2. Trigeminal neuralgia.
3. Post herpetic pain.

Adverse reactions

1. Nausea and vomiting.
2. Diplopia and blurred vision.
3. GIT: Nausea, vomiting and abdominal pain.
4. Liver damage.
5. Increase in body weight.
6. Hair loss.

Nursing care

1. Advise patient to get liver functions done at monthly intervals.
2. Inform the patient regarding ADR's specially increase in body weight and hair loss.

Lamotrizine: It is useful in refractory cases of petitmal epilepsy. It is long acting drug therefore it is given on alternate days.

Adverse drug reactions

1. Ataxia and dizziness.
2. Nausea and vomiting.
3. Stevens-Johnson syndrome.
4. Disseminated intravascular coagulation.

Felbamate: It is effective in intractable epilepsy in children (Lennox-Gastant syndrome) consisting of convulsions, and mental retardation. This condition is resistant to other anticonvulsants.

Zonisamide, oxycarbazepine, vigabartin, stirepentol and milacemide all have been lately introduced in management of epilepsies.

Amphetamine: It is added to other drugs, e.g.

(a) With phenobarbitone in grandmal epilepsy, it reduces drowsiness.
(b) In petitmal it is given with suximides.
(c) Given alone it corrects hyperkinetic epilepsy in children.

NEWER ANTIEPILEPTIC DRUGS

Vigabatrin, topiramate, tiagabine, levetiracetam.

Vigabatrin: It preserves GABA by inhibiting GABA transaminase. It is effective in patients with refractory epilepsy. It is used as an adjuvant.

Topiramate: It acts by various mechanisms (by Na^+ channel inactivation, GABA potentiation, antagonism of glutamate receptors and inhibition of carbonic anhydrase).

It has broad spectrum of anticonvulsant activity. It is used to treat grandmal, petitmal and myoclonic epilepsy.

Tiagabine: If potentiates GABA mediated neuronal inhibition. It is used to treat partial seizures not controlled by standard antileptic drugs.

Nursing care of epileptic patient

1. Therapy should be started after proper evaluation—single drug in minimal dosage should be given.
2. The dosages can be gradually increased to degree of efficacy or tolerance.
3. Combinations should be employed when necessary.
4. Phenobarbitone, phenytoin, primidone and ethosuximide can be given once a day at night. All other drugs should be given in divided doses.
5. Relatives of the patient should be instructed to note the frequency of attacks. This gives an indication whether treatment is effective or not.
6. Treatment should be continued for at least two years after the last attack and drugs withdrawn gradually.
7. Patients and his relatives must be made aware of the toxicity of these drugs. They must report signs of toxicity.
8. Patient must be warned against sudden stoppage of the drugs.
9. Nurse must examine urine of patients on trimethadione on every visit for the presence of albumin.

STATUS EPILEPTICUS

It is a condition in which convulsions occur at short intervals. If patient is allowed to continue in this state, he gets exhausted, develops hyperpyrexia and may die.

Treatment of Status Epilepticus

1. This condition is treated by controlling convulsions by:

   (A) **Diazepam** given intravenously in the dose of 10 mg in adults and 3–10 mg for children of over 6 months of age. Dose may be repeated after 15 minutes till the convulsions stop.

   or

   5–10 ml paraldehyde is given intramuscularly. This can be repeated after 60 minutes. Phenobarbitone is injected along with it.

   Phenytoin is given 13–18 mg/kg by slow IV infusion..

   Lidocaine infusion is used to control convulsions.

   If the above fails and the facility of general anaesthesia is available **thiopentone sodium** can be administered.

   After the convulsions have been controlled patient is nursed the way unconscious individual is done. Intravenous fluids, input/output charts and patency of airway are the factors that need attention of the attending nurse.

   Appropriate anti-epileptic agent should be started in these patients. Patients should be maintained on oral antiepileptic agents and discharged.

   Convulsions due to other causes are managed on similar lines.

Pregnancy and antiepileptic agents: Most antiepileptic drugs produce fetal damage, hence advise the patients against pregnancy. If this is not possible keep the patient on minimal dosage of one drug.

30

Antianxiety Drugs

Following drugs are used in treatment of anxiety.

Benzodiazepines

1. Ultrashort acting: Triazolam and midazolam.
2. Short acting (12–24 hrs): Alprazolam, oxazepam, nitrazepam, lorazepam, halazepam and temazepam.
3. Long acting: Diazepam, clonazepam, flurazepam, clobazam and chlordiazepoxide.

All there drugs act on GABA receptors and produce calmness, sedation, amnesia. In addition these drugs reduce BP and nocturnal gastric acid secretion.

Aprazolam: It is short acting anti-anxiety drug and can be administered 8 hourly. It is effective in mild depression associated with insomnia.

Clonazepam: It is useful in manic depression as well as acute and recurrent anxiety.

Diazepam: It is one of the most commonly used benzodiazepines.

1. It produces calmness without inducing sleep—a daytime sedative.
2. Given at night it produces sleep resembling normal sleep. It does not suppress REM sleep. Orally administered diazepam has better anti-anxiety effect than parenterally administered.
3. It has anticonvulsant effect.
4. Relaxes skeletal muscles.

Dose: 2–5 mg twice daily. It is useful in generalised anxiety disorders as well as acute and recurrent anxiety.

Oxazepam: It is an active metabolite of diazepam.

Disadvantages

1. It is short acting
2. It is not well absorbed.

Chlordiazepoxide (Librium): Though it is a benzodiazepine, its actions resemble barbiturates.

1. It produces calmness.
2. It also produces sedation.
3. It produces skeletal muscle relaxation.
4. It stimulates appetite.

Adverse reactions

1. Drowsiness, lethargy and ataxia.
2. Hypotension is produced in a few.

Disadvantages

1. Tolerance develops.
2. It induces physical dependence. Withdrawl symptoms are produced on its stoppage.

Uses

1. Anxiety and neurosis.
2. It is used to suppress withdrawal symptoms of alcohol.
3. As preanaesthetic medication.

Precautions to be observed during its administration:

1. Patients should be instructed to avoid alcohol with this drug.
2. It should not be given to patients with depressed respiration.
3. Response to this drug varies among patients.

Dose: 110 mg two to three times a day.

Busipirone: It has good anxiolytic activity but onset is delayed (2 weeks). It has no muscle relaxant activity.

Propranolol: Reduces symptoms due to anxiety and can be used in combination with benzodiazepines.

Nursing care of anxious patient

1. It is important for the nurse to remember that anxious and neurotic patients are those who have failed to adjust to environment. Drugs can only help relieve symptoms but cure lies in helping the individual to adjust to his circumstances. Sympathetic attitude is of greater help than drugs.
2. It is duty of the nurse to educate the relatives of patients in this direction.

31

Antidepressants

Depression could be reactive (due to some cause and is treated by psychotherapy) while endogenous depression is due to biochemical abnormalities and needs drug therapy.

Depression may alternate with mania (bipolar depression).

These drugs are found to be useful in relieving endogenous depression. These are classified as:
1. Tricyclic antidepressants — Imipramine, amitryptyline.
3. Selective serotonin reuptake inhibitors (SSRIs) — fluoxetine, trazadone, maprotiline.
2. Monoamine oxidase inhibitors — isocarboxazid, iproniazid, tranylcypromine.
4. Miscellaneous — lithium and mianserum.
5. Newer antidepressants.

TRICYCLIC ANTIDEPRESSANTS

Imipramine and Amitryptyline: These drugs
1. Reduce suicidal tendencies.
2. Produce improvement in behaviour — patients become less withdrawn, take interest in surroundings and feel energetic.

Disadvantages
1. It takes 3–4 weeks before the effects are seen.
2. Produce sedation.
3. Patients experience difficulty in concentrating and thinking.
4. Produce drug dependence.

Adverse reactions
1. Due to anticholinergic effects: dry mouth, glaucoma is precipitated and urinary retention can occur.
2. Due to alpha blockade produces postural hypotension, tremors and hallucinations.
3. With large doses cardiac arrhythmias are produced.

Dose: Amitryptyline: 50 mg/day, imipramine: 50–150 mg/day.

Drug interactions
1. Thyroid and phenothiazines increase the effect of these drugs.

2. Imipramine increases the effect of phenylephrine and noradrenaline.

3. Antihypertensive effects of guanethedine and mecamylamine are blocked by these drugs.

Uses

1. For treatment of depression.
2. Bed wetting.

Newer tricyclic antidepressants (doxepin and iprindole) are no way superior to the older drugs.

MONOAMINE OXIDASE INHIBITORS

(i) **Non-selective** — isocarboxazide, nialamide, phenelzine and tranylcypromine.

(ii) **Selective–MAO A inhibitors** — clorgyline.

MAO B inhibitors — selegiline (deprenyl), rasagiline, meclobamide.

These drugs produce improvement in the patient. Suicidal tendencies are reduced.

Non-selective MAO inhibitors are usually not preferred because:

1. These produce many adverse reactions.
2. They interact with drugs and food items and produce serious adverse reactions.
3. It have late onset of action.
4. It have low therapeutic index.

Adverse reactions

1. May induce excitement.
2. Tremors, twitching and ataxia.
3. Constipation and dry mouth.
4. Allergic reactions.
5. Severe hypertension is produced when given along with cheese.

Interactions: Patient taking MAO inhibitors should avoid following drugs.

Alcohol, barbiturates, morphine, pethidine, amphetamine, atropine and tricyclic antidepressants.

Dose

1. Isocarboxazide: l0 mg/day.
2. Nialamide: 75–150 mg/day.
3. Phenelzine: 45–60 mg/day.
4. Tranylcypromine: 10–30 mg/day.

NEWER ANTIDEPRESSANTS
Doxepin
Advantages

1. Causes less complications associated with CNS, therefore preferred in elderly patients.
2. It has quicker onset of action.

Mianserin: It blocks α_2 presynaptic receptors. It does not inhibit uptake of 5-HT or noradrenaline, therefore does not block activities of clonidine and guanethidine.

It has sedative activity and relieves anxiety and panic attacks.

It has quick onset of action.

Disadvantages

1. Increases proneness to convulsions.
2. Blood dyscrasias are produced.

Amoxapine

Advantages

1. It has antidepressant and neuroleptic actions hence useful in psychotic depression.
2. It has quicker onset of action.

Disadvantages

1. It is cardiotoxic.
2. Produces Parkinsons' syndrome.
3. In overdose it produces status epilepticus.

SELECTIVE SEROTONIN UPTAKE INHIBITORS (SSRIs)

Advantages of SSRIs

1. It have low anticholinergic effects therefore adverse effects (urinary retention, constipation and dry mouth) are limited.
2. Cause less sedation.
3. Cardiovascular effects are minimal.
4. Safer because of high therapeutic index.

Trazadone: It selectively blocks 5-HT uptake and has sedative activity.

Advantages

1. Less prone to precipitate cardiac arrhythmias is therefore useful in the elderly patients.
2. It has no anticholinergic activity. It produces bradycardia.

Fluoxetine: It is a selective 5-HT uptake blocker. It is longest acting.

It has no sedative and hypotensive effects.

Does not produce cardiac arrhythmias.

It is used as first line drug. **It is slow acting therefore not used in acute attack.**

Adverse drug reactions: Headache, insomnia, anxiety and diarrhoea.

Maprotiline: It is selective 5-HT uptake blocker with weak dopaminergic (D_2) blocking effect. It is effective in neurotic depression.

Disadvantage: It is cardiotoxic and can precipitate epilepsy.

LITHIUM CARBONATE

This drug is useful in mania and manic depressive psychosis.

Advantages

1. It causes less sedation.
2. It is highly effective in mania.

It effectively controls psychomotor overactivity of these patients.

Disadvantages

1. All patients do not respond to this drug.
2. **Chronic use produces severe renal toxicity.**
3. Gain in body weight.

Adverse reactions (mild toxicity)

1. Muscular weakness, tremors and ataxia.
2. Allergic reactions.
3. Hypothyroidism.
4. Increase in body weight.
5. Abnormal ECG.

Severe Toxicity (acute)

1. Parkinson-like syndrome.
2. Hypotension.
3. Coma.

Uses

1. Maniac episodes.
2. Manic depressive psychosis.

Precautions

1. Watch for adverse reactions.
2. Body weight, serum levels of T_3 and T_4 should be done every 6 months.
3. Renal function should be done every 6 months.
4. Serum lithium level should be checked at least once a month.

Other drugs used in depression: Caffeine, amphetamine and methylphenidate are helpful in exogenous depression but have no role to play in endogenous depression.

Nursing care of patient of depression

Everyone experiences depression during bereavements in family circle or failures. In fact to fail to be depressed at such times would be abnormal. Some individuals may get more depressed (exogenous depression) and for a longer time. These individuals need **psychotherapy** rather than drugs.

There are individuals, who become deeply depressed for no obvious reason—this is referred to as endogenous depression which needs treatment. Many of these patients take their own lives.

Nurses must make efforts to win the confidence of these patients.

Try to prevent giving them a feeling of guilt.

These patients usually avoid taking drugs. Nurses must ensure drug compliance.

32

Psychotomimetic Agents

As the name indicates these drugs produce symptoms which resemble psychosis.

LYSERGIC ACID DIETHYLAMIDE (LSD)

It is an alkaloid derived from ergot.

Actions: It is highly potent—20–25 microgram of this drug is capable of producing:

1. Fear psychosis and emotional outbursts.
2. There is disorientation of time and space.

Adverse reactions

1. LSD may produce suicidal tendencies.
2. Permanent psychosis may develop. Produces chromosomal damage.

Mescaline: It is an alkaloid obtained from Mexican cactus. It produces tremors and hallucinations, disturbances in thought process and mood changes. It is not much abused in India.

Cannabis (Marihuana): It is obtained from a plant Cannabis sauva or Cannabis indica.

Resinous exudate of the female plant is called *Charas*.

Dried leaves and flowering shoots are used as *Bhang*. *Ganja* is resinous mass obtained from brackets of female inflorescence.

Marihuana is the common name.

It produces following effects:

(a) Euphoria—dysphoria may be produced in few individuals.
(b) Perceptions of sense is increased but they become vivid.
(c) Visual hallucinations are common.
(d) Sense of time and space is lost.

It has low toxicity. Aggressive behaviour is not common. Tolerance and dependence both develop.

COCAINE

Cocaine is obtained from plant called *Erythroxylum coca*.

Actions

1. It produces local anaesthesia as it blocks conduction in nerves.
2. It prolongs and enhances sympathetic nerve activity.
3. In the central nervous system it produces stimulation (euphoria, excitement) followed by depression.
4. It constricts blood vessels and raises blood pressure.
5. It dilates pupils but does not produce cycloplegia.
6. If taken through nose repeatedly it produces perforation of septum.

Uses

1. Not used now as it is toxic and habit forming (drug abuse).
2. When used as local anaesthetic on skin or mucous membrane, it does not require addition of vasoconstrictors.

AMPHETAMINE (FOR DETAILS REFER ANS SYSTEM)

Actions

1. Euphoria.
2. Increased mental and muscular power.
3. It produces resistance to fatigue.

Chronic use leads to:
1. Weight loss.
2. Insomnia.
3. Mental and physical deterioration.

KHAT AND BETEL NUT (SUPARI)

These are plant derivatives similar to cocaine.

Actions: Both these agents produce stimulation of central nervous system and euphoria. Use of betel stains teeth, saliva, urine and faeces red. Betel increases the risk of cancer. A squamous cell carcinoma is frequently seen on the inside of the cheek of betel chewers.

Nursing care of patients taking hallucinogens

1. Patients should be placed in quiet environment.
2. Reassure the patient and provide emotional support.
3. Monitor patient constantly until the acute reaction subsides.
4. Protect the patient from accidental or self inflicted injuries.
5. These patients should be advised to seek medical help.
6. Parents of young patients should be advised on developing confidence in these children.
7. Keep them occupied by providing recreational activities.

33

Central Nervous Stimulants

Central nervous stimulants are therapeutically not much exploited. This is because:

(a) Excessive CNS stimulation produces long lasting depression of CNS.

(b) No drug specifically stimulates only one area of brain. Generalised CNS stimulation produces convulsions and death.

Following CNS stimulants are used clinically:

(a) Xanthine alkaloids (caffeine, theophylline and theobromine), amphetamine, methylamphetamine and piperadrol.

(b) Sympathomimetic agents.

(c) Medullary stimulants — nikethamide, picrotoxin, camphor and carbon dioxide.

(d) Drugs causing reflex stimulation of CNS — lobeline, ammonia and nicotine.

XANTHINE ALKALOIDS

Caffeine, theophylline and theobromine.

Tea leaves contain caffeine and theophylline, coffee contains only caffeine. Theobromine is contained in cocca.

The knowledge about these drugs is essential as they are consumed by a large population.

Actions

1. CNS: Cerebral cortex is stimulated

   (i) Fatigue is delayed.

   (ii) Mental alertness is produced.

   (iii) Caffeine improves reflex activity.

   Higher concentrations of these agents produce confusion, nervousness and tremors.

2. By acting on medulla, larger doses of caffeine stimulate respiratory, vasomotor and vagal centers. Heart rate is reduced but blood pressure is raised.

3. Effect on spinal cord — still higher doses of these drugs are needed to stimulate spinal cord.

4. By a direct action, these drugs increase heart rate, force of contraction and oxygen consumption. High doses may lead to tachycardia and arrhythmias. Blood vessels are dilated. Systolic blood pressure is increased.

5. Smooth muscles—small concentration of caffeine increases motility of gut while higher doses produce relaxation.

   Theophylline relaxes smooth muscles. Effect on bronchi is very marked. This drug is therefore used in bronchial asthma.

6. Kidney: All these agents increase the urinary output.
7. Voluntary muscles: Contraction of the skeletal muscles is improved.
8. These drugs increase the acidity of the stomach. Caffeine has greater effect on CNS. Theophylline has maximum effect on smooth muscles. Theobromine has predominant diuretic effect.

Adverse reactions: They usually do not produce toxic effects. Consumption of high quantities of tea or coffee for long duration predisposes to peptic ulceration. Tolerance and habituation develops.

Uses

1. Coffee and tea are often consumed to relieve fatigue.
2. Early morning cup of these beverages is taken to move bowels.
3. Caffeine is combined with ergotamine to treat migraine.
4. Aminophylline (theophylline ethylene diamine) is used in bronchial asthma including status asthmaticus and acute left ventricular failure, it is employed as diuretic in certain conditions.

AMPHETAMINE AND METHYLAMPHETAMINE

These are sympathomimetic agents. These drugs produce following effects:

(a) Wakefulness and alertness.
(b) Delay fatigue.
(c) Skeletal muscular function is improved.
(d) Appetite is suppressed. Amphetamine is usually added to commercial preparations meant for reducing body weight.

Disadvantages

1. Sleep is only postponed.
2. Judgement is impaired.
3. Tolerance develops to anorexic effect.

Uses of amphetamine

1. For treatment of narcolepsy.
2. For treating brain dysfunction.
3. It is given as adjuvant in epilepsy.

Dextroamphetamine: It has actions and uses similar to amphetamine.

DRUGS USED IN TREATMENT OF OBESITY

Amphetamine, phenylpropanolamine, diethylpopion, fenfluramine, mazindol, methylphenidate, phendimetrazine, phenmetrazine and phenmetraphentermine.

All these drugs act on the satiety center in brain and suppress appetite.

Nursing care

Except fenfluramine all the above mentioned drugs produce stimulation of the central nervous system.

1. These drugs should not be given to patients suffering from hypertension, hyperthyroidism, cardiac problems and anxiety states.
2. Patients receiving these drugs should be under constant medical supervision.
3. Patients should be monitored closely for adverse reactions due to these drugs.
4. Use of amphetamines to eliminate fatigue and for keeping awake at night should be condemned. These drugs are often misused by medical and paramedical students.

RESPIRATORY STIMULANTS

Picrotoxin: It stimulates respiration, salivation and emesis. It increases blood pressure.

Disadvantages

1. This stimulation is followed by depression.
2. Higher doses produce clonic convulsions.

Nikethamide (Coramine): It is less potent than picrotoxin. Unlike the previous drug, in therapeutic doses, it has no effect on BP. Stimulates respiration alone.

Higher or toxic doses produce hypertension, tachycardia, vomiting, tremors, hyperpyrexia, arrhythmias and convulsions.

Doxapram: It is used to stimulate respiratory center in the postanaesthetic period.

Advantage: It is considered safer than other drugs. Toxic doses produce effects like nikethamide.

Dose: 0.5–1.5 mg/kg intravenously at the rate of 5 mg/min.

Bemegride, pentylenetetrazol and camphor are all non-specific CNS stimulants and are rarely used for clinical purposes.

Camphor is made use of as counter irritant in liniment turpentine.

Combination of Ethyl and Propylbutamide

Used in treatment of:

1. Drowning.
2. Suffocation.
3. Acute ventilatory insufficiency.
4. Postoperative pulmonary complication.

Carbon Dioxide: It is used to stimulate respiratory center.

Uses of analeptics: For stimulation of respiratory center in:

(i) The newborn
(ii) Patients of narcotic poisoning
(iii) Post anaesthetic respiratory depression
(iv) Drowning

(v) Respiratory failure due to overdose of oxygen

(vi) Chronic lung disease.

Stimulants of Spinal Cord: **Strychnine** is of no therapeutic interest. Strychnine is used as rat poison. Accidental poisoning of this drug is treated by diazepam (10 mg IV).

Ammonia and lobeline reflexly stimulate respiratory center. Ammonia is often employed to treat syncope (home remedy).

Local Anaesthetic Agents

34. Local Anaesthetic (LA) Agents

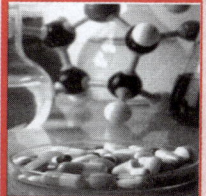

34

Local Anaesthetic (LA) Agents

Sensory nerves carry impulses for pain, touch, cold, warmth and deep pressure.

Local anaesthetic (LA) reversibly inhibit generation as well as conduction in nervous tissue. Their main site of action is the cell membrane and there is little action on the axoplasm.

Local anaesthetic action is achieved through inhibition of Na^+ entry into the cell (depolarisation). This blocks conduction. The sensitivity of the nervous fiber to these agents depends on their diameter. Smaller nerve fibers are more susceptible to their action than large fibers.

Pain sensation is the first to be lost followed by the sensations of cold, warmth, touch and deep pressure.

These drugs are marketed as hydrochloric salts which increases their stability and solubility.

These drugs lose their effect in alkaline medium, e.g. pus.

Classification of local anaesthetics

1. Surface anaesthetics—lignocaine, tetracaine, benzocaine and oxethazine (ointments, creams and eye drops and dusting powers).

2. Injectables
   (a) Short acting—procaine and chloroprocaine.
   (b) Intermediate acting—lignocaine, prilocaine.
   (c) Long acting—tetracaine (amethocaine) bupivacaine, dibucaine, ropivcaine and etidocaine.

Types of local anaesthesia

1. **Surface or topical anaesthesia:** Local anaesthetic agent is applied to the skin or mucous membrane (eye, nose, throat) to be anaesthetised, e.g. lozenges are used for throat.

2. **Infiltration anaesthesia:** This causes paralysis of sensory nerve endings and small cutaneous nerves. Injection of the drug is made in subcutaneous tissue close to the nerve endings.

3. **Regional anaesthesia:** Nerve block:

   (a) Local anaesthetic is injected around the nerve or nervous plexus. This blocks both sensory and motor nerves and produces relaxation of muscles supplied by this nerve. It is used in causalgia. Sympathetic nerves can also be blocked by this technique and used in peripheral vascular diseases.

   (b) **Intravenous regional anaesthesia:** Local anaesthetic is injected intravenously into the limb, (which is cut off from the systemic circulation by application of a cuff) thus effect of LA gets localised to this limb alone. This is done in cases where general anaesthesia is contraindicated and surgery needs to be performed on the limb in emergency.

(c) **Epidural block:** LA is injected into the lumbar epidural space. It is used in women during labour. Technique is difficult.

4. Spinal anaesthesia: Local anaesthetic agent is injected into subarachnoid space.

Advantages of spinal anaesthesia

1. General anaesthesia can be avoided.
2. This technique is useful for surgery on the abdomen as well as lower limbs.
3. It is commonly employed for performing cesarean section. Patient's co-operation is available throughout surgery.
4. Postoperative complications are less as compared to general anaesthesia.

Disadvantages

1. Hypotension may develop.
2. Headache is common during postoperative period.
3. Local neurological problems may be produced.
4. Haemorrhage and infection of meninges may occur if care is not exercised during injections.

During delivery: In the initial stages pethidine can be given but when the cervix gets fully dilated nitrous oxide inhalations are found to serve the purpose.

Nursing care of patient during labour and receiving local anaesthesia

1. Foetal heart rate should be checked frequently and a chart maintained.
2. Look for the signs of foetal distress.
3. Blood pressure of the patient should be checked every 30 minutes.
4. Dilatation of the cervix and contraction of the uterus should be watched for assessing the progress of labour (0.25–0.75%).

Adverse reactions of local anaesthetics

1. CNS excitability followed by respiratory depression.
2. Nausea, vomiting and abdominal pain may occur.
3. Cardiovascular and respiratory failure may occur.
4. Allergy is likely to be produced in susceptible cases.

Systemic uses of local anaesthetic agents

1. For treatment of cardiac arrhythmias (lidocaine is used intravenously in digitalis induced arrhythmias as well as those occurring during surgery).
2. These agents can be given as intravenous infusion in generalised pain (due to intensive burns).
3. In malignancy during last stages.

Nursing care and preparations of patients to receive local anaesthesia

1. Routine tests for allergy or intolerance should be performed.
2. Patient is advised to fast overnight.

3. Patient is given preanaesthetic medication 2 hours before the administration of local anaesthetic. Sedation with barbiturate provides protection against convulsions and immediate complications of local anaesthetic.

4. Appropriate LA should be used for the condition. Care should be exercised whether the ampule contains a vasoconstrictor or not.

Lidocaine (Lignocaine, Xylocaine): Can be used both for surface (2–4% drops, ointment) and injection anaesthesia (1–10% infiltration, nerve block, epidural, spinal and intravenous regional block).

Uses: In addition to LA it is used to treat cardiac arrhythmias.

Disadvantage: It can produce convulsions, which can be prevented by giving barbiturates before LA and treated by diazepam.

Prilocaine: It has actions like lignocaine but is less toxic. It is used as 5% cream locally and 4% injection for nerve block anaesthesia. It can cause methaemoglobinaemia.

Amethocaine (Tetracaine): It is used for topical (1–2%) as well as spinal anaesthesia (0.5% mg). It has greater systemic toxicity.

Procaine (Novocaine): It has to be given by injection, **it cannot be used for surface anaesthesia.**

Chlorprocaine: It is more potent but less toxic. Since, it destroys nerve roots it is not used as spinal anaesthesia.

Bupivacaine and ropivacaine (2–10% mg) used as infiltration, nerve block, spinal and epidural anaesthesia.

Local anaesthetics for eyes: Tetracaine — 1–2% ointment, benoxinate — 0.4% drops

For mucous membrane of nose and ear: Lidocaine and tetracaine.

Vasoconstrictors are added to local anaesthetics, because vasoconstrictor:

1. Reduces absorption of LA therefore reduces its systemic toxicity.
2. Prolongs the duration of the LA.
3. Makes area under surgery blood less and bleeding is reduced during surgery.

Disadvantages of addition of vasoconstrictor to local anaesthetic

1. Enough of these agents (vasoconstrictors) get absorbed to show effects on heart and blood pressure.
2. Healing is delayed.

Precautions

1. Local anaesthetic containing vasoconstricting agent **should not be injected in fingers, toes, nose and penis.**
2. This combination should not be used in patients of heart diseases.
3. Vasoconstrictors containing local anaesthetic should not be given in patients taking antidepressant drugs.

On absorption local anaesthetics also produce:

(a) Stimulation of the central nervous system which may manifest in the form of anxiety, tremors and even convulsions.

(b) quinidine like effect on the heart (reduces contractility and conduction of impulse is blocked) and severe bradycardia is produced. **Bupivacaine** is more cardiotoxic.

(c) Smooth muscles are relaxed.

For skin: Benzocaine, cyclomethycaine.

Urethra: Lidocaine and cyclomethycaine.

Spinal anaesthesia: Lidocaine for short periods, bupivacaine for medium and tetracaine for surgeries requiring long duration.

Section

V

Cardiovascular System

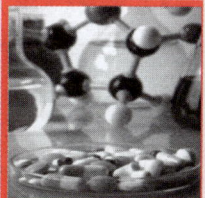

35

Cardiovascular System

PHYSIOLOGY OF HEART

Heart is a muscular pump. Its function is to move the blood through vascular system. Circulating blood provides body cells with oxygen, nutrients and other chemicals necessary for functions of life. Blood also carries away the waste products of cell metabolism. Heart therefore, is vital to life.

Heart has two pumps, right side of the heart (right atrium and right ventricle) receives blood from the veins and pumps it to the lungs for oxygenation. Left side of the heart pumps out oxygenated blood to the body against arterial resistance. Arteries are formed of thicker musculature. The musculature of right ventricle is less developed as it functions against low resistance.

Cardiac tissue has ability to generate spontaneous impulses called automaticity The automaticity differs in different areas of the heart. Heart rate is controlled by pace maker situated in SA node. If SA node fails to generate impulses AV node takes up this function, should the AV node not function properly, bundle of His can initiate impulses. Even cardiac cells outside the specialised conduction tissue can initiate stimuli specially if they are injured or irritated.

Heart rate (chronotropic effect) is influenced by various factors.

Cholinergic activity reduces rate while sympathetic stimulation increases it. Eating and exercise tend to increase heart rate.

Ionotropic effect: Strength of contraction of cardiac muscle is called ionotropic affect. Degree of contraction of the myocardium depends upon its tone. Calcium and sympathomimetic agents increase contraction.

Reduction in contractile strength of the heart produces congestive cardiac failure.

Chemicals increasing contractile strength are called cardiotonic or positive inotropic agents. Those reducing cardiac contraction are referred to as negative inotropic drugs.

Clinically three types of problems are associated with heart.

1. Congestive cardiac failure which is due to the failure of pumping action of the heart.
2. Cardiac arrhythmias which are due to disturbances in either the generation of impulses or its conduction in the heart.
3. Angina pectoris or myocardial infarction which are due to deficiency in supply of oxygen to heart.

CARDIOTONIC DRUGS

Digitalis: William Wuthering in 1785 discovered the use of leaves of foxglove (a plant called Digitals in Latin) in dropsy (oedema). Digitalis contains a number of active glycosides (lanatoside and digoxin). These preparations have similar effect but differ in their onset and duration of action.

Digitalis glycosides increase the ability of the myocardial proteins to convert chemical energy into useful mechanical energy without requiring extra oxygen that is the contractile strength of the myocardium is improved. Digitalis by Na^+ K^+ ATPase inhibition increases intracellular Ca^{++} that enhances myocardial contraction. Excessive inhibition of Na^+ K^+ ATPase produces arrhythmias. **Potassium protects this enzyme against glycosides as it reduces their effects**. Loss of potassium therefore will increase toxicity of digitalis.

Pharmacological actions of digitalis glycosides (digitoxin, gitoxin, digoxin and ouabain)

All glycosides ae equally effective but differ in pharamacokinetics.

1. These glycosides increase force of contraction of heart which brings about reduction in the size of failing or failed heart. This in turn increases cardiac output, thus making the heart to perform more efficiently.

2. Vagal activity is increased by digitalis that leads to bradycardia. In addition has antiadrenergic effect. Digitalis increases refractory period of conducting tissue (bundle of His) leading to ventricular bradycardia and complete heart block in high doses.

3. These drugs **increase excitability and automaticity** (capacity to generate impulse) of myocardium leading to cardiac arrhythmias. Multiple extrasystole — ventricular tachycardia and fibrillation are all produced by digitalis overdose. Refractory period of the atria is reduced which is responsible for conversion of auricular flutter to auricular fibrillation.

4. Digitalis associated glycosides exert **diuretic activity** by increasing cardiac output which increases glomerular filtration.

5. Digitalis has direct vasoconstrictor effect. **In patients of congestive cardiac failure digitalis counters the reflex vasoactivity.** It has no effect on coronary circulation.

6. Cause **decrease in peripheral resistance** and decrease in venous tone.

7. Increase PR interval, shorten QT interval, depression of ST segment and **widening of QT complex (toxicity)**.

8. Therapeutic doses of digitalis do not exert any effect on other systems.

9. Toxic doses cause nausea and vomiting as CTZ is stimulated.

Changes in signs and symptoms brought about by digitalis in congestive cardiac failure.

1. Because of improvement in cardiac output back pressure in the veins is reduced. This lessens the distension in the neck veins and causes improvement in breathing. Sacral oedema is reduced. Body weight is reduced.

2. Substantial diuresis is produced.

3. Auricular flutter is converted into auricular fibrillation by digitalis, this is advantageous as conduction in bundle of His is reduced which reduces ventricular rate. This improves ventricular filling and cardiac output.

Conduction becomes irregular in the bundle of His which is responsible for irregular pulse (sign of toxicity).

Preparations

1. **Digoxin:** It is the commonly used preparation. It is absorbed when given orally and is excreted through kidneys. Blood levels of this drug are higher in kidney failure as 80–85% is excreted in urine in unchanged form.

   It is preferred in all conditions **except renal failure.**

2. **Digitoxin:** It is absorbed from the gut and is metabolised in liver and little is excreted unchanged in the urine. **Blood levels of this drug are influenced by liver functions.** It has longer half life (170 hours). This drug is **preferred in renal failure**.

	Digitoxin	*Digoxin*
Oral absorption	Very good	Good
Administration	Oral	Oral + IV
Onset of action	1/2 hrs	15–30 minutes
Duration of action	2–3 weeks	1–2 days
Enterohepatic circulation	+	–
Elimination	Metabolised	Excreted unchanged
Status in renal failure	Can be given	Not given
Potency	Lowest	Medium

Uses

1. To correct systolic dysfunction in ischaemic heart disease, tachyarrhythmias and dilated cardiomyopathy. Digitalis helps by improving contractility of myocardium.

2. Dystolic dysfunction as seen in patients of hypertension of long standing, coronary heart disease, AV shunt, aortic stenosis.

   Most CHF patients have both dysfunctions.

3. Atrial flutter: Digitalis is drug of choice for controlling atrial fibrillation. It acts by reducing number of impulses that are able to pass down AV node to bundle of His. It directly acts and by its antiadrenergic effect reduces ventricular rate.

Relatively smaller doses of digoxin/digitoxin are required in:

(a) Elderly patients.

(b) Renal impairment.

(c) Patients of hypothyroidism.

(d) In patients with low serum potassium.

(e) In patients with fresh myocardial infarct.

Digitalis is ineffective in correcting congestive failure associated with

(a) Severe degree of cardiac damage.

(b) Rheumatic heart failure.

(c) Cardiac failure with primary lung infection.

Ouabain: It has actions similar to digitalis. It is poorly absorbed from gastrointestinal tract. It can be given intravenously in emergencies. Action starts within 3–10 minutes.

This drug has narrow therapeutic range—that is the effective dose and toxic doses are close to each other, therefore nurses are not given the responsibility for dosage management.

Dosage of digoxin: Digoxin is given in the dose of 0.25 mg four times a day (as loading dose) for a period of two to four days. Dose is less in the elderly and is given only twice a day. Maintenance doses are proportional to daily loss of digitalis dependent on kidney and liver function.

Maintenance dose varies from 0.25 mg once daily to 0.25 mg three times daily.

Adverse drug reactions

1. GIT: Anorexia, nausea and vomiting
2. CNS: Headache, fatigue and drowsiness, disorientation and confusion.
3. Cardiac: Irregular heart rate (this is a serious reaction and may prove to be fatal). **Doctor should immediately be informed.**

Anorexia, nausea and vomiting occurring in patient receiving digoxin are indicative of digitalis toxicity. These symptoms may be the first indication of intoxication due to this drug and should not be ignored by the nursing staff.

Headache and drowsiness occur much less often than anorexia. Side effects of digitalis on heart are numerous. **Any irregularity of rhythm or rate may occur and is worth reporting to treating physician.** Most commonly occurring ECG abnormalities in the heart due to overdose of this drug are:

1. Bradycardia.
2. Ventricular extrasystoles.
3. Coupled beats.

Ventricular Tachycardia: If ECG shows extrasystoles, drug should be immediately stopped and corrective measures started. Ventricular fibrillation can be easily prevented at this stage or death occurs in matter of minutes.

Treatment of digitalis toxicity:

1. Stop digitalis preparations.
2. Give potassium chloride 5–7 g/day in divided doses with frequent monitoring of serum K^+.
3. **Phenytoin or lidocaine are given to treat arrhythmias.**
4. Atropine is given to treat bradycardia.
5. **Fab fragments** of digitalis binding antibody can be given.

Patient should not be given following drugs with digitalis:

1. Calcium salts.
2. Diuretics which cause K^+ loss.
3. Methyldopa as it increases blood levels of digitalis.
4. Nifedipine as it reduces clearance of digitalis from kidneys.
5. Thyrotoxin as patients are more prone to arrhythmia.

Nursing care

1. Watch for the development of anorexia, nausea and vomiting.
2. Watch for irregularities in pulse specially coupled beats.
3. Digitalis should be withheld if

  (a) the pulse rate is below 60 beats/min.

  (b) If patients of atrial flutter are being treated with digitalis, pulse rate and heart beat should be counted. Any difference (pulse deficit) in the two should be immediately brought to the notice of the treating physician.

Higher degree of difference between ventricular rate and pulse rate can prove fatal.

4. Input/ouput chart should be maintained in congestive cardiac failure being treated with digitalis. Higher degree of renal output must be there if the patient is responding to therapy.

5. Diet should be low in sodium but rich in potassium.

6. Drug should be administered after meal at the same time each day.

7. Parenteral preparation should be given by deep intramuscular injection.

8. Bradycardia, prolongation of PR interval and shortening of QT interval in ECG are characteristics of digitalis toxicity.

Other drugs given in congestive cardiac failure:

1. Diuretics (K^+ sparing diuretics are preferred with digitalis).

2. Alpha-adrenergic blocking drugs.

3. Vasodilators.

4. Amrinone.

DIURETICS

1. Cause decrease in circulating blood volume, therefore, reduce preload on heart and improve cardiac functioning.

2. Decrease pulmonary congestion and peripheral oedema.

These drugs are first line treatment for mild-to-moderate degree of congestive cardiac failure.

Furosemide 40 mg is given IV for rapid action. This treatment has replaced rapid digitalisation as well as the use of digitalis.

IV frusemide causes prompt increase in systemic venous capacitance vessels and decreases left ventricular filling pressure even before exerting diuretic action, is therefore helpful in left ventricular failure.

ALPHA-ADRENERGIC BLOCKERS

These drugs produce vasodilatation that reduces preload and helps improve the cardiac functioning.

BETA-ADRENERGIC RECEPTOR BLOCKERS

Dobutamine is used to treat acute but potentially reversible heart failure (e.g. as a cardiogenic and septic shock).

Carvedilol a non-selective blocker is being tried.

Advantages

1. It increases myocardial contraction.

2. Produces less tachycardia as compared to other β_1 agonists.

It is given IV.

Uses

(a) In idiopathic dilated cardiomyopathy.

(b) In ischemic cardiomyopathy.

If used in severe cardiac failure these drugs are likely to worsen the condition.

Glucagon: It increases myocardial contractility (increases cAMP) and is used in patients with acute cardiac failure resulting from over dose of β-blockers.

PHOSPHODIESTERASE III INHIBITORS

Amrinone, milrinone, pimobendan and vesnarinone.

Amrinone: It has positive inotropic effect and is a vasodilator.

It reduces afterload thereby improving inotropic activity.

It is used in refractory cases of CHF.

Milrinone

Advantages

(a) It is more potent than amrinone.

(b) It has less toxicity.

(c) It is better tolerated.

Disadvantages

1. It is toxic to liver and produces GIT upsets.

2. Causes arrhythmias.

VASODILATORS

Hydralazine, prazosin, ACE inhibitors and other arteriolar dilators (nifedipine, etc.) reduce afterload and improve efficacy of left ventricle. Vesodilators such as glyceryl trinitrate (IV) reduce preload.

(a) Increase local tissue blood flow.

(b) Reduce arterial pressure.

(c) Reduce central venous pressure.

These three actions result in net reduction of cardiac preload and afterload and hence reduction of cardiac output.

Uses

(a) As antihypertensives (angiotensin converting enzyme inhibitors).

(b) Treatment of angina.

(c) Congestive cardiac failure.

ACE Inhibitors: Captopril, enalapril, lesinopril, perindopril, romipril and benazepril.

Angiotensin I $\xrightarrow[\text{ACE}]{}$ Angiotensin II → Angiotensin III → Inactive

Cause: Reduction in peripheral resistance (arterioles fragments dilate and compliance of large arteries is increased).

1. K$^+$ is retained and if given with K$^+$ sparing diuretics hyperkalaemia is produced.
2. Antacids reduce bioavailability and should be avoided.

Adverse effects

1. Most common — **cough**, hypotension and hyperkalemia.
2. Less common — headache, rashes, nausea, renal failure and granulocytopenia.

Treatment of congestive cardiac failure: Combination of drugs (diuretic and digitalis) is commonly used. Vasodilators are lately being preferred over digitalis. In addition to medicines the diet has to be salt free. **Nurse must advise the patient against the use of salt in diet.**

36

Antiarrhythmic Agents

In cardiac arrhythmia rhythm of the heart is disturbed. Arrhythmias can be due to either:
   (a) Increased rate of spontaneous discharge in conducting tissue.
   (b) Impaired conduction in part of the conducting system due to drug or diseases.

Classification of antiarrhythmics:

Class I: Sodium channel blockers

   (a) Quinidine, procainamide and disopyramide.
   (b) Lidocaine, phenytoin, mexiletine, tocainide.
   (c) Encainide, lorcainide, flecainide.

Class II: Beta adrenoreceptor blockers — propranolol, sotalol, metoprolol.

Class III: Potassium channel blockers — bretylium, amiodarone, (increase effective refractory period).

Class IV: Calcium channel blockers — verapamil and diltiazem.
Class V: Miscellaneous drugs — adenosine.

CLASS I

Quinidine: Pharmacological actions:This drug has **membrane stabilising, anticholinergic** and **alpha blocker** activities.

   1. It decreases automaticity of pacemaker cells.
   2. Reduces responsiveness of cardiac cells to excitation.
   3. Reduces conduction velocity of impulses in atria, ventricles and conducting tissues.
   4. Refractory period of atria, AV node and bundle of His are prolonged.
   5. Contractility of myocardium is reduced.
   6. Vagal activity on the heart is reduced.
   7. Dilates veins and reduces blood pressure. It is absorbed when given orally.

Uses

   1. It is used for prevention and treatment of paroxysmal ventricular tachycardia and ventricular extrasystoles.
   2. Used for prevention and treatment of atrial flutter, atrial fibrillation, tachycardia and atrial extrasystoles.

It should not be used for treatment of atrial fibrillation of more than 6 weeks standing.

Adverse reactions: High incidence of side effects

1. Allergic reactions are common.
2. Tinnitus, vertigo and blurring of vision.
3. Nausea, vomiting and diarrhea is common.
4. Thrombocytopenia.
5. Cardiac arrest.
6. Depresses myocardium and can produce cardiac failure.

Quinidine displaces digitalis from its binding sites and increases its toxicity.

Nursing care

(i) In patients allergic to quinidine, administration of this drug will produce hypotensive shock. Therefore, it is advisable to test sensitivity to this drug by initially giving small dose of 120 mg. If patient feels faint or complaints of ringing in the ears (tinitus) or dizziness (vertigo) or double vision (diplopia) further administration of the drug should be stopped.

(ii) Quinidine reduces platelet count (thrombocytopenia) which manifests itself in the form of bleeding from gums or skin (purpura). Nurse must look for these bleeding spots and discontinue the treatment.

(iii) Cardiac arrest occurs when excess of quinidine is given. Quinidine should therefore be temporarily withdrawn if pulse rate is less than 60/min.

Procainamide: It is an amide of procaine a local anaesthetic. It differs from procaine as it can be given orally, has longer half-life than procaine and has more selective cardiac effects.

Pharmacological actions of this drug are the same as those of quinidine but duration of action is less.

It reduces automaticity, reduces excitability and conduction velocity as this drug too has membrane stabilising activity.

Uses: In treatment of ventricular arrhythmias when quinidine has failed.

It is not used for atrial arrhythmias as these are less sensitive to this drug.

Adverse effects

1. Lupus like syndrome (20%) — slow acetylators are more likely to suffer.
2. Hypotension.
3. Nausea, vomiting and diarrhea.
4. Giddiness and mental depression or hallucinations.
5. Allergic reactions occur.
6. Can precipitate cardiac failure.

Nursing care

When injection of procainamide is being given to detect development of hypotension constant blood pressure should be recorded. Control the rate of infusion carefully.

Phenytoin: This drug is used to treat ventricular tachycardias produced by overdosage of digoxin. However, lignocaine is preferred as phenytoin is less safe.

Adverse reactions: Intravenous injection produces hypotension, bradycardia and cardiac arrest.

Same precautions should be taken as with procainamide.

Lignocaine: It is a local anesthetic agent and is safest antiarrhythmic agent.

Pharmacological actions: It reduces automaticity and also reduces excitability. It differs from quinidine in that:

(a) It reduces the effective refractory period and duration of action potential.

(b) **Conduction velocity** in bundle of His and AV node **is not reduced**.

(c) **Force of contraction of heart is not reduced.**

Because of these effects it is found to be effective even when other drugs (quinidine and procainamide) have failed.

Use: In treatment of ventricular arrhythmias specially after myocardial infarction and digitalis over dose.

Adverse reactions

1. Hypotension, dizziness.
2. Blurred vision, agitation and confusion.
3. Convulsions.
4. Increased sweating.

Nursing care

(a) Intravenous lignocaine is a frequent medication in ICU. If excess of lignocaine is going—cardiac monitor may show cardiac asystole. Watch for this finding.

(b) Convulsions can also be produced by high doses of lignocaine and they should be prevented.

Dose: 2 mg/min

Disopyramide

Pharmacological actions

(i) It is a class IA drug as it has membrane stabilising activity

(ii) In addition like class II agents it prolongs the effective refractory period and duration of action potential.

(iii) Like quinidine it reduces contractility of myocardium.

(iv) **It has atropine like activity and tends to produce urinary retention.**

Uses

1. Supraventricular tachycardia.
2. Ventricular tachycardia.
3. Wolff-Parkinson-White syndrome.
4. It is given to maintain normal rhythm after DC shock.

Adverse reactions

1. Urinary retention.
2. Can precipitate glaucoma.
3. Dry mouth and blurred vision.
4. May precipitate cardiac failure.

Nursing care

If patients complain of hesitancy in passing urine report the event to the treating physician specially in elderly patients as they may go into urinary retention.

Mexiletine and Tocainide: These drugs are like lidocaine.

Pharmacological actions:

(a) These drugs reduce automaticity and excitability but the velocity of impulse conduction is less affected.

(b) Like lignocaine these drugs produce uniform reduction in effective refractory period and action potential duration.

Uses

(a) Ventricular arrhythmias after myocardial infarction.

(b) In treatment of digitalis overdose.

Adverse reactions

1. Nausea, vomiting, hiccup and hepatoxicity.
2. Drowsiness and confusion.
3. Diplopia.
4. Peripheral neuropathy.
5. Sinus bradycardia and atrial fibrillation.
6. Hypotension.

Nursing care

Not commonly used in Indian medical practice. If patient is on these drugs nurse should routinely look for signs of bradycardia or atrial fibrillation.

Encainide, Lorcainide and Flecainide: These drugs depress conduction in AV node, ventricles and accessory pathways. Reduce antegrade as well as retrograde conduction.

Uses

In treatment of:

(a) Ventricular extrasystoles.

(b) Sustained ventricular tachycardia.

(c) Wolff-Parkinson-White syndrome.

Aropafenone: It can cause bronchospasm. It is most potent Na^+ channel blocker. It is not used commonly because it can cause arrhythmia.

BETA ADRENORECEPTOR ANTAGONISTS

In treating arrhythmias they are useful because:

(a) They counteract arrhythmogenic activity of catecholamines.

(b) Few of these agents (propanolol, oxprenolol, acebutanol) have membrane stabilising activity which contributes to their antiarrhythmic effect.

These drugs are used in all the following conditions:

(a) Treatment of angina pectoris.

(b) Treatment of hypertension.

Pharmacological actions

1. Reduce contacitility of the cardiac muscle therefore this group can precipitate congestive cardiac failure.
2. Reduce excitability.
3. Reduce oxygen demand of the myocardium and are useful in treating angina pectoris.
4. Heart rate is reduced and are useful in treating tachycardia.
5. Conductivity is reduced therefore produce heart block.
6. Refractory period is increased.

Uses

1. Cardiac arrhythmias associated with thyrotoxicosis and anxiety.
2. Paroxysmal atrial tachycardia.
3. Wolff-Parkinson-White syndrome.

Adverse reactions

1. Bronchoconstriction leading to precipitation of asthma. There is no such danger in the non-asthmatic patient. This occurs only in the asthmatic patients.
2. Left ventricular failure may be precipitated during treatment with these agents.
3. Defects in conduction block are produced.

Propranolol: This agent is commonly employed for the treatment of angina pectoris, cardiac arrhythmias and hypertension. It is usually given orally but in emergencies in small doses can be given intravenously. In addition to precipitating cardiac failure and asthmatic attacks, it also causes drowsiness. Allergy is also reported.

Sotalol: It is a non-selective beta adrenoreceptor blocker. It is less toxic therefore can be used.

Adverse drug reactions: If serum K^+ is low it can cause prolongation of QT interval (Torsades de pointes).

Oxprenolol: Pharmacological actions are similar to propranolol except it is less likely to cause bronchoconstriction.

Nursing care

1. Attacks of wheezing should be looked for which suggests the beginning of asthmatic attack. Cardiospecific beta blockers less often produce this problem.
2. Swelling of ankles or complain of breathlessness suggests the onset of cardiac failure. Beta blocker must be withdrawn.

K^+ CHANNEL BLOCKER

Amiodarone

It prolongs the effective refractory period and duration of action potential. Therefore it is the drug of choice in resistant re-entrant supraventricular tachycardia, e.g. Wolff-Parkinson-White syndrome.

Adverse reactions

1. Corneal opacities.
2. Nausea.
3. Skin disorders.

Contraindications

1. Serious bradycardia and AV block.
2. Any thyroid disorder.
3. **Should not be given with verapamil or beta blocker.**

Nursing care

It can produce serious adverse reactions like visual defects. Nurse must elicit history regarding this feature and inform the physician accordingly.

CALCIUM CHANNEL BLOCKERS

Calcium is needed for the initiation of impulse as well as for contraction of myocardium. These drugs interfere with the slow calcium influx hence block generation of impulse, its conduction and myocardial contraction. Decrease cardiac work therefore decrease oxygen demand of heart. They prevent coronary spasm.

These are latest drugs in the management of cardiac diseases such as:

(a) Angina.
(b) Cardiac arrhythmias.
(c) Hypertension.
(d) Vasospastic diseases.

Verapamil: It effects heart more than blood vessels.

Uses

1. AV nodal tachycardia.
2. Wolff-Parkinson-White syndrome.
3. Angina pectoris.
4. Supraventricular tachycardia.

Adverse reactions

1. Hypotension.
2. Asystole.
3. Constipation.

Hypotension and asystole are seen on intravenous administration.

Dose: 40–80 mg three times a day orally.

Perhexiline Maleate: It is a calcium channel blocker. It reduces incidence of ventricular ectopic beats but has no effect on atrial arrhythmias.

Adverse reactions

1. Allergic reactions.
2. Liver damage.
3. Hypoglycemia.

Use: It is preferred in asthmatic patients suffering from arrhythmias.

Bretylium: As it increases effective refractory period it abolishes re-enterant arrhythmias. It may increase cardiac output for short time. Not used because of toxicity.

Nursing care of patient on antiarrhythmic drugs

1. Disopyramide is administered with caution to persons with a history of urinary retention and in males with prostatic hypertrophy.
2. When bretylium is administered intramuscularly injection site should be changed regularly.
3. Barbiturates must be kept ready to counter convulsions produced by lignocaine.
4. Sensitivity should be checked for quinidine and procainamide.
5. Preparation of lignocaine used for controlling arrhythmias should not contain vasoconstrictors.
6. Beta adrenergic blockers should preferably be avoided in asthmatics, patients taking hypoglycemics and hypothyroid patients.
7. Dosage of most drugs needs reduction in persons with renal and hepatic impairment.
8. Control the rate of infusion carefully if the drug is administered intravenously.
9. Treatment with these drugs should be started in special cardiac unit with monitor.
10. Patients as well as their relatives must be instructed about strict drug compliance.
11. Inform patients about the cardiac emergencies that can arise.

Treatment of paroxsymal supraventricular tachycardia

Stimulation of the vagus nerve produces:
   (a) Bradycardia.
   (b) Slowing in conduction in the bundle of His.
   (c) Reduced force of contraction of heart.
   (d) Shortening of refractory period of atria.
   (e) Decrease in excitability of the myocardium.

Thus, stimulation of vagus nerve can stop arrhythmias of short duration. Vagus nerve can be stimulated by:
   (a) Tingling of fauces
   (b) Valsalva's maneuver
   (c) Pressure on the eyeballs
   (d) Pressure over one of the carotid sinus for 30 seconds.
   (e) Swallowing ice cream

Atrial tachycardia: Verapamil is given provided there is no AV block. Should not be given if there is congestive cardiac failure or hypotension.

Atrial flutter: Digitalis followed by quinidine or verapamil or propranolol.
Atrial fibrillation: Digitalis.

Ventricular ectopic beats: propranolol lidocaine or procainamide **ventricular tachycardia:** Lidocaine or IV procainamide or IV phenytoin.

DRUGS USED IN TREATMENT OF HEART BLOCK

Heart block is a condition where the impulse from the atria does not pass on to ventricles. This is a serious condition as ventricles come to a stand still. Drugs are therefore, to be given urgently.

1. Isoprenaline (isoproterenol) increases automaticity thereby enhancing rhythmicity of the SA node as well as AV nodal and ventricular pacemakers.

2. **Adrenaline and ephedrine** have similar effects but are less effective.

3. **Corticosteroids** are helpful only when the heart block is due to inflammatory process such as in rheumatic fever.

4. **Atropine** by reducing the inhibitory influence of vagus also helps in this condition.

AC and DC depolarisation in arrhythmias are found helpful.

37

Drugs used in Angina Pectoris

Heart muscle gets its blood supply from aorta via coronary arteries. Coronaries get their blood supply during diastolic phase. Whenever there is increase in oxygen demand (as occurs during stress, excessive exercise) or blood supply is reduced (as occurs in atherosclerosis) pain in chest is manifested called **angina**.

Factors responsible for angina pectoris (cardiac pain): Lactic acid is produced as a metabolite of the cardiac muscle activity. If the blood supply to heart is poor as happens in atheroma or thrombus formation these metabolites get accumulated and pain is produced.

Classification of drugs used in angina pectoris:

1. *Direct vasodilators:* Nitrites.
2. *Beta adrenergic blockers:* Propranolol.
3. *Calcium channel blockers:* Verapamil and nifedipine.
4. *Miscellaneous drugs:* Trimetazidine, nicorandil and molsidomine.

NITRATES AND NITRITES

Short acting: Amyl nitrate and glyceryl trinitrite.

Long acting: Erythrityl tetranitrite, pentaerythitol, mannitol hexanitrate, isosorbide dinitrate and isorbide mononitrate.

Pharmacological actions

1. On heart and coronary blood vessels:
    (a) Nitrates produce intense vasodilation resulting in venous pooling of the blood. This reduces preload on the heart resulting in reduction in end diastolic size of heart thereby reducing oxygen demand. The improvement in the left ventricular function outlasts its pharmacological actions.
    (b) The advantageous effect of nitrates is due to redistribution of coronary blood flow with improved perfusion in ischemic subendocardial areas in the myocardium.
    (c) Chronic administration of nitrates increases intra-arterial anastomoses within myocardium. This increases survival rate.
    (d) Nitrates produce some arteriolar dilatation resulting in slight reduction in peripheral resistance.
2. Blood pressure is reduced — systolic more than diastolic.

3. Nitrites and nitrates produce relaxation of smooth muscles of gallbladder, biliary ducts, sphincter of Oddi and the bronchi. Motility of the gastrointestinal tract is reduced. Ureteral and uterine muscles are also relaxed.

4. Intracranial tension is increased due to dilatation of blood vessels giving headache to patient. Tolerance develops to this effect.

Nitrates are not well absorbed when given orally hence these **are given sublingually**. The absorbed drug reaches coronaries directly and does not go through liver.

Amyl nitrite is effective when inhaled.

Adverse reactions

1. Headache is common.
2. Glaucoma may be precipitated.
3. Excess of this agent produces methemoglobinaemia. Oxygen carrying capacity of the blood is reduced. Cyanosis will be observed.
4. Giddiness occurs because of fall in blood pressure. Patients may collapse.

Uses of nitrites and nitrates

1. Angina pectoris.
2. Nitroglycerine produces immediate relief in paroxysmal nocturnal dyspnoea of left ventricular failure.
3. They are being used in chronic heart failure associated with myocardial infarction.
4. Amyl nitrite inhalation and sodium nitrite are drugs of choice in cyanide poisoning.
5. Biliary colic.

Nitrates should not be given if patient is suffering from:
1. Glaucoma.
2. Severe anemia.
3. Hypotensive state.
4. Increased intracranial pressure.

Adverse drug reactions

1. Tolerance develops.
2. Methaemoglobinaemia.
3. Acute fall in BP leading to syncope.
4. Headache.
5. Can aggravate myocardial ischemia.

Nursing care

1. Any patient who complaints of angina pectoris can be given sublingual glyceryl trinitrate. Instruct patients to allow the sublingual tablets to dissolve under tongue.
2. Nurse must keep a watch on blood pressure. Patient should be instructed to keep in bed during this time.
3. Instruct patient to throw out the tablet if relief is obtained.
4. Monitor the amount of drug used and response to treatment.
5. Analgesics can be given to relieve headache. Assure the patient that headache will disappear on constant use of drug.

6. Warn patient against syncope. Instruct patient to rest during headache and faintness.

7. Educate patient to avoid activities that precipitate angina.

8. Nitroglycerine may be taken before undertaking activities likely to precipitate anginal episodes.

9. Apply nitroglycerine ointment on chest at night.

10. **Nitroglycerine is sensitive to air, light, heat and moisture.** It should be stored in small brown tightly stoppered glass bottles.

Instruct patient to discard nitroglycerine if it fails to produce relief when placed under the tongue.

Glyceryl Trinitrate: Tablet contains 0.5 mg of the drug. It is available as sustained release tablets and also as ointment. The drug is unstable in plastic containers. Tablets must be stored in tightly closed amber glass bottles without cotton plugs preferably in fridge.

Sublingual tablets give immediate relief. Capsules, oral tablets and ointments are used for prophylaxis. Isosorbide dinitrate (sorbitrate) tabs are of 5 and 10 mg. These are useful in providing immediate relief as well as in prophylaxis of angina.

BETA ADRENERGIC BLOCKING AGENTS

These drugs benefit angina by:

(a) Reducing the sympathetic cardiac stimulation produced during exercise, anxiety or excitement. In all these conditions (exercise, anxiety and excitement) there is increased sympathetic discharge resulting in increased heart rate, increased blood pressure and therefore increase in the preload and afterload of heart.

(b) These drugs decrease oxygen demand of the heart. These drugs are considered basal preventive medicaments for angina pectoris. Long-term studies have shown that these drugs reduce the incidence of myocardial infarction.

Adverse reactions

(a) Severe bradycardia, hypotension, heart failure.

(b) Bronchospasm.

Uses: Prophylactically given in patients of stable and unstable angina. Propranolol is preferred.

Precaution: These drugs should not be withdrawn suddenly.

Combination of beta blockers and nitrates is better in treatment of angina because

1. Tachycardia due to nitrates is countered by beta blockers.

2. Nitrates counter ventricular dilatation produced by beta blockers.

3. Nitrates counter reduction in coronary flow that is produced by beta blockers.

4. Beta blockers reduce oxygen demand by the heart.

CALCIUM CHANNEL BLOCKERS

Verapamil, diltiazem and perhexilene — these drugs exert antianginal action by:

(a) Reducing left ventricular filling pressure which reduces workload of the heart. **This reduces oxygen demand of myocardium.**

(b) These drugs reduce exercise induced tachycardia which reduces frequency of anginal attacks.

Adverse reactions

1. Allergic reactions.
2. Liver damage.
3. Sodium retention resulting in weight gain and oedema.
4. Peripheral neuropathy.
5. Raised intracranial pressure and impotence.
6. Negative inotropic effect on heart and conduction block on heart.

Nursing care

Development of allergic symptoms should be watched for.

Uses

1. Prinzmetal angina and classical anginas.
2. Systemic hypertension.
3. Paroxysmal supraventricular tachycardia.
4. Prophylactic treatment of migraine.
5. Cinnarizine is useful in vertigo.

Disadvantage: Late onset of action.

Adverse reactions

1. Diarrhea
2. Lethargy
3. Problems associated with central nervous system.

Dose: 60–240 mg three times a day.

Nifedipine: Nifedipine though calcium channel blocker is not used in angina as it causes tachycardia. Cardiac output is increased thereby increasing oxygen demand and worsening ischaemia.

Verapamil: It is a calcium channel blocker.

(a) It depresses SA node producing bradycardia.
(b) Cardiac contractility is reduced therefore oxygen demand is reduced.
(c) Produces reduction in atrioventricular conduction.
(d) Produces peripheral vasodilation.
(e) It selectively depresses nodal tissue therefore found effective in arrhythmia.

Adverse reactions

1. Confusion
2. Vertigo
3. Bradycardia
4. Nervousness and hypotension.

Prenylamine (Segontin): It acts by depletion of catecholamines from the heart. It is used only for prophylaxis of angina.

Nursing care

Severe constipation should be avoided in these patients as this precipitates and aggravates angina.

Pulse rate of less than 60/min is indicative of excess dose of this drug and requires reduction in dosage.

Dipyridamole though coronary dilator is not used as it causes coronary steal.

MISCELLANEOUS DRUGS

Molsidomine: It is a new drug and resembles nitroglycerine in mode of action but acts more slowly.

Nicorandil: It is potassium channel activator and has nitrate like activity. On chronic dosing tolerance is produced.

Trimetazidine: It acts by reducing intracellular acidosis. Accumulation of Na^+ and Ca^{++} is avoided and K^+ loss from intracellular spaces is reduced thus it improves availability of oxygen.

Platelet aggregation is inhibited.

In addition it improves ventricular functioning.

Dose: 20 mg three times a day.

Levocarnitine: It is a natural constituent of myocardium. This is being tried.

Summary of treatment of angina pectoris:

1. Body weight should be reduced.
2. Cause of angina like anaemia should be removed.
3. Glyceryl trinitrate should be taken before any physical exercise.
4. **Beta adrenergic blocking agents** are given for long-term prophylaxis. **These drugs should not be suddenly withdrawn**.
5. **Calcium channel blockers** are advocated as first choice of drug in uncomplicated mild-to-moderate cases of angina.
6. Smoking should be stopped.
7. Sedation helps in relief of anxiety.
8. **Nifedipine is contraindicated.**

38

Antihypertensive Agents

Factors controlling the blood pressure:

There are three factors that control blood pressure.

(a) Cardiac output.

(b) Peripheral resistance.

(c) Viscosity of the blood — this factor is not changed in diseases producing hypertension and except in polycythemia vera does not contribute towards hypertension.

Cardiac output is determined by

(a) Venous return

(b) Heart rate

(c) Cardiac contractility.

The last two factors depend on sympathetic activity. Increase in sympathetic activity increases heart rate, cardiac contractility, peripheral resistance and therefore blood pressure.

Pheripheral resistance is a major factor determining blood pressure. It depends on the lumen of the arterioles, which in turn is regulated by sympathetic and angiotensin activity. The state of contraction or relaxation of the arterioles is under the control of vasomotor center in the brain and exerts its influence on the arterioles via autonomic nervous system.

In case of cardiovascular system acetylcholine produces bradycardia and decreases conduction velocity in bundle of His (negative chronotropic effect) as well as decreases contractility of heart (negative inotropic effect).

Blood vessels are not innervated by parasympathetic system but acetylcholine dilates them and the blood pressure is reduced.

The sympathetic system on the other hand has two transmitters — and two types of receptors on this side namely alpha (α) and beta (β). Alpha receptors when stimulated produce intense vasoconstriction thereby increasing peripheral resistance. Stimulation of beta receptors produces tachycardia and increase in cardiac output. Both these factors increase blood pressure. On the other hand drugs which block the release of catecholamines or their synthesis interfere only with sympathetic nervous system.

Drugs which block the receptors of sympathetic system (alpha and beta receptor blocking agents) selectively lower the blood pressure and the adverse reactions get limited.

Fall in the peripheral resistance causes pooling of blood in periphery that reduces venous return to the heart. The maximum fall in the blood pressure occurs when the patient taking these drugs suddenly from lying down position stands errect. This is called **postural hypotension**.

171

Direct vasodilators, diuretics, drugs reducing sympathetic outflow by acting in the central nervous system also exert antihypertensive effect.

Angiotensin and calcium antagonists also lower blood pressure by causing vasodilatation.

CLASSIFICATION OF ANTIHYPERTENSIVE AGENTS

1. **Drugs acting in the brain,** e.g. clonidine and methyldopa

2. **Drugs blocking autonomic ganglia,** e.g. hexamethonium, trimethaphan and mecamylamine.

3. **Drugs depleting catecholamines** by acting on postganglionic sympathetic nerve endings—guanethidine, reserpine, debrisoquine.

4. **Drugs blocking adrenergic receptors.**

   Alpha blocking drugs: Phentolamine, phenoxybenzamine and prazosin.

   Beta blocking drugs: Propranolol, metoprolol.

   Alpha and beta blocker: Labetalol.

5. **Direct vasodilators:** Hydralazine, diazoxide, sodium nitroprusside, minoxidil.

6. **Antagonists of renin-angiotensin system:** Captopril, enalpril, lisinopril and saralasin.

7. **Calcium channel blockers:** Verapamil, nifedipine diltiazem (arteriolar dilators).

8. **Diuretics:** Thiazides.

9. **5-HT antagonists:** Ketanserin.

10. **Miscellaneous:** Sedatives, pargyline.

DRUGS ACTING ON CNS

Clonidine (Catapres, Arkamine): **It is slow acting, therefore, it is not for emergencies.** It stimulates α_2 receptors.

Pharmacological actions

(i) It is partial agonist of α_2 receptors in the brain thereby reduces the sympathetic outflow from the brain. This reduces release of NA from nerve endings in the periphery that contributes to antihypertensive effect. It produces prolonged fall in systolic as well as diastolic blood pressure. Fall in the blood pressure is accompanied by bradycardia.

(ii) At higher doses the antihypertensive activity is less marked. Blood levels of 0.2–2.0 ng/ml concentration of this drug produces maximum fall in blood pressure.

(iii) Reduces plasma levels of noradrenaline

(iv) Postural hypotension is not produced.

(v) It also reduces plasma renin activity.

(vi) Does not affect plasma lipids.

(vii) It has antihistaminic activity. Sedation is produced by this drug which contributes to its antihypertensive effect.

(viii) It decreases insulin secretion but increases level of growth hormone.

Disadvantages

1. **On sudden withdrawl it causes rebound hypertension.**
2. Causes bradycardia.

Adverse reactions

1. Excessive drowsiness.
2. Dry mouth and dry eyes.
3. Vertigo.
4. Constipation.
5. Impotence.
6. Allergic reactions.
7. Gynaecomastia can occur in males.

Uses

1. For treatment of hypertension
2. For management of opioid withrawal
3. In diagnosis of pheochromocytoma
4. It is used to control diarrhoea in diabetic neuropathy (as it helps Na^+ absorption).

Nursing care and precautions

1. It should not be given parenterally initially.
2. If patient develops drowsiness, or becomes depressed this drug must be gradually withdrawn. Sudden stoppage of the drug produces hypertensive crisis and therefore patient should be warned against this danger.
3. Drug schedule must be strictly followed.
4. Increase in dose may not increase effect.

Dose: Initial 0.05 mg — 0.1 mg two to four times daily.

Maximum daily dose — 2.4 mg per day.

Alpha Methyldopa (Aldomet):

It is a prodrug and its metabolite acts like clonidine by stimulating α_2 receptors in the brain which reduces sympathetic outflow in the periphery. Antihypertensive effect is exerted in 3–6 hours. Peak effect comes in 2–3 days.

Pharmacological actions

1. (a) It reduces total peripheral resistance.
   (b) Does not affect cardiac output.
   (c) Bradycardia is produced.
2. Reduces plasma renin activity.
3. It increases serum prolactin level.

Advantages

1. It is considered safe in persons with renal failure
2. Methyldopa has been **used during pregnancy without apparent adverse effects on the fetus**, however, the possibility that the drug may cause foetal injury cannot be ruled out.

Adverse reactions

1. Produces fever accompained by derangement of liver functions.
2. Drowsiness and forgetfulness.
3. Changes in sleep rhythm.
4. Mental depression and Parkinsonism.
5. It may cause hemolytic anaemia.

Dose: 20 mg twice or thrice daily.

Nursing care

1. Same as with clonidine.
2. It should not be given to patients with liver diseases.

ACE INHIBITORS

Captopril, Lisinopril, Enalpril, Perindopril and Ramipril: **Angiotensin plays an important role in maintaining vascular tone. Inhibitors of this enzyme inhibit formation of angiotensin II and increase bradykinin.** Peripheral resistance is reduced, hence used in treatment of hypertension. All are metabolised in the liver to their active forms except lisinopril and excreted through kidneys. All are effective in hypertension **but not in renal artery stenosis.**

Advantages

(a) No change in HR, cardiac output or myocardial contraction.
(b) Ventricular afterload is reduced, hence used in treatment of congestive cardiac failure.
(c) Renal blood flow is increased and renal vascular resistance is reduced.
(d) Left ventricular hypertrophy gets reversed.
(e) No hyperuricaemia, no deleterious effect on plasma lipid.
(f) No postural hypotension.

Uses: In cases of hypertension specially if associated with increased renin activity.

ACE inhibitors are first line drugs nowadays because:
(a) Reduce cardiovascular mortality.
(b) Increase life expectancy.
(c) Greatest potential for remodelling of cardiac muscles.

Captopril

(a) Effective even in cases of hypertension associated with normal renin activity.
(b) It is effective in hypertension resistant to other drugs.
(c) It acts as antihypertensive because:
   (i) It decreases secretion of aldosterone.
   (ii) It exerts diuretic activity which contributes to antihypertensive effect.
  (iii) Enhances the diuretic activity of diuretics and hence smaller doses of diuretic may be required.

Uses

1. Hypertension, specially diabetic hypertension.
2. Congestive cardiac failure.
3. Rheumatoid arthritis.

Adverse drug reactions: Loss of taste, renal impairment and neutropenia.

Dose: 25–50 mg twice daily on an empty stomach.

Enalapril: It is ACE inhibitor and causes lowering of BP.

It is better than captopril because
(a) Needs to be given once daily as has long duration of action. It has better compliance.
(b) It has lesser side effects.
(c) Absorption not affected by food.

Disadvantage: Onset of action is slower.

Perindopril

1. It is more potent.
2. Less chance of first dose hypotension.
3. Restores elasticity of vessel wall, hence used in arteriosclerosis.

Ramipril: It has most extensive tissue distribution due to greater tissue binding, has long half life.

Nursing care for patients on ACE inhibitors

1. Serum creatinine may be slightly elevated.
2. Fetal growth is affected, advise the patient against pregnancy.
3. There is blunting of compensatory mechanisms involved in volume depletion. Hence, keep the patient hydrated.
4. Diuretic should not be given along with it.

ANGIOTENSIN II RECEPTOR ANTAGONISTS

Losortan: Blocks AT_1 receptors. It is prodrug.

Actions

1. Reduces peripheral resistance.
2. Increases excretion of salt and water.
3. Relaxation of vascular smooth muscles is produced.
4. Decreases ventricular hypertrophy.

Advantages

1. Reduces BP without causing increase in heart rate.
2. Action lasts for 24 hours.
3. Cardiovascular reflexes are not interfered.
4. **Does not cause cough.**

5. It has uricosuric effect.
6. Causes less angioedema.
7. Causes less proteinuria.

Adverse reactions

1. Hypotension
2. Hyperkalaemia
3. Gastrointestinal discomfort.

Candesartan: It dissociates slowly from the receptors therefore has long duration of action. It is used to the treat:

(a) Hypertension.
(b) Portal hypertension.
(c) Congestive cardiac failure.
(d) For prophylaxis of cardiovascular diseases.
(e) As alternative to ACE inhibitors.

GANGLIONIC BLOCKING AGENTS

Drugs blocking the release or actions of acetylcholine in the ganglion interfere with the activity of both parasympathetic and sympathetic nerve fibers and produce adverse reactions related to disturbances of both systems. These drugs inhibit both parasympathetic and sympathetic ganglia. Good effects (antihypertensive) are due to inhibition of sympathetic ganglion. Adverse reactions are due to inhibiting parasympathetic activity.

Trimethaphan: It stabilises postsynaptic membranes against the action of acetylcholine. In addition it probably has a direct vasodilatory effect. It releases histamine. When given intravenously it produces immediate effect.

Advantage: It is preferred by clinicians for the initial control of hypertension in persons with dissecting aneurysms of the aorta as it produces immediate effect.

Dose: Initial dose is 3–4 mg/min intravenously. The rate of flow is subsequently adjusted according to blood pressure.

Mecamylamine: It acts like trimethaphan.

It is absorbed when given orally but it crosses blood brain barrier and produces additional adverse reactions in the form of mental confusion, tremors, convulsions and psychological disturbances.

Use: This drug is reserved for hypertension refractory to other antihypertensives.

Precautions: Alkalinisation of the urine increases the risk of toxicity of this drug. **The urine should therefore be maintained on acidic side.**

Adverse reactions: Salivary glands, ciliary muscles of the eye, the sweat glands, the smooth muscle of arteriolar walls, sphincters of bladder and bowel and the male sex organs are all innervated by autonomic nervous system. Inhibiting the ganglion therefore, produces the following adverse reactions.

1. Reduction in sweating and dry mouth.
2. Loss of accommodation due to interference with the function of ciliary muscles.
3. Constipation and retention of urine. These two effects limit the use of these agents in the elderly patients.
4. Inhibition of errection and ejaculation.
5. Postural hypotension.

Nursing care

1. Postural hypotension can lead to serious problems. The patient while getting up from the bed due to extreme hypotension may suddenly become unconscious. Nurse must prevent this mishap by informing her patient regarding such a possibility.
2. These drugs are usually employed in emergency and constant blood pressure recordings must be made.

DRUGS ACTING ON THE POSTGANGLIONIC SYMPATHETIC NERVE ENDINGS

Guanethidine: It depletes the stores of noradrenaline at the endings. In the first phase there is reduction in the release of noradrenaline followed by inhibition of reuptake mechanism leading to ultimate depletion of catecholamine stores. **Large doses of this drug initially produce transient hypertension (specially on intravenous administration).** It produces bradycardia.

Adverse reactions

1. Postural hypotension, as well as hypotension with exercise.
2. Diarrhea.
3. Failure to ejaculate.
4. Nasal congestion resulting in nasal block.
5. Marked Na^+ retention occurs.

Precautions: Guanethidine should be discontinued 2 to 3 weeks before elective surgery requiring a general anaesthetic.

Dose: 25–50 mg/day initially in the hospitalised patients while only 10 mg/day should be given to ambulatory patients. Step up the dose every 3rd day. It is used to treat refractory hypertension.

Bethanidine: It has shorter duration of action, therefore the dosage can be easily adjusted.

Diarrhea is rare.
Debrisoquine, guanoxan and guanadrel are similar to guanethidine.

Nursing care

1. Blood pressure should be taken in bed as well as in standing position. Difference of 10 mm in two positions is normal but diiference of over 30 mm in the two blood pressures indicates potential postural hypotension. Patient should be instructed to leave bed gradually.
2. If the patient complains of dry mouth or blurring of vision these should be reported to the treating physician.
3. Constipation and hesitancy in passing urine should also be reported to the superior.

BETA BLOCKING DRUGS

Propranolol, Atenolol, Metoprolol and Carvedilol: These drugs exert anti-hypertensive effect by:

(a) Reducing cardiac output.

(b) **Reducing release of renin.**

(c) Initially peripheral resistance is increased but on chronic administration this returns to basal level.

Adverse effects

1. Increase LDL/HDL ratio — an undesirable effect.

2. Work capacity is reduced.

3. Reduced libido.

Propranolol

Precautions

1. It is cummulative in nature therefore doses should be carefully monitored.

2. **It is not substantially removed by dialysis.**

Dose: 40 mg twice a day.

Adverse reactions and nursing care same as explained under antianginal drugs.

Atenolol: In low doses it selectively inhibits β_1 receptor activity (cardiac depressant and lipolytic activities).

Disadvantage: Mesenteric thrombosis and ischaemic colitis have been reported in patients receiving atenolol. Not used in renal failure.

Advantages

1. Does not reduce renal blood flow and GFR.
2. Does not cross BBB therefore does not produce CNS associated ADRs.

Dose: 50 mg/day. Single dose a day is sufficient. Maximum dose is 100 mg/day.

Metoprolol: This drug too is a selective β_1 receptor blocker. It have same action as atenolol.

Actions

(a) It improves left ventricular ejection fraction.
(b) Increases exercise tolerance.

Dose: 50 mg twice a day up to 450 mg/day orally.

Nadolol behaves like propranolol.

Pindolol, oxprenolol and alprenolol are partial agonists with membrane stabilising activity.

Advantages

1. Reduce peripheral resistance more effectively.
2. Do not reduce renal blood flow or GFR.
3. Effect on lipid profile is less marked.

Disadvantage: All cross BBB and produce CNS associated adverse reactions like propranolol.

Uses of beta blockers

(a) Hypertension associated with coronary disease (except prinzemetal angina).
(b) Hypertension associated with increased cardiac output.
(c) Hypertensive patients who suffer from anxiety.
(d) Hypertension associated with increased renin.
(e) It is added to other drugs likely to cause tachycardia. **These drugs are not good for elderly patients.**

ALPHA BLOCKING DRUGS

Prazosin, Tetrazosin, Doxazosin, Trimazosin and Indoramin

Adverse reactions of all non-specific alpha receptor blocking agents
1. Postural hypotension.
2. Nasal stuffiness.
3. Red sclerae.
4. Failure of ejaculation in males.

Prazosin: It selectively blocks α_1 receptors.

Actions: It dilates resistance as well as capacitance vessels. Reduces total peripheral resistance and mean blood pressure. Postural hypotension occurs but reflex tachycardia does not occur.

(a) Causes mild tachycardia.
(b) Mild reduction in cardiac output.
(c) Renal blood flow is maintained.
(d) Fluid retention may occur.

Advantages

1. Improves carbohydrate metabolism and insulin resistance and can be used in diabetic patients.
2. Increases HDL and lowers LDL.
3. Does not reduce contractility of myocardium and can be given in patients with left ventricular failure.
4. It is of benefit in patients with peripheral vascular diseases.

Precautions

(a) Causes excessive hypotension leading to **syncope with first dose** therefore start the patient on small doses given at bed time.
(b) Use with caution in patients of angina pectoris.
(c) **In renal insufficiency dose of this drug should be reduced.**
(d) **Diuretics enhance its anti-hypertensive effect** hence caution to be exercised when combination is given.

Disadvantage: Postural hypotension and impotence.

Uses

1. Hypertension.
2. Congestive cardiac failure.

3. Raynaud's phenomena.

4. **Benign prostatic enlargement** causing renal obstruction.

Tolazoline (Priscol)

Pharmacological actions

1. Blockade of alpha receptors produces vasodilation.
2. In addition it **has direct vasodilatory effect.**
3. **Heart rate is increased.**

Adverse reactions

1. Peptic ulcer.
2. Nausea and vomiting.
3. Diarrhea.

Phenoxybenzamine (Dibenzyline): Onset of action is slow, duration of action is very long.

Uses

It is used to control hypertension associated with:

(a) Pheochromocytoma.

(b) Clonidine withdrawal.

(c) Cheese reaction.

DRUGS CAUSING BOTH ALPHA AND BETA BLOCK

Labetalol: It has both alpha and beta receptor blocking effects. Works faster than beta blockers.

Pharmacological actions

1. Dilates arterioles.
2. Increases heart rate, and causes increase in oxygen demand.
3. Causes retention of fluid.

Uses: It quickly controls blood pressure and is useful in emergencies and in pheochromocytoma, clonidine withdrawl and cheese reaction.

Adverse reactions

1. It can precipitate angina pectoris.
2. Headache and flushing.
3. Nasal and conjunctival congestion.
4. Palpitations and vomiting.
5. Systemic lupus erythematosus.

Carvedilol: It has actions similar to labetalol ($\alpha_1 + \beta$ blockade). It has antioxidant properties.

It is long acting.

Advantages: **It is used in patients with congestive cardiac failure.** It can be given to asthmatic and CHF patients.

Dose: 100 mg/day as single or in divided doses.

CALCIUM CHANNEL BLOCKERS

This class includes drugs like **nifedipine, verapamil and diltiazem**.

These drugs inhibit the entry of calcium into the heart and vascular smooth muscles. This results in reduction of contractility of the cardiac as well as vascular smooth muscles.

These drugs do not alter the serum calcium levels.

Actions

1. Decrease cardiac output.
2. Dialate blood vessels and lower blood pressure (systolic as well as diastolic).
3. Decrease oxygen demand of myocardium.

Adverse reactions

1. Hypotension and congestive cardiac failure.
2. Headache.
3. Fatigue and drowsiness.
4. Hepatic damage.

Diltiazem: In addition to above effects it inhibits cardiac conduction which can produce AV block.

Dose: 30 mg/day initially.

Nifedipine: It is most potent vasodilator of this group. This drug has little effect on conduction in the heart or on the myocardium causes tachycardia.

Dose: 10 mg three times a day.

Verapamil: It has greater effect on heart than blood vessels. It inhibits cardiac contractility and conductivity.

It is used in:
1. Angina pectoris.
2. Cardiac arrhythmias.

Adverse reactions

1. It can produce AV block.
2. It can **precipitate congestive cardiac failure** or **pulmonary oedema.**
3. It produces constipation.

Dose: 320–480 mg/day.

DIURETICS

Thiazides: These drugs increase excretion of sodium and water through kidneys thereby reducing blood volume. Chronic administration of these drugs by reducing sodium content of the arterial wall reduces peripheral resistance and BP. Salt restrictions aids antihypertensive effect while salt loading has opposite effect. Fall in BP develops over 2–3 weeks. Thiazides are more effective in elderly.

Advantages

1. Potentiate the effect of other antihypertensive drugs.
2. Prevent development of tolerance to other antihypertensives.

3. No CNS side effects.

4. Low cost.

Disadvantages

1. Effective in 30% patients.

2. Antihypertensive action is slow to develop.

3. Effect on blood pressure is mild.

4. Tend to precipitate diabetes and gout.

5. Increase LDL.

Frusemide and Ethacrynic Acid: Frusemide and ethacrynic acid are not recommended for long-term treatments except in the following:

(a) Hypertension with acute heart failure.

(b) Hypertension with marked fluid retention as happens with use of vasodilators.

Uses

1. Mild hypertension can be treated by diuretic (chlorothiazide) alone.

2. For treating moderate and severe hypertension these agents are combined with other drugs, e.g. hydralazine and beta blockers.

DIRECT ACTING VASODILATORS

Diazoxide

Actions

1. Acts by opening K^+ channels. It has direct vasodilatory effect on the peripheral arterioles. It has no effect on veins.

2. Inhibits the secretion of insulin from the pancreas and precipitates diabetes.

3. Inhibits uterine contraction.

4. Increases HR and cardiac output.

Adverse reactions

1. Precipitates diabetes mellitus.

2. Produces Parkinsonism like syndrome.

3. Hirsutism is produced in females.

4. Causes Na^+ and water retention.

Uses

1. Useful in hypertensive emergencies such as hypertensive encephalopathy and eclamptic toxaemia of pregnancy.

2. In treatment of hypoglycemia.

3. Insulinoma.

4. Alopecia.

Precautions

1. Monitor blood glucose for hyperglycemia.
2. Serum uric acid levels in patients predisposed to gout.

Dose: 300 mg intravenously rapidly.

Sodium Nitroprusside: **It is short acting direct vasodilator. It is drug of choice for hypertensive emergencies with immediate effect.** It is highly effective in lowering blood pressure.

Decreases preload and afterload on heart. Increases stroke volume. Effect comes on immediately and lasts for 1–5 minutes after discontinuation of the drip, therefore, it is **given as continuous drip**. No reflex tachycardia therefore there is no myocardial ischaemia.

Adverse reactions

1. Delirium and psychotic symptoms.
2. Acidosis.
3. Cyanosis.

Precautions

1. Do not mix sodium nitroprusside with other drugs in the IV solution.
2. **Protect nitroprusside containing solution bottles from light.**
3. Watch for signs of toxicity:
   (a) Metabolic acidosis
   (b) Dyspnoea
   (c) Rash
   (d) Tinnitus
   (e) Blurred vision, headache and confusion.
4. It should not be given in patients suffering from:
   (a) Renal impairment
   (b) Hypothyroidism
   (c) Hyponatremia.

Uses

1. Controlled hypotension.
2. Refractory CHF.
3. Acute mitral valve regurgitation.

Dose: 0.25–1.5 ug/kg/min.

Nursing care

1. Blood pressure should be checked repeatedly and rate of infusion adjusted according to blood pressure.
2. Look for signs of cyanosis as this gives indication of toxicity. In case of cyanosis drip should be stopped and the treating physician informed.

Hydralazine: This drug causes relaxation of the smooth muscles of the arterial walls. It does not affect veins. Reduces total peripheral resistance.

Adverse reactions

1. Angina can be precipitated.
2. Blood dyscrasias.
3. Peripheral neuritis associated with pyridoxine deficiency.
4. **Reaction resembling lupus erythematosus is produced.**
5. **It produces retention of sodium and water.**
6. Postural hypotension.

Precautions

1. Hydralazine should either be avoided or used with caution in patients of renal failure.
2. It undergoes acetylation in the body. **Dose has to be reduced in slow acetylators.**
3. Discontinue the drug if systemic lupus is developing.

Dose: Start therapy with 10 mg given three times a day. Maximum of 400 mg/ day can be given.

Uses

1. It is drug of choice for hypertension in pregnancy.
2. Used in moderate hypertension.
3. In combination with beta blockers and diuretics, it is used in severe hypertension.

DRUGS ACTIVATING K⁺ CHANNEL

Minoxidil: This drug too is a direct vasodilator, effect on arterioles is more than on veins. It is prodrug. It acts by increasing K^+ influx.

Adverse reactions

1. It produces severe cardiac complications including pericardial effusion.
2. It produces ST changes in ECG.
3. Breast tenderness and gynaecomastia.
4. Allergic reactions.

Uses

1. Severe hypertension.
2. Male baldness — 2% solution applied on scalp for 6 months.

Precautions

1. Treatment with this drug should be started in a hospital with ECG monitoring.
2. Care needs to be exercised in patients with history of myocardial infarction.

Ketanserin: It is $5\text{-}HT_2$ receptor blocker.

Actions: Lowers blood pressure. Lowers serum lipids. It is more effective in elderly patients. It is usually given in combination with a thiazide (diuretic) or a beta blocker.

Advantages of combination therapy in hypertension

1. Most of the antihypertensive drugs cause sodium and water retention. Diuretics counter this effect and promote their efficacy.

2. Fall in blood pressure produces reflex tachycardia. Combination with beta blockers stops tachycardia.

3. A few of these drugs increase renin release, beta blockers stops this increase.

MANAGEMENT OF HYPERTENSIVE CRISIS

Diazoxide, sodium nitroprusside and trimethaphan are given intravenously in treatment of hypertensive crisis.

1. Though rapid reduction of blood pressure is desired, abrupt excessive fall in blood pressure is not desirable. The treatment should be monitored.

2. Cardiac monitoring is required.

3. Vital signs should be watched carefully.

Nursing care of patients of hypertension

1. Early and vigorous treatment of hypertension reduces the risk of death from cardiovascular diseases. Early detection of hypertension is important.

2. If hypertension is secondary to thyrotoxicosis and pheochromocytoma the treatment should be aimed at primary disease.

3. Obesity should be controlled.

4. Instruct patients to take low sodium diet.

5. Lack of exercise and excess of stress should be avoided by the patients.

6. Promotion of sleep at night by hypnotics or sedatives helps the patient.

7. Nurse must emphasise the need for drug compliance.

8. Patients should be informed about the expected adverse drug reactions. Nurse must educate her patients regarding handling of these agents.

39

Drugs used to Treat Shock

Shock is characterised by fall in blood pressure (both systolic and diastolic) weak and rapid pulse. Tissue perfusion is reduced which is probably responsible for high mortality. Shock can be of following types.

   (a) **Hypovolemic shock:** Loss of blood due to any cause (injury, surgery or even burns—where plasma is lost) produces shock. Initially, compensatory mechanisms such as increase in sympathetic activity leading to acceleration of heart rate, and vasoconstriction maintain tissue perfusion but when this compensation becomes inadequate shock sets in.

   (b) **Cardiogenic shock:** In conditions like myocardial infarction and ventricular arrhythmia heart fails to pump blood. Peripheral vascular failure adds to above component and produces shock.

   (c) **Septic shock:** Severe infections specially due to gram-negative organisms (endotoxic shock) produce sudden peripheral vascular failure due to release of certain mediators such as histamine, kinins, endorphins, interleukins and prostaglandins. There is neutrophil aggregation, microthrombi formation and metabolic block.

   (d) **Peripheral vascular failure:** Decrease in sympathetic activity (spinal anaesthesia or after ganglionic blocking agents and adrenergic neuron blocking drugs) results in pooling of blood in vessels producing reduction in cardiac output and fall in blood pressure.

   (e) **Anaphylactic shock:** Antigen-antibody combination produces histamine and other substances **which produce bronchospasm, laryngospasm and fall in blood pressure.**

Treatment of Shock

   1. **Plasma expanders** are substances that can increase circulating blood volume when they are administered intravenously. These agents are capable of maintaining increased blood volume for long time in contrast to sodium chloride or glucose.

   These agents have high molecular weight that restricts their distribution and they stay in intravascular compartment. These agents in addition have following qualities:

   (a) These are pharmacologically inert.

   (b) These are completely removed from the body either through excretion or by metabolism.

   (c) Do not produce either allergic reactions or have pyrogenic activity.

   (d) Do not interfere in laboratory procedures such as cross-matching of blood.

   (e) It have long shelf life.

Plasma expanders commonly used are:
 (i) Pooled human plasma.
 (ii) Concentrated human albumin.
(iii) Dextran.
(iv) Polyvinylpyrrolidone and gelatin polymers.

Human Plasma: Human plasma and albumin are the best substances for this purpose but they may not be easily available. It is available in 50, 100 and 250 ml ampoules.

Disadvantages

1. It is expensive.
2. It can transmit serum hepatitis and AIDS.

Human Albumin: It is available as 20% solution in 20 and 50 ml ampoules. It is the drug of choice in hypoproteinemia but in shock it has to be diluted with 0.9% sodium chloride (5 times dilution is needed, i.e. 20 ml is made 100 ml). It is expensive but it does not transmit viral diseases. It is used in burns, edema, hypovolemic shock, acute liver failure and in dialysis. Allergic reactions can occur.

Dextran: It is available in various forms — dextran 70 and dextran 40, the latter is called low molecular weight dextran.

Dextrarn 70 is available as 6% solution and 40 as a 10% solution in isotonic saline or 5% dextrose.

Dextran 40 acts more rapidly. It decreases viscosity of blood and prevents sludging of RBCs. Dextran 70 has delayed onset but long effect.

Advantages

1. Efficacy is good.
2. Does not interfere with cross-matching of blood or Rh determination.
3. Half-life is 10 hours and they maintain blood volume for at least 24 hours.
4. Dextran 40 acts more rapidly than dextran 70.

Disadvantages

1. Produces allergic reactions.
2. If given in excess it can precipitate cardiac failure.
3. Dextran 70 inhibits roulex formation by RBCs and also interferes with coagulation factors.
4. Can cause widespread hemorrhages.
5. Dextran 40 can produce acute renal failure.

These should not be given in patients
 (i) of congestive cardiac failure,
 (ii) of renal diseases,
(iii) of hypofibrinogenemia.

Nursing care to be exercised in the use of crystalloids

1. The bottle should not be used if there is any suspended matter present in the bottle
2. The bottle is to be discarded if it is leaking.
3. Bottle of crystalloid is to be stored in cool place. It can be used only once. Remaining portion of the fluid is discarded.

4. Do not add sulphonamides, barbiturates, methicillin and novobiocin to dextrose or fructose solution.

5. Noradrenaline cannot be added to normal saline. For intravenous infusion of this drug **dextrose** is needed.

6. Penicillin, ampicillin, heparin and aminophylline are unstable in these solutions.

Polyvinylpyrrolidone: It is synthetic water soluble compound with molecular weight of 35,000 to 40,000. It is available as isotonic solution in bottles of 100 and 500 ml.

Disadvantages

1. It interferes with blood matching and typing.

2. It remains in body for very long time producing foreign body reactions.

Advantage

It lacks antigenicity.

Gelatin Polymers: Haemaccel commercially available has molecular weight of 30–35,000. Its action lasts 12 hours.

Advantages

1. It has long shelf life of 3 years.

2. It does not interfere with cross-matching or typing.

Disadvantage: Antigenicity is present which may produce flushing, urticaria, rigors and bronchospasm.

Hydroxyethyl Starch: It maintains blood volume for long period. Allergic reactions are rare and it does not interfere with cross-matching.

Disadvantage

Releases histamine therefore not much used.

Contraindications of plasma expanders — cardiac failure, pulmonary oedema, renal failure and severe anaemia.

BLOOD AND BLOOD PRODUCTS

Collection and storage of blood and blood products.

420 ml of ACD whole blood is preserved with solution containing 2.5 g of disodium monohydrogen citrate and 3.9 g of dextrose in 120 ml.

Blood is stored at temperatures ranging between 2 and 6°C.

Stored blood should be utilised within 21 days.

A bottle of blood which is taken out of fridge once and kept at room temperature for over 30 minutes should be used or discarded and not kept back for storage. Pink or red stained plasma in the bottle indicates haemolysis. Such a bottle should not be used.

If the blood has not been used within 21 days then the plasma contained in this bottle should be separated and used but the whole blood cannot be used as the degree of haemolysis increases after 21 days.

Indications for whole blood transfusion

1. Acute blood loss.
2. Anaemia of moderate degree (in severe anaemia packed red blood cells should be given instead of whole blood).
3. Aplastic and haemolytic anaemias.
4. Agranulocytosis.
5. **Fresh blood** is given to supply clotting factors in haemorrhagic disorders.
6. **Fresh blood** to be given to patients with low resistance and suffering from severe infections. This is done to infuse antibodies.
7. In newborn — if Rh incompatibility.

Complications of blood transfusion

1. **Air embolism:** This is because of carelessness.
2. **Allergic reactions:** Antihistaminics and adrenaline should be immediately administered.
3. **Pyrexial reaction:** Patient complains of rigor. It is due to the use of infective perfusion device.

   Immediate attention is needed:
   (a) Drip should be immediately discontinued.
   (b) Give morphine.
   (c) Give antihistaminics.
   (d) Glucocorticoids should be given.
4. Following **diseases can be transmitted** through blood transfusion.
   (i) Acute viral hepatitis.
   (ii) Malaria.
   (iii) AIDS.
   (iv) Syphilis (rare).
5. Haemolytic reaction due to **mismatched blood.**

   It is characterised by pain in renal area, jaundice and oliguria. It needs immediate treatment:
   (a) Stop the transfusion.
   (b) Initiate diuresis by giving normal saline or mannitol (20%).
6. Citrate intoxication occurs in patients who receive many bottles of blood. It is characterised by cardiac irregularities and metabolic acidosis.

Packed Red Cells: Packed red cells are given in cases of severe anaemia where there is need to improve oxygen carrying capacity of blood without increasing blood volume, e.g. in severe anaemia or anaemia associated with congestive cardiac failure and pregnancy.

Plasma: It is used in

(i) Hypovolemic shock.
(ii) In burns.

CRYSTALLOID FLUIDS

Normal Saline: It is 0.95% salt solution of sodium chloride. It is used in conditions where the deficiency of water or salt occurs.

Uses

1. To correct dehydration (isotonic dehydration).
2. As vehicle for giving drugs intravenously.
3. In cases of shock where hypovolemia occurs due to loss of fluid from gut, e.g. vomiting or diarrhea. It does not expand blood volume for a long time as it is rapidly excreted through kidneys.

1.8% sodium chloride solution

Hypotonic dehydration occurs when there is disproportionately greater loss of sodium chloride than water as occurs in salt losing nephritis and adrenocortical insufficiency. Treatment of this condition lies in giving excess of sodium chloride, e.g. 1.8% sodium chloride solution (double the isotonic concentration).

Hypertonic dehydration occurs when there is excess water loss without the proportionate loss of salts. This is seen in the following conditions.

(i) Diabetes insipidus.
(ii) Diabetes mellitus.
(iii) Heat stroke.

These conditions are treated by giving **5% glucose solution intravenously along with 0.9% sodium chloride.**

Dextrose — 5% in water. One litre of dextrose in water raises blood volume by about 100 ml only. It is useful when kidney function is impaired. In addition it supplies energy. **Noradrenaline** can be given in this infusion.

SYMPATHOMIMETICS are used to raise BP in shock

(A) Dopamine: 1–2 mcg/kg/min is given IV. It increases blood perfusion to kidneys, coronaries and mesentery. In moderate doses: 2–10 mcg/kg/min it increases:

(a) Cardiac output.
(b) Systolic and diastolic BP.
(c) HR.

Nursing care

(a) Careful monitoring of dose is required depending upon the response on **BP, ECG and urinary output.**
(b) The site of infusion should be changed every 12 hours
(c) Leakage of fluid should be prevented as it causes necrosis.

(B) Dobutamine: Consists of two isomers dextroisomer has alpha antagonistic and beta agonist activity while levo isomer has predominant α_1 agonist activity with very little beta activity. It may help in a few patients only.

Uses

Cardiogenic shock

(C) Noradrenaline is used if dopamine/dobutamine fail.

(D) Corticosteroids: These are used in all types of shock. The exact mechanism is not known. **These are life saving in anaphylactic shock.**

(E) PGI$_2$, eoprostenol have positive inotropic activity.

DRUGS UNDER STUDY

1. Naloxone in septic shock.
2. Antagonists of PAF (platelet activating factor).

TREATMENT OF DIFFERENT TYPES OF SHOCKS

Cardiogenic Shock

(i) Morphine 15 mg IM.

(ii) Oxygen and rest.

(iii) 5% dextrose solution IV.

(iv) Vasopressors such as **phenylephrine, methoxamine, metaraminol** can be given. **Dopamine** is the drug of choice. It raises blood pressure and increases blood flow to kidneys. It does not induce arrhythmias easily.

(v) **Plasma expanders** should be used with caution as they can precipitate congestive cardiac failure. The rate of infusion of plasma expanders should be slow.

(vi) **Thrombolytic agents** IV.

(vii) Arrhythmias should be corrected by **lignocaine** (1–2 mg/min) or **procainamide** (50 mg/IV every 5 minutes) or DC shock.

(viii) **Vasodilator drugs** are found useful in cardiogenic shock but require careful monitoring which is not possible in every hospital.

(ix) **Isoproterenol should never be given.**

HYPOVOLEMIC SHOCK

In case of hypovolemic shock blood volume should be replaced. Cross-matched blood is the best fluid for replacement. In burns, plasma is a better choice as there is no loss of blood cells. In case of non-availability of plasma or whole blood, plasma expanders should be used. Isotonic solution of glucose or sodium chloride may be rapidly administered before treatment with blood is initiated. Sodium chloride is the drug of choice if fluid loss has occurred through gastrointestinal tract.

(a) Stop loss of fluids.

(b) Replace fluid volume by suitable fluids.

(c) Metabolic acidosis is corrected by alkalies (sodium bicarbonate solution 1.3% which is isotonic with plasma) or 1.9% sodium lactate solution.

(d) Morphine is given if pain is there.

(e) Vasopressor agents are employed if treatment with above agents fails.

(f) Oxygen administration helps the patient.

NEUROGENIC SHOCK

Treated like hypovolemic shock. **Vasopressors** produce definite improvement.

ANAPHYLACTIC SHOCK

(a) **Adrenaline** (1 ml) given intramuscularly reverses few of the symptoms of anaphylactic shock such as hypotension, bronchospasm and laryngeal oedema. It can be repeated at intervals of 15–20 minutes.

(b) Administer fluids as in hypovolemic shock

(c) Chlorpheniramine (10 mg IV) is given to counter histamine.

(d) 100 mg of **hydrocortisone hemisuccinate** is given intravenously. The onset of action of steroids sets in late, therefore, treatment must start with adrenaline and not with steroids.

(e) Specific antidote if available should be given to neutralise the antigen, e.g. penicillinase is given if allergic to penicillin.

(f) Antihistaminic drugs are not very useful but they can be tried.

(g) Oxygen should be continuously administered and artificial respiration given if necessary.

ENDOTOXIC SHOCK

Identify the focus of infection and treat it with antimicrobials and surgically if necessary. **Sympathomimetics** are used to raise BP in shock.

SEPTIC SHOCK

(a) This condition is treated by giving **specific antibiotics**.

(b) Associated acidosis should be corrected by giving appropriate alkalies.

(c) Fluids and plasma expanders are given.

(d) Vasopressors are given.

(e) Heavy doses of steroids are helpful.

PERIPHERAL VASCULAR FAILURE

It is treated by giving:

(a) Plasma expanders.

(b) Dopamine is given, this shows good results.

(c) Oxygen flow should be maintained.

(d) Angiotensin is tried if the patient is not responding to noradrenaline or dopamine.

Nursing care

Patient should be placed in supine position or a head low position. He should be kept warm. Oxygen should be administered (4–6 liters per minute) through intranasal tube. In case of pain (neurogenic shock) morphine can be given. Airway should be maintained by sucking out the secretions at frequent intervals.

PERIPHERAL VASCULAR DISEASE

1. Aspirin and other antiplatelet aggregators are helpful in reducing chances of thrombosis.
2. Simvastatin and ramipril (ACE 1) reduce risk of ischaemic coronary artery disease.
3. In Raynaud's
   (a) Smoking should be stopped
   (b) Avoid cold.
   (c) Nifedipine
   Beta blockers are contraindicated.

40

Drugs used to Treat Migraine

Migraine is a type of headache characterized by throbbing pain on one side of the head. It is caused by dilation of the cerebral blood vessels (specially branches of external carotid artery). In certain individuals certain food items such as cheese and chocolates can trigger migraine.

DURING ACUTE ATTACK

Ergotamine: It is obtained from poisonous parasitic fungus that contaminates reye (claviceps purpurae). It constricts cerebral arteries and in slightly higher doses the peripheral blood vessels are also constricted. The drug is given orally or sublingually. For rapid action it can also be given intramuscularly and as suppository (per rectum).

Adverse reactions

1. Nausea and vomiting.
2. It precipitates angina in patients predisposed to this condition.
3. Produces gangrene in fingers and toes specially if septic.

Uses

Migraine: Moderate to severe degree. It is given with 100 ml of caffeine citrate for prophylaxis.

Nursing care

1. Oral ergotamine takes 5–6 hours to produce relief. You must inform the patient accordingly.
2. 10 mg/day is the maximum dose. **This dose should never be exceeded**.
3. Patients with septic lesions of the extremities should not be given this drug.
4. Advise patient to try to abort an attack of migraine rather treat it when it is full blown.

Sumatriptan: It blocks 5-HT$_{ID}$ receptors and prevents development of neurogenic plasma outflow into dura mater.

Adverse reactions: Coronary spasm leading to angina. It should not be given to patients of angina and MI.

Steroids have been tried and found useful.

Methysergide: It prevents attacks of migraine. On chronic use it may reduce both the frequency and severity of attacks.

Three month course of this drug is recommended.

Adverse reactions: Serious problems of retroperitoneal fibrosis can develop. In this condition kidneys, ureters and other retroperitoneal structures become enmeshed in thick layer of fibrous tissue and the patients may die of renal failure.

DRUGS USED TO PREVENT MIGRAINE

Clonidine: Small doses of clonidine (smaller than required for antihypertensive effect) reduce number and the severity of episodes of migraine. It prevents changes in the blood vessels. For details please refer chapter on 'Antihypertensive Drugs'.

Propranolol: A beta adrenoreceptor blocking agent has been found to be useful in this condition. It is required to be taken for long times. It is not helpful in acute attacks.

Calcium Channel Blockers: Flunarizine is the most commonly used drug in this group. It reduces frequency of attacks. Constipation and orthostatic hypotension are the major side effects.

Tricyclic Antidepressants: Amitriptyline is effective.

41

Drugs used for Prevention and Treatment of Atherosclerosis

It is a condition characterized by narrowing of the blood vessels due to deposition of lipids, fibrous tissue and calcium. Cerebral and coronary arteries are specially prone to this malady. Chylomicrons and lipoproteins are responsible for this problem.

Lipoproteins are of three types:
1. Very low density lipoproteins (VLDL)
2. Low density lipoproteins (LDL)
3. High density lipoproteins (HDL)

Chylomicrons and VLDL are made of triglycerides and LDL is basically cholesterol.

DRUGS WHICH LOWER SERUM LIPIDS

1. Fibric acids — clofibrate, gemfibrozil, fenofibrate.
2. Bile acid binding resins — cholestyramine and colestipol.
3. Antioxidants — probucol.
4. HMG–COA reductase inhibitors — lovastatin, simvastatin, provastatin.
5. Miscellaneous — nicotinic acid, neomycin, thyroxine D, gugulipid, omega-3 fatty acid.

Clofibrate: It effectively lowers both cholesterol and triglyceride levels in blood. It inhibits the synthesis of cholesterol and transfer of triglycerides from liver to plasma.

It causes increase in **lipoprotein lipase activity** thereby causing
1. Reduction in free fatty acids in plasma.
2. 20–50% reduction in triglycerides.
3. 10–15% increase in HDL.

Adverse reactions
1. Nausea, vomiting and flatulence. There is blunting of taste.
2. Dizziness.
3. Cardiac arrhythmias.
4. Hepatic damage.
5. Renal damage.
6. Decrease in libido.

Nursing care

1. It increases effect of oral anticoagulants (coumarin derivatives) the dose of oral anticoagulants should be reduced when given along with these drugs.
2. Liver function tests and complete blood counts should be done regularly.
3. Patients should be monitored for signs and symptoms of gallbladder disease.
4. **It should not be given during pregnancy.**

Gemfibrozil and Benzafibrate, Fenofibrate:
These drugs enhance activity of the enzyme lipoprotein lipase which causes breakdown.

1. Reduce small dense LDL and protect against atherosclerosis.
2. Reduce platelet aggregation.
3. Reduce plasma fibrinogen.

Uses: Effective in type II, III, IV and V types of hyperlipidemia.

Fenofibrate:
Among this group it is most effective. It lowers LDL as well as triglycerides.

Bile Acid Binding Resins:
Bile acids are required for absorption of cholesterol these resins bind bile acid and do not allow absorption.

Cholestyramine and Colestipol

(a) These drugs reduce absorption of cholesterol from food and this leads to breakdown of endogenous cholesterol into bile acids.
(b) Causes **increase in LDL receptors** on liver cells leading to removal of LDL from the blood.

Uses

1. Heterozygous familial hypercholesterolemia.
2. Relieves itching in biliary obstruction.

Adverse reactions

1. These drugs reduce absorption of fats and fat soluble vitamins (A, D and K).
2. Nausea, vomiting and diarrhea.
3. Colestipol in addition produces headache, fatigue and pancreatitis.

Drug interactions

These drugs reduce absorption of:

(a) Digoxin.
(b) Oral anticoagulants.
(c) Phenylbutazone.
(d) Thiazides.
(e) Barbiturates.

Probucol:
It is antioxidant.

It reduces serum cholesterol but has no effect on triglycerides.

It is used to treat familial hypercholesterolemia.

It causes regression of xanthomas.

Adverse reactions: Headache, dizziness, paraesthesia and eosinophilia.

HDL is reduced.

Cardiac arrhythmias may occur.

HMG-COA REDUCTASE INHIBITORS

Lovastatin, simvastatin, pravastatin, atorvastatin and fluvastatin these drugs inhibit HMG-COA enzyme that is needed for synthesis of cholesterol.

These drugs:

(a) Inhibit synthesis of cholesterol in the liver.

(b) Deplete intracellular pools of sterols.

(c) Increase LDL receptor transcription thereby increasing removal of plasma LDL.

(d) Reduce production of VLDL.

(e) **Increase HDL cholesterol.**

Adverse drug reactions: Myositis and myalgia.

OTHER DRUGS

Dextrothyroxine (D-thyroxine): It produces increase in basal metabolic rate and oxygen consumption, though much less than with L-thyroxine. By increasing degradation lowers serum cholesterol. Triglycerides are not much affected.

Sitosterols: It is obtained from plants. It is not very effective and produces diarrhea.

Estrogens: Reduce LDL cholesterol by 15% however triglycerides may increase. Large doses of estrogens are required for producing hypolipidemic action. These doses are undesirable in male as they exert feminizing effect.

Heparin: It is physiological agent which produces hydrolysis of triglycerides but to following **disadvantages** it cannot be used.

1. Repeated IV injections are required as it is not effective orally.

2. There is inherent danger of bleeding.

3. Allergic reactions are known to occur.

4. Cannot be give IM as it may cause haematoma.

Vitamin C, neomycin and aminosalicylic acid are known to affect lipid metabolism.

Role of vitamin C in hyperlipidemia is ambiguous.

Neomycin lowers plasma cholesterol concentration. It can be used to treat **refractory type II hypercholesterolemia**. It is too toxic for routine use.

Nicotinic Acid (Niacin): It has only mild effect. Not used.

Actions

1. It reduces cholesterol as well as triglycerides (VLDL, IDL and LDL) in the blood.

2. It reduces hepatic production of triglycerides.

3. It increases HDL.

Adverse reactions

1. Flushing and skin rash.
2. Impairment of liver functions.
3. Hyperglycemia and hyperuricemia may occur.
4. Precipitates peptic ulcer.

Precautions

1. Increase dose gradually.
2. Avoid its use in pregnancy, liver and kidney disease.

Omega-3-unsaturated Fatty Acids: Omega-3 is present in fish oil while omega-6 is found in oils of soya bean, sunflower and safflower and black gram. These oils lower LDL as well as HDL. Omega-3 reduces serum triglyceride level.

Gugulipid: It is a preparation from gum-guggal.

(i) Causes moderate reduction in plasma cholesterol and triglycerides.

(ii) Increases serum fibrinolytic activity.

(iii) Decreases platelet adhesiveness.

Nursing care

1. Dietary care is most important. Diet should contain less fats.
2. Obesity and stress should be discouraged.
3. Certain diseases which produce hyperlipidemia (diabetes mellitus and hypothyroidism) should be treated appropriately.
4. Drug treatment should be supplemented by diet and exercise.
5. Patient should be informed about the adverse reactions.
6. Anion-exchange resins should never be ingested dry. These should be taken before meals.
7. Anion-exchange resins reduce the absorption of various drugs (thyroid hormones, digoxin, vitamins A, D, K and E, iron, phenylbutazone and thiazides). These drugs should be given one hour before or 4 hours after ingestion of these drugs.
8. Constipation should be prevented by giving high fiber diet.
9. Niacin should be taken with meals to prevent irritation of the gut.

42

Sclerosing Agents

These agents are used to treat varicose veins. Varicose veins is a condition characterised by tortuous, distended veins with incompetent valves. These drugs when injected into the veins produce irritation and fibrosis so as to cause their closure.

Following drugs are used for this purpose

Sodium morrhuate

Quinine and urea hydrochloride

Sodium tetradecyl sulphate

Sodium morrhuate is a solution of fatty acids of cod-liver oil. It is injected into localised segment of vein.

Quinine and urea hydrochloride are used to treat piles.

Uses of sclerosing agents

1. To treat varicose veins in the leg.
2. Piles.
3. For removal of condylomata accuminata.
4. For closure of hernial rings.

Adverse reactions

1. Pain at the site of injection.
2. Sloughing of the area may occur if injection leaks out of vein.
3. Hypersensitivity is seen to sodium morrhuate.

Nursing care

1. Predisposing factors should be avoided, e.g. obesity, long periods of sitting or standing.
2. Advice patients to raise legs frequently to promote drainage.
3. Plastic hose or bandage can be applied to reduce distention.
4. **Surgical removal should be advised as it gives better results.**

Patient should be aware of the adverse reactions which are likely to be produced when treated with sclerosing agents.

43

Histamine and Histamine Antagonists

Histamine is present in animals as well as plants. Venom of bees and wasps contains histamine. Mast cells release large quantities of this agent. Tissue injury causes release of histamine. It is said to be responsible for symptoms of allergy and anaphylactic shock.

Histamine is released:

1. By drugs such as morphine, d-tubocurarine and chlortetracycline.
2. By cold and chemical injury.
3. Allergic conditions — antigen-antibody reactions.
4. By proteolytic enzymes.

There are three types of receptors on which histamine acts: H_1 and H_2 and H_3 receptors.

Actions

(A) Due to stimulation of H_1 receptors

1. Histamine dilates the smaller blood vessels.
2. It constricts larger blood vessels.
3. Produces fall in blood pressure of short duration.
4. When injected into skin it produces itching, pain and various other changes collectively called triple response: vasodilation producing flush or reddening of the area followed by redness and oedema formation.
5. Smooth muscles of the bronchi and gut are contracted by this agent.

(B) Due to stimulation of H_2 receptors

1. It produces cardiac irregularities — ventricular tachycardia.
2. Secretions of gastric juice is increased.
3. Secretions of all exocrine glands — pancreatic, bronchial, salivary and lacrimal glands are increased.

HISTAMINE AGONIST

Betazole: It is a histamine substitute.

Advantages

1. It can be given orally while histamine has to be injected subcutaneously.
2. The effect of this drug lasts longer.
3. Effect on gastric secretion is more marked than other effects, therefore, the adverse reactions are limited.

Disadvantages

1. Effect of gastric secretion is slow in onset. Dose 0.5 mg/kg.
2. It has to be given IV.

Adverse reactions

1. Bronchial asthma.
2. Headache and visual disturbances are common. It is used only for diagnostic purposes.

Uses

1. For diagnose of achlorhydria and pernicious anaemia.
2. In diagnosis of leprosy.
3. Rarely it is employed for diagnosis of pheochromocytoma.

Betahistine Hydrochloride: It is histamine substitute found useful in Meniere's syndrome.

Disadvantages

1. It aggravates peptic ulcer.
2. It precipitates bronchial asthma.

ANTIHISTAMINES

These drugs block the effect of histamine at its receptors. There are therefore, three types of antihistaminic drugs.

1. H_1 blockers.
2. H_2 blockers.
3. H_3 blockers.

H_1 receptor antagonists or blockers were discovered in 1933. Effect of histamine on H_1 receptors are inihibited by these drugs.

CLASSIFICATION OF H_1 BLOCKERS

(a) **Highly sedative:** Diphenhydramine, dimenhydrinate, promethazine, hydroxyzine

(b) **Moderately sedative:** Pheniramine, antazoline, trimeprazine, cyproheptadine, meclizine, buclizine.

(c) **Mild sedative:** Chlorpheniramine, methdilazine, mepyramine (pyrilamine), dimethindene, triprolidine, mebhydroline, cyclizine, clemastine.

(d) **Newer compounds**
  (i) **Non sedating-antiallergic** terfenadine, astemizole, loratidine, cetrizine, fenofenadine and azelastime.
  (ii) Antivertigo-cinnarizine

Advantages of newer compounds

1. Cause relatively less sedation.
2. They have higher selectivity and do not cause anticholinergic effects.
3. Possess additional antiallergic mechanisms such as inhibition of platelet activating factor.

Actions due to H_1 receptors:

(a) These drugs have anticholinergic activity therefore inhibit salivary secretions and produce dryness of mouth.

(b) Motility of the gut is inhibited—leading to constipation.

(c) Urinary retention is produced.

(d) Most of these agents produce sedation and induce sleep.

Terfenadine, cetrizine and loratadine do not cross BBB and therefore lack sedative effect. Have no anticholinergic effect. Degree of sedation varies from one drug to another.

(e) Few may precipitate epilepsy (phenendamine).

(f) **Vomiting due to motion sickness is inhibited.**

(g) A large number of these drugs possess local anaesthetic activity.

(h) Cyproheptadine in addition has anti-5-HT effect.

(i) Promethazine has alpha blocking activity.

Adverse reactions

1. Dryness of mouth.

2. Sedation (except with cetrizine, terfenadine and loratidine).

3. Blurring of vision.

4. **Allergic reactions may be produced by these agents**

5. **Nausea and vomiting are also possible as adverse reactions**.

Toxicity of these agents produces drowsiness, delirium and convulsions. Diazepam is given to treat convulsions. Rest of the symptoms of toxicity are treated through supportive measures.

Uses

1. Allergic conditions—hay fever, vasomotor rhinitis and common cold.

2. May be used as hypnotic.

3. Few of these drugs (diphenhydramine and orphenadrine) are used to treat Parkinsonism.

4. Promethazine in combination with pethidine and chlorpromazine (lytic cocktail) is given to bring down fever and in treatment of eclampsia.

5. They are used to prevent motion sickness. These agents should be given half an hour before the start of journey. Driving is not possible after taking these drugs.

H_1 receptor antagonists do not block the following actions of histamine

(a) Gastric acid secretion.

(b) Bronchospasm.

(c) Hypotension associated with anaphylactic shock.

(d) Cardiac irregularities produced by histamine.

Precaution: Driving and handling of machinery is to be avoided.

HISTAMINE RECEPTOR BLOCKERS

Cimetidine, burimamide and metiamide block H_2 receptors

Cimetidine: It reduces gastric acid secretion but is not preferred due to adverse reactions and interactions.

Adverse reactions

1. Liver damage, diarrhoea, drowsiness.
2. Sexual impotency, gynaecomastia.
3. Serious reduction in WBC count.

Ranitidine

1. It has actions like cimetidine but the effect produced by the drug is longer lasting.
2. It produces lesser number of adverse reactions. It does not produce endocrinological disturbances.

Burimamide: It too reduces gastric acid production.

Famotidine

Advantages

(a) It is 20 times potent than cimetidine and 8 times potent than ranitidine.
(b) It is well tolerated.
(c) It has fewer side effects.

Nizatidine, roxatidine and ebrotidine are like ranitidine but with fewer side effects.

Precautions in the use of H_2 receptor blocking agents

1. These agents should be used with caution in patient with hepatic or renal failure.
2. Dosage of these drugs needs to be reduced in renal failure.
3. Predisposition to gastric carcinoma by cimetidine is reported.
4. They are not recommended during pregnancy and should not be given to children or lactating mothers.
5. Ranitidine reduces secretion of intrinsic factor therefore patients receiving this drug for long periods should be monitored for vitamin B_{12} deficiency.

HISTAMINE H_3 RECEPTOR

It is a presynaptic receptor in brain.

It regulates synthesis and release of histamine.

R-alpha methyl histamine is specific agonist.

Actions

1. CNS — sedative effect.
2. GIT — reduces HCl secretion.
3. Respiratory — bronchodilatation.
4. CVS — negative chronotropic effect in atria.

H_3 blockers: Thioperamide is under study for its therapeutic effects.

44

Serotonin (5-HT) and its Antagonists

90% of total amount of 5-HT is present in gut and remaining (10%) is in platelets and brain.

Bananas, pineapples and tomatoes are rich source of 5-HT. There are 3 types of receptors $5\text{-HT}_{1\,(A,\,B,\,D)}$, $5\text{-HT}_{2\,(B,\,C)}$ and $5\text{-HT}_{3,\,4,\,5,\,6,\,7}$.

Actions: Physiological

CNS: 5-HT is involved in sleep, BP, mood, sexual functions and temperature regulation.

CVS: Exerts positive inotropic and chronotropic effects on heart. Constricts blood vessels (except those of skeletal muscles).

GIT: Increases acid secretion, increases motility.

Blood: It is a weak platelet aggregator.

Nerve endings: Stimulates pain mediating nerve endings.

5-HT is not clinically used.

Urinary excretion of 5-HIAA provides measure of 5-HT turnover.

Metoclopramide stimulates 5-HT_4 and increases peristaltic activity and is used for treatment of nausea and vomiting.

Ketanserin: It blocks 5-HT_2, alpha-adrenergic and dopaminergic receptors.

Actions

1. Inhibits 5-HT induced vasoconstriction, platelet aggregation and bronchoconstriction.
2. Produces fall in BP.

Adverse reactions: Dry mouth, headache, sedation and dizziness.

Ondansetron, granesetron and tropisetron block 5-HT_3 receptros and are used to prevent/treat vomiting in cancer patients during chemotherapy.

Methysergide, dihydroergotamine, ketotefen block 5-HT_2 receptors. These are used to treat migraine.

Cyproheptadine: Blocks histamine (H_1), cholinergic (M), 5-HT and calcium channels.

Uses

1. Antiemetic.
2. Stimulator of appetite causing increase in body weight.

Drugs Acting on the Respiratory System

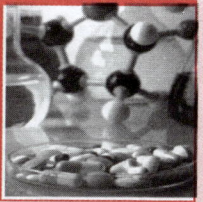

45

Drugs Acting on the Respiratory System

Drugs used for respiratory system belong to one of the following groups:

1. **Anti-tussive** — for suppression of cough.
2. **Expectorants and mucolytics** for liquefying and removal of the secretions from the respiratory passages.
3. For reducing secretions of the respiratory tract as is required during anaesthesia and surgery.
4. **Analeptics** — for stimulation of the respiration.
5. **Anti asthmatics** — for dilatation of bronchi.

ANTI-TUSSIVE AGENTS

Cough is a protective reflex aimed at removing irritant from the respiratory tract (pharynx, larynx, trachea or bronchi). There is a cough center in the brain that is responsible for co-ordination of efferent and afferent impulses that bring about cough.

Cough is said to be useful if it removes accumulated secretions from the lungs as it serves to clear respiratory passages. Cough is non-productive when no useful action is performed — this type of cough needs treatment specially if it causes sleepless nights and restless days.

Productive cough needs suppression when it is likely to precipitate other health problems, e.g. after surgery on abdominal wall, cough may hinder healing of the wound. Cough may precipitate congestive cardiac failure in failing heart. It can produce haemorrhage in the eye after cataract surgery.

Anti-tussives are used to suppress dry and unproductive cough.

Steam Inhalation

(a) Steam increases humidity of the inspired air which reduces irritation of the mucous membranes.
(b) The irritant in the air gets diluted.
(c) Inhalations liquefy the secretions and help in their removal.
(d) Inhalations pass with ease down the smallest bronchioles to reach the site of obstruction and inflammation.

Techniques of administering steam inhalations

Boiling water is poured over menthol crystals. The patient is instructed to cover the top of the jug with towel or cloth to prevent burns from boiling water and to cover his head and face and inhale through this jug for about 10–15 minutes in a sitting posture.

COUGH SUPPRESSANTS

Locally acting agents such as **lozenges or syrup or linctus** can remove irritation in the pharynx and can stop dry cough of pharyngitis. All these agents produce demulcent effect.

Drugs acting on the cough center in the brain reduce its sensitivity to incoming impulses and are used to treat dry cough.

(A) Codeine: It is a natural alkaloid of opium. Codeine is the active ingredient of most of the medicaments available in the market. It partly gets converted in the body to morphine.

It is given orally as syrup. For adults two teaspoonfuls are given four times a day. For infants quarter of teaspoon four times a day is sufficient.

For older children half to one teaspoon can be given 4 times daily.

Advantages

1. It is highly effective.
2. Taste is good, therefore can be easily administered even to children.

Disadvantages

1. It is addicting in nature.
2. It produces constipation.

(B) Dihydrocodeine: This drug has actions like codeine but is long acting—10 mg twice a day is sufficient.

(C) Noscapine: It is a good anti-tussive. It does not produce sleep or addiction or any other CNS effect, but worsens asthma. It does not cause constipation. 10–30 mg dose is given three or four times a day.

(D) Pholcodeine: It is synthetic opioid. It is comparable to codeine.

(E) Dextromethorphon and Levopropoxyphen: Like noscapine they do not suffer from bad effects of morphine. Anti-tussive effect lasts for 6–8 hours.

(F) Benzonatate: It is non-opoid, chemically similar to procaine.

It suppresses cough center as well as the pulmonary stretch receptors. It is given orally in the dose of 50–100 mg three to four times a day.

(G) Methadone: It is a synthetic drug with morphine-like activity. It is used in patients who do not respond to codeine. It is long acting and is used for deaddiction.

Morphine has anti-tussive activity but is rarely used for this purpose. Derivatives of morphine are not preferred as they produce addiction. However, they can be effectively **used in patients with terminal illness such as cancer.**

(H) Carbetapenatane: This drug has anti-tussive effect. It is given in the dosage of 15–30 mg orally.

DRUGS ACTING PERIPHERALLY

(A) Antihistamines (Chlropheneramine, Diphenhydramine, Promethazine, Astemezole): When the cough is due to allergic reaction, antihistaminics are used as anti-tussive agents. These drugs produce drying of secretions and are **not appreciated in asthma. Expectorants or mucolytic agents may be combined with these drugs to counter this drying effect.**

(B) Soothing Agents, Demulcents: These agents reduce the viscosity of pharyngeal secretions. Liquid cough mixtures containing alcohol, propylene glycol or expectorants such as guaifenesin are used to suppress cough. Water, cough drops and lozenges act through this mechanism.

(C) Local Anaesthetics: Benzocaine containing lozenges are used to treat minor throat irritation. Lidocaine is used for suppression of cough during bronchoscopy.

EXPECTORANTS AND MUCOLYTIC AGENTS

Mucolytic agents **bromhexine, iodides and streptokines and acetylapteine** produce liquefaction of the mucus (by breaking disulfide chains) making expectoration easier. These are used for liquefying expectoration in weak patients who cannot cough out thick secretions. Expectorants help in removal of secretions of the respiratory tract.

Smaller doses of these agents stimulate mucus secretion in lungs while larger doses irritate gastric mucosa and produce vomiting, e.g. ipecac, iodides.

Volatile oils of menthol, eucalyptus, cresote, terpine hydrate and benzoin act through this route.

Iodides: The salts of iodine such as potassium iodide, are used in chronic productive cough due to chronic bronchitis.

Disadvantages

1. Produces adverse reactions in the form of allergic reactions.
2. Iodism is produced.

Dose: 0.3 to 0.6 g three times a day.

Ipecac: It is used to treat dry cough associated with acute respiratory diseases.

Ammonium Salts: Produce gastric irritation and reflexly increase bronchial secretions. 0.3 g ammonium chloride or citrate or its carbonate salt are used.

Volatile Oils: Tincture benzoin is added to steam inhalation. Oils of eucalyptus or balsam and tolu are common ingredients of cough mixtures.

Terpine hydrate and Vasaka syrup are also useful.

Bronchodilators relieve cough due to bronchospasm and are given if patient has wheeze along with cough.

DRUGS USED FOR REDUCING SECRETIONS OF THE RESPIRATORY TRACT

The patient is incapable of coughing out the secretions during anaesthesia. The secretions tend to accumulate and are source of trouble in the postoperative period. In addition certain anaesthetic agents (e.g. ether) increase respiratory secretions. These drugs are therefore used before administering general anaesthesia, to counter these effects.

Atropine or hyoscine are preferred for this purpose.

Antihistaminic drugs produce dryness of nasal as well as respiratory tract. These drugs are therefore used in allergic conditions effecting these areas (rhinitis, allergic bronchitis). (For details refer chapter on antihistaminics.)

46

Drugs used in Bronchial Asthma

Bronchial asthma is characterised by **dyspnoea and wheeze**. Individuals suffering from asthma have bronchial smooth muscles which are hypersensitive to constricting agents normally present in the body, e.g. **acetylcholine, histamine**. **Slow reacting substance A**, **prostaglandins** and **kalikreins** that are released due to antigen and antibody interaction on mast cells. Reversible contraction of smooth muscle of the bronchi and inflammation of the bronchial mucosa results in constriction of air passages which produces a wheeze when patient exhales.

There are three different ways to relieve bronchial obstruction.

1. By use of bronchodilators
   - (i) β_2 agonists — salbutamol, salmetrol, terbutaline, adrenaline
   - (ii) Direct smooth muscle relaxants, e.g. aminophylline
   - (iii) Anticholinergics — ipratropium
2. By preventing the allergic reaction through use of glucocorticosteroids.
3. Mast cell stabilizers — by preventing the release of chemical agents in response to antibody-antigen reaction which cause muscle contraction, e.g. **sodium chromoglycate, nedocromil and ketoprofen**.

BRONCHODILATORS

Adrenaline hydrochloride: It is used during acute attack of bronchial asthma not responding to conventional treatment. It has no prophylactic role.

Method of Injection: A BCG syringe is filled with 1.0 ml of 1:1000 solution of adrenaline. The needle is placed subcutaneously and the syringe strapped on the forearm. Solution is injected at a time till the patient feels relieved.

Dose 0.2 to 0.5 ml of 1:1000 aqueous solution subcutaneously can be repeated 20–30 minutes later if attack does not subside.

Adverse reactions: Adrenaline produces serious side effects.

- (i) Ventricular tachycardia.
- (ii) Ventricular fibrillation.

Hence, it is advisable that **doctor must give this drug**. If nurse is asked to give this injection, then it should be under the supervision of a senior member of medical faculty.

Adrenaline should not be given in:
1. Cardiac asthma (pulmonary oedema).
2. Hypertension.
3. Thyrotoxicosis.
4. In older patients.

Isopropylnoradrenaline (Isoprenaline): It acts like adrenaline but has the advantage that it can also be given through an aerosol. Not used now.

Advantages of aerosol

1. Drugs given through the aerosol show quicker results.
2. The administered drug gets localised and maximum concentration of drug is delivered at the large bronchi and trachea. This minimises the systemic adverse reactions.
3. The dose and frequency of administration can easily be monitored by the patient.

Disadvantage: Drug does not reach small bronchi.

Nursing care of patient on aerosol

1. For maximum effect two puffs should be inhaled at an interval of one minute each.
2. Release of aerosol should coincide with the start of deep inspiration.
3. Frequent use of aerosol at short intervals should be discouraged. In such a condition patient must be advised to see his physician.

Salbutamol: It stimulates β_2 receptors and has no or very little effect on β_1 receptors. Available as tablet, inhaler and nebuliser.

Advantages over isoprenaline

(i) It is more selective bronchodilator. Bad effects on heart are not frequently seen.
(ii) It has longer duration of action.
(iii) It is safe.
(iv) It can be given orally as well as through aerosol.

Disadvantages

(i) Onset of action is slow.
(ii) Tremors usually occur.

It is ineffective in asthma produced by propranolol.

Terbutaline: This drug has actions similar to salbutamol. It can be given SC.

Salmeterol: It acts selective on β_2 receptors. Its onset is delayed but has long duration of action (12–14 hrs). It is given by inhalation. In children and elderly, spacer can be used for better delivery. It can also be given by nebuliser, and as dry powder (rotacaps).

Formoterol: Longest acting (14 hours) β_2 agonist.

Disadvantages of β_2 agonists

1. Some degree of tachycardia may occur.
2. On constant use — tolerance develops, therefore cannot be given alone for long-term use as in chronic asthma.

Rimiterol: It is more specific β_2 agonist. It has rapid onset of action and is effective on inhalation.

Ephedrine: It is a weaker bronchodilator. It was used in between asthmatic attacks. It prevents sleep, therefore the last dose should be given at least four hours before bed time.

It is for prophylaxis and not for acute attack.

30–60 mg orally 3–4 times daily.

Aminophylline: This is a salt of theophylline (xanthine) a direct smooth muscle relaxant.

Advantages

1. It is drug of choice during acute attack of asthma specially when it is not possible to differentiate cardiac from bronchial asthma.
2. It is used in emergency in bronchial asthma after adrenaline has failed to relieve the attack.

It is given as slow intravenous injection (10 mg). If it is given too quickly there is a risk of acute peripheral collapse. The drug can be repeated every four hours.

Adverse reactions

1. Specially in cardiac patients deaths have been reported after quick intravenous injection of this drug.
2. Epileptiform fits may occur.

PREVENTING ANTIGEN/ANTIBODY REACTION

Corticosteroids: These drugs are dealt in detail in chapter on endocrinology. All these drugs produce many undesirable adverse reactions.

(a) These drugs are used for their immunosuppressant and anti-inflammatory effects.
(b) These reduce bronchial oedema and **reactivate beta receptors** in patients who become resistant to beta agonists. Steroidal drugs are therefore, used only in cases where the patient has ceased to respond to common drugs.

Prednisolone may be life saving in these patients—60 mg/day orally may be given initially. The drug is gradually withdrawn.

Hydrocortisone hemisuccinate may be given intravenously in doses of 100 mg every 6 hours. **Corticosteroids may be considered for chronic treatment only in cases that fail to respond to rest of the drugs.**

For nursing care and precautions refer endocrinology.

Inhalational Steroids

Beclomethasone

This is a corticosteroid given in the form of aerosol.

It relieves asthma by acting locally on the tracheobronchial tree.

Systemic adverse reactions are not seen.

Adverse reactions: It can lead to localised infections with Candida albicans in the mouth and throat.

Advantages

1. No systemic effects.
2. No systemic toxicity.
3. Dose can easily be monitored.
4. In chronic asthma is preferred over oral glucocorticoids.

Budesonide: It is preffered drug because

1. It is long acting.
2. Does not suppress growth in children as it does not affect cartilage.
3. Causes less suppression of adrenocortical axis.

ANTICHOLINERGICS

Ipratropium: It is cholinergic blocking agent. **It prevents exercise induced asthma.** It is given through inhalation.

PREVENTION OF RELEASE OF MEDIATORS OF ALLERGY

Trotropium: It is inhalational drug acts like ipratropium but is longer acting and more potent. Side effects are less.

MAST CELL STABILISERS

Sodium Cromoglycate: This drug prevents asthmatic attacks. **It is of no value during the attack.**

Interaction of antigen and antibody produce certain substances (serotonin, SRA-A, etc.) which produce bronchoconstriction and inflammation in the bronchial mucosa. This drug allows the interaction of antigens (allergens like dust, pollen or bacteria) with antibody but does not allow the release of chemical mediators.

It is available as 20 mg capsule for aerosol. It is also available as powder for nasal insufflation.

Uses

1. Allergic bronchial asthma.
2. Other respiratory allergies.
3. In allergic rhinitis.
4. Allergic conjunctivitis.

Ketotifen: It is serotonin antagonist. It has actions similar to cromoglycate but can be given orally. Drowsiness is the main side effect.

Antimicrobials (Ampicillin or Cotrimoxazole): Can be started to prevent infection.

To improve respiratory functions

(a) Establish patent airway
(b) Provide oxygen therapy
(c) Supply humidified oxygen

(d) Decrease airway resistance by:
   (i) Removing secretions.
   (ii) Reducing viscosity of secretions by using mucolytic agents.
   (iii) Reducing bronchial secretions by using expectorants.
(e) Decrease anxiety of the patients by:
   (i) Reassuring them.
   (ii) Providing comfortable surroundings.
(f) Train your patients to perform breathing exercises.
(g) Prevent infections.

Nursing care of patients of asthma

1. Patients of asthma must be advised on prevention of the attack. If the provocative agent is known, it should be avoided or the patient asked to get desensitisation done.

2. These patients usually come to causality and visit more frequently during change of season. Nurse in emergency must keep her kits ready to meet these emergencies.

3. Patient is kept in reclined posture with the hand rest provided. Head end of the bed should be raised to a degree convenient to the patient.

4. Patient is encouraged to cough out secretions as far as possible and bring out the mucus plugs.

5. Aminophylline or adrenaline is given as described earlier.

6. The rate of drip needs close monitoring. Blood pressure should be taken at short intervals.

7. Patient should be advised against the use of the drugs which precipitate asthma, e.g. histamine, beta adrenoreceptor blockers and opiates.

8. If your patient needs sedation avoid the use of morphine and its substitutes as they precipitate asthma. Diazepam or chloral hydrate can be safely used in these patients.

Patient of **status asthmaticus** needs special attention as it is a serious medical emergency. As these are unsafe drugs are best handled by the doctors. But in case no doctor is around (as in Primary Health Center) you can start the treatment with nebulisation salbutamol or 0.4 mg IM/SC and watch for tachycardia.

Hydrocortisone hemisuccinate in dose of 100 mg can be given intravenously initially and repeated every four hours. According to responses to hydrocortisone—replace it with prednisolone (20 mg/6 hourly) by mouth. Aminophylline 25 mg is given by slow IV injection keeping an eye on heart rate.

Antibiotics to be started to prevent infections.

Humidified O_2 reduces distress due to dyspnoea.

Respiratory secretions are to be handled with care. Excess as well as deficiency of these secretions worsens condition. In cases of dried up secretions administration of IV fluids is helpful.

47

Respiratory Gases

OXYGEN THERAPY

Treatment with oxygen is required during its deficiency. Brain cells are highly sensitive to lack of oxygen and are permanently destroyed if hypoxia lasts for more than 4 minutes.

Deficiency of oxygen can arise in any one of the following ways.

1. When there is impairment of oxygen carrying capacity of the blood, e.g. anaemia, methaemoglobinaemia and in carbon monoxide poisoning, etc.
2. In diseases of heart and lung resulting in reduction in passage of oxygen from air to blood, e.g. pneumonia, congestive cardiac failure and pulmonary oedema or when air is deficient in oxygen (high altitude).
3. When the blood flow to the tissue is reduced there is localised hypoxia and the damage becomes localised, e.g. coronary artery thrombosis produces myocardial infarction.
4. When the respiratory enzymes in the tissue are non-functional, e.g. cyanide poisoning.

1. Impairment of the Oxygen Carrying Capacity of Blood

Oxygen in blood is carried by haemoglobin. In case there is deficiency of haemoglobin or when haemoglobin of blood is incapable of carrying oxygen hypoxia results. This condition is seen in severe anaemia and in carbon monoxide poisoning, etc.

Carbon monoxide poisoning occurs in persons involved in fire fighting. In this condition Hb combines with CO (because Hb has greater affinity for CO than O_2) and not with oxygen. Toxicity is directly proportional to the duration of exposure.

To treat carbon monoxide poisoning the patient (a) should be removed from the atmosphere containing this gas. (b) **Oxygen should be given under pressure.** This reduces hypoxia. Availability of oxygen in high concentrations dislodges carbon monoxide from Hb.

2. Diseases of the Heart and Lungs

In (congestive cardiac failure, pneumonia, pulmonary oedema), due to poor diffusion of alveolar oxygen into the blood there is deficiency of O_2. These patients develop central cyanosis that manifests as bluing of lips, ear lobes and tips of fingers.

In all these conditions oxygen is administered to the patient with caution as in these patients blood normally contains high levels of CO_2 which keeps the respiratory center in stimulatory state. **Respiratory Center is Depressed by O_2.** On administration of 100% oxygen, CO_2 is quickly removed from blood and hypoxia disappears. High O_2 and low CO_2 depress respiration. Such patients may stop breathing and die in coma. **Excessive oxygen therapy in these individuals can therefore be dangerous (carbon dioxide narcosis).**

These patients therefore **are treated with low oxygen concentration** in the breathing air. This gradually corrects blood as well as tissue hypoxia without inhibiting respiratory center. Special oxygen masks are available for this purpose.

Impairment of Oxygen Flow to Tissues:
This is seen commonly in cold weather when to reduce heat loss the peripheral arterioles get constricted. **Finger tips get blue (peripheral cyanosis), but there is no bluing of lips.** Myocardial infarction and hypovolemic shock produce similar condition.

Oxygen therapy is given in these patients to improve the oxygenation of tissues.

Cyanide Poisoning:
The respiratory enzymes in the tissue (cytochromes) have greater affinity for cyanide radical than O_2. 100% oxygen under pressure is administered in these individuals.

TECHNIQUES OF ADMINISTRATION OF OXYGEN

Oxygen cylinders have black body and white neck. Oxygen can be administered in various ways.

1. Tents.
2. Nasal catheters.
3. Face masks.
   (a) Poly mask.
   (b) MC mask.
   (c) Ventimask.

Tents:
Humidified oxygen is administered through a tubing into airtight tent fitted over the patients head and the chest.

Uses

1. It is useful in paediatric practice.
2. This technique is required in patients of cardiothoracic surgery.

Disadvantages

1. Cumbersome to use.
2. There is danger of fire.

Nasal Catheter:
This is commonest mode of administration of oxygen in chronic lung diseases.

A soft, fine rubber catheter lightly covered with local anaesthetic is passed through nostril into the nasopharynx. **Humidified oxygen** is blown through this catheter at the rate of 3–6 liters per minute.

Advantages

1. It is well tolerated by the patient.
2. Flow rate of oxygen can be easily adjusted.

Face Mask:
Polymasks are made of plastic, are cheap and can be used for many years.

Disadvantages

1. It is cumbersome and patients (elderly and confused) usually do not tolerate this device.
2. If the mask is ill fitted much of the blown oxygen gets lost to the atmosphere.
3. Sterilization of these masks is a problem.

MC Mask (Henley): This mask delivers oxygen in high concentrations provided it is carefully fitted to the patient. Ventimask has the advantage that the flow of O_2 can be well regulated. This is specially desirable in patients who have chronically excessive carbon dioxide.

Hyperbaric Oxygen (Oxygen at high pressure)

Hyperbaric oxygen is administered to patient in a pressure chamber. This is useful in patients of **pulmonary oedema** and in infections produced by **anaerobic bacteria,** e.g. gas gangrene and tetanus.

Uses of hyperbaric oxygen

1. Respiratory diseases of the newborn.
2. Carbon monoxide poisoning.
3. Decompression sickness.
4. Anaerobic infections (gangrene and tetanus).
5. For open heart surgery.

Hazards of hyperbaric oxygen

1. Danger from fire.
2. Carbon dioxide narcosis.
3. Retrolental fibroplasia in infants.
4. CNS stimulation, e.g. restlessness, tremors and convulsions.

Nursing care of the patients receiving oxygen therapy

1. Nurses must ensure that no fire comes near the oxygen, e.g. through smoking or by way of lighting match sticks.
2. Mask must be fitted properly round the contours of cheeks of the patients and nose. Nurse must observe whether patient is tolerating this mask.
3. Flow rate of oxygen must be checked frequently specially in chronic patients with high levels of carbon dioxide.
4. In chronic bronchitis and emphysema watch for the signs and symptoms of carbon dioxide wash out and development of failure of respiratory center (Cheyne stokes breathing).

CARBON DIOXIDE

This gas is produced in the body and is thrown out through the lungs. **In higher concentrations it decreases heart rate and myocardial contraction.** In smaller concentrations it stimulates central nervous system while higher concentrations depress it.

It increases both the rate and depth of respiration. It produces fall in blood pressure.

Adverse reactions: 7% and concentrations higher than this produce headache, dizziness, mental confusion, palpitations, dyspnoea and high blood pressure.

Uses

1. 5–10% of carbon dioxide is mixed with oxygen and administered in patients of respiratory depression.
2. Same concentration is used in carbon monoxide poisoning.
3. Hiccups.
4. For treatment of anxiety neurosis.
5. It is applied on warts.

HELIUM

This is a very light gas

1. It is used for treating prolonged asthmatic attacks not responding to other therapy.
2. It is used for the treatment of laryngeal oedema and larygospasm.

TREATMENT OF ACUTE RESPIRATORY FAILURE

Respiratory failure is defined as a condition in which there is abnormality of blood gases (there is excess of CO_2 and deficiency of O_2) and occurs at rest.

Acute respiratory failure can result either from cardiac or pulmonary diseases or it can be due to inhibition of the central nervous system (narcotic poisoning, stroke, head injuries, etc.).

Acute respiratory failure due to respiratory cardiovascular diseases is treated in following ways:

1. Oxygen therapy is started at the earliest. In chronic lung conditions to avoid carbon dioxide narcosis low concentration of oxygen (25–30%) are given.
2. Patient should be made to cough out mucus plugs. Inhalations of humidified oxygen helps in this direction.
3. Bronchodilators including large doses of glucorticoids are given.
4. Supportive therapy is given to maintain blood pressure and electrolyte balance.
5. Respiratory stimulants can be given if patient does not improve after oxygen or if reduction in ventilation occurs after oxygen therapy. These drugs in addition stimulate cough.
6. Intensive nursing care is the mainstay of treatment.

Nikethamide and doxapram (stimulants of respiratory center) are commonly used for this purpose. These drugs are also employed in comatosed patients (for details please refer CNS).

Disadvantages of these drugs

(a) None of the drugs available in this group selectively stimulates respiration. All these drugs produce adverse reactions—including convulsions.
(b) The efficacy of these drugs is poor therefore they cannot be relied upon completely.
(c) All these drugs initially stimulate respiration but ultimately depress it. This depression may add to the depression caused by drugs and disease of CNS.

In case of poisoning by drugs attempt is made to increase their excretion, e.g. in case of barbiturate—fluids are given intravenously in excess along with sodium bicarbonate.

In morphine poisoning **naloxone** (nalorphine is given if naloxone is not available) counters the inhibition of respiratory centre. It is a specific antidote. Similarly, **flumezonil** specifically antagonises respiratory depression due to benzodiazepines.

Nursing care of patient of acute respiratory failure

1. If patient has difficulty in getting air in and out of his lungs it is necessary to use mechanically assisted ventilation.

2. No time should be lost in clearing the airways. Aspirate secretions and administer bronchodilators.

3. Rate of oxygen must be closely monitored—25–30% can be given in chronic obstructive lesions of the lung. High concentrations are given in other conditions. Carbon dioxide narcosis can be avoided by exercising care in this direction.

4. In unconscious patient—to avoid aspiration pneumonia he should be put on one side.

5. Intravenous fluids should be given. A life line is maintained for drugs to be given intravenously.

6. Input/output chart to be maintained.

Section

VII

Endocrinology

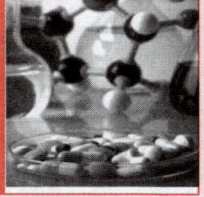

48

Endocrinology

Hormone is defined as a substance secreted by ductless gland (endocrine) transported to a distant tissues where it produces its effect.

Endocrine glands in the body
1. Hypothalamus
2. Pituitary gland
3. Thyroid gland
4. Parathyroid gland
5. Pancreas
6. Adrenal glands.

HYPOTHALAMIC RELEASING HORMONES

Hypothalamus secretes specific releasing or release inhibiting factors/hormones which are carried via portal system to adenohypophysis where they act. **There are six releasing hormones namely**.
 (a) Corticotropin releasing hormone (CRH).
 (b) Follicle stimulating hormone releasing hormone (FSH-RH).
 (c) Luteinising hormone releasing hormone (LH-RH).
 (d) Thyrotropin releasing hormone (TRH).
 (e) Growth hormone releasing hormone (GH-RH).
 (f) Melanocyte stimulating hormone releasing hormone (MSH-RH).

Inhibitory hormones from hypothalamus are

1. Prolactin release inhibitory hormone.
2. Growth hormone release inhibitory hormone (somatostatin).
3. Melanocyte stimulating hormone release inhibitory hormone.

LH-RH and FSH-RH are probably identical and the combined abbreviation LH FSH RH is therefore used.

PITUITARY GLAND

It is termed as master gland as it regulates the functioning of most other glands in the body. It consists of
 (a) Adenohypophysis (anterior lobe)
 (b) Neurohypophysis (posterior lobe)
 (c) Pars intermedia.

225

Following hormones are secreted from anterior pituitary

(a) Corticotropin (ACTH)

(b) Thyroid stimulating hormone (TSH)

(c) Follicle stimulating hormone (FSH)

(d) Luteinizing or interstitial cell stimulating hormone (LH or ICSH)

(e) Growth hormone (GH)

(f) Prolactin

Hormones from posterior pituitary (neurohypophysis)

(a) Oxytocin

(b) Antidiuretic hormone (ADH)

Hormones from pars intermedia

(a) Melanocyte stimulating hormone (MSH)

Corticotropin (ACTH): Regulation of ACTH secretion

(a) Release of ACTH is stimulated by corticotropin releasing factor (CRF) released from hypothalamus.

(b) Feedback inhibition by ACTH.

Physiological Actions: It increases the size of adrenal gland. It stimulates adrenal cortex to secrete

hydrocortisone, corticosterone and androgens. To a lesser extent it increases the release of aldosterone.

Most of the actions of ACTH (metabolic and anti-inflammatory) are due to the release of glucocorticoids.

Pharmacological Actions

(a) Causes hyperglycemia.

(b) Hyperpigmentation of skin.

(c) Lipolysis.

(d) Enlarges adrenal gland.

Due to similarity in chemical structure with melanocyte stimulating hormone in large doses, it causes hyperpigmentation of skin.

Uses

1. To stimualte adrenal cortex after it is suppressed—due to prolonged steroid therapy.

2. For diagnosing primary from secondary adrenal insufficiency.

Adverse reactions

(a) Allergic reactions.

(b) Hypokalemic alkalosis.

(c) Pituitary suppression.

(d) Acne.

Pituitary gonadotropins are

(a) FSH (follicular stimulating hormone)

(b) LH (luteinising hormone)

Non-physiological sources

(a) Human chorionic gonadotropins.

(b) Human menopausal gonadotropins.

(c) Gonadotropins from pregnant mare serum.

Regulation of Secretion: Positive reinforcement is exerted by the releasing hormones from the hypothalamus.

Feedback inhibition is exerted by the hormones of target organs which regulate the secretion of these hormones.

Follicle Stimulating Hormone

Actions: In **males** it stimulates spermatogenesis. In **females** it

(a) Produces maturation of graafian follicle.

(b) Stimulates graafian follicles to secrete estradiol.

(c) Induces development of ovum.

Luteinising Hormone (LH): In **males** it stimulates Leydig cells to secrete testosterone.

In **females** it causes rupture of the mature follicle to cause ovulation.

It initiates and maintains secretion of progesterone from corpus luteum.

HCG and human menopausal gonadotropin (HMG) have actions similar to LH and are therefore used in

1. Amenorrhoea and infertility due to hypopituitarism.

2. Cryptorchidism.

3. Hypogonadotropic hypogonadism.

4. Making a few diagnosis

(a) HCG for detection of pregnancy.

(b) differentiating cause of undescending testis from defects other than hormonal.

Adverse effects

1. In women these agents (gonadotropins) produce enlargement of ovaries with cyst formation

2. Multiple pregnancies may result

3. Produces precocious puberty in children.

Tests used for detection of pregnancy are based on the release of HCG in urine, which can be detected immunologically or biologically (on rats, frogs or rabbits).

Clomiphene: It is commonly employed for inducing ovulation. It has anti-estrogenic activity, i.e. it inhibits the inhibitory influence of oestrogen on the anterior pituitary thereby causes release of LH. It enlarges ovaries and induces cyst formation. Multiple pregnancies frequently occur.

It is also used in metropathia hemorrhagica.

Dose is 50–100 mg daily from 5th to 10th day of the mensturation.

Growth Hormone (Somatotropin-GH)

Actions

1. It regulates tissue growth in conjunction with other hormones, e.g. thyroxine, adrenal and testicular androgens.

2. It promotes linear growth of the long bones as well as viscera.

3. It causes retention of nitrogen, calcium, phosphorus, sodium and potassium (it is anabolic in nature).

4. It promotes entry of amino acids and increases protein synthesis (like insulin).

5. On **chronic use it increases blood glucose level** (anti-insulin) by increasing release of glucose from the liver and also by reducing glucose uptake but **acute administration produces hypoglycemia**.

6. Increases lipolysis.

Uses: In dwarfism due to pituitary failure.

Growth hormone obtained from human source alone should be used.

Synthetic growth hormones

(a) Somatrem

(b) Somatotropin.

Adverse drug reactions

(a) Increase in intracranial tension.

(b) Hyperglycemia.

Contraindications

(a) Active malignancies.

(b) Unhealed intracranial lesions.

(c) After epiphysis have closed.

Thyrotropin (TSH): Release of this hormone is regulated by:

(a) Releasing hormone of hypothalamus that stimulates its release.

(b) Thyroxine that inhibits its release.

It acts on the thyroid gland where it

(i) Increases vascularity and the size of the gland.

(ii) Increases uptake of iodine by this gland.

(iii) Increases release of thyroxine from the gland.

Uses: It is used to differentiate primary thyroid failure from thyroid failure due to pituitary (secondary). In primary thyroid failure TSH does not increase iodine uptake by the gland while in secondary failure it does.

Prolactin: Regulation of secretion.

Hypothalamus has inhibitory effect on prolactin secretion.

Breastfeeding stimulates prolactin secretion.

Certain drugs increase the release of prolactin, e.g. antipsychotic drugs (**chlorpromazine and haloperidol**), antianxiety drugs (**diazepam and chlordiazepoxide**), hormones (**estrogens, testosterone and thyrotropin releasing hormone**), **opiates, phenobarbitone, alpha methyl dopa**, and **cimetidine**.

Bromocriptine, cabergoline, pergolide and quinagolide inhibit prolactin.

Actions

(a) In certain animals it is necessary for initiation and maintenance of corpus luteum and lactation.

(b) Promotes development of mammary tissue during pregnancy.

(c) Stimulates milk production after delivery.

(d) Suppresses ovulation.

POSTERIOR PITUITARY

It consists entirely of nerve endings and neuroglial cells. Oxytocin and antidiuretic hormones are released from it. These hormones are synthesised in the supraoptic and paraventricular nulcei of anterior hypothalamus and are carried along nerves to posterior pituitary from where they are released.

Antidiuretic Hormone (ADH, Vasopressin): Release is stimulated by

(a) Acute loss of water and Na^+.

(b) Chronic conditions leading to effective reduction in blood volume (CHF, cirrhosis and diuretics).

(c) Stress.

(d) High temperature.

(e) Pain and trauma.

(f) Drugs—morphine and colchicine.

Drugs reducing ADH: Alcohol and steroids.

Actions

1. The primary effect is exerted on the distal and the collecting ducts of renal tubules where it inhibits the water loss. It increases water reabsorption at this level thereby concentrating urine. In diabetes insipidus (deficiency of ADH) urine cannot be concentrated and water loss is increased.

2. In higher doses it constricts smooth muscles producing hypertension, abdominal colic and ecobolic effect.

3. Tachyphylaxis to pressor effect is seen with this drug.

4. Increases release of ACTH.

5. Plays role in learning and behaviour.

Uses

1. Diabetes insipidus.

2. It is used to concentrate urine for certain radiographic studies.

3. Esophageal varies.

4. Rarely used in paralytic ileus.

Adverse reactions: In coronary heart it may precipitate angina and myocardial infarction.

Preparations

(i) Vasopressin tanate (IM or SC)–2.5 IU

(ii) Felypressin

Oxytocin: It is a polypeptide (8 amino acids) and is secreted from posterior pituitary during coitus and suckling.

Actions

1. It stimulates uterine muscle. It increases the tone as well as rhythmicity of uterus. Estrogen sensitises uterus to the effect of oxytocin while progesterone reduces it. Thus pregnant uterus is more sensitive to its action than the nonpregnant uterus. Sensitivity to oxytocin increases with gestation period. It differs from ergometrine in that it allows complete relaxation of the uterus between two contractions thus allowing the blood to flow into placenta. Ergometrine produces spasmodic contraction of uterus thus restricting blood flow to fetus.

2. It expels milk from smaller to larger ducts.

3. In high doses it causes.
   (a) Increase in BP
   (b) Decrease in urine output
   (c) Increase in HR.

Uses

1. It is used for induction of labour. Slow IV drip (5 units in 500 ml of glucose saline) is given for this purpose.

2. Used to prevent postpartum bleeding, however ergometrine is better for this purpose.

Care should be exercised in administering this drug. There should not be any disproportion between foetal head and maternal pelvis.

Nursing care of patient receiving oxytocin

1. Oxytocin solution for intravenous infusion is prepared by adding 10 units of the drug to a liter of 5% dextrose (or 5 units of oxytocin to 1 bottle of 5% dextrose).

2. Infusion should go at a very slow rate initially (2 drops/minute). The rate can be increased if there is no response (maximum of 8 drops per minute can be given).

3. If large doses are required synthetic preparation of oxytocin should be given to patients.

4. Uterus should be observed carefully for force and rate of contractions. If uterine contractions are too forcible, drip should be discontinued. Infusion can also be disconnected after normal uterine contractions have set in. Record must be maintained of the uterine contractions.

5. Foetal heart rate should be counted regularly and recorded. If signs of foetal distress appear (e.g. increase in foetal heart rate over 160/min or below 120/min) the drip may be stopped.

6. Progress of labour should be recorded and the chart maintained.

7. Blood pressure of the patient should be taken every 30 minutes and recorded. In case of hypertension drip should be discontinued.

49

Thyroid and Antithyroid Drugs

Thyroid gland concentrates iodine and forms thyroxine and triiodothyronine. Iodine is essential for synthesis of thyroxine. In iodine deficiency (as is seen in certain areas of our country) thyroxine is not formed and goiter is produced.

Thyroid is essential for health because it produces 3 hormones. Thyroxine, triiodothyronine and calcitonin.

Thyroid mainly secrets T_4 (**thyroxine**), which in periphery is converted to T_3 (**triiodothyronine**). Both these hormones have similar actions but T_3 is more active.

Actions of thyroid hormones: Triiodothyronine (T_3) and tetraiodothyroxine (T_4)

1. Are essential for normal growth and development of fetus and infants. These promote synthesis of proteins and promote growth. Deficiency of thyroxine in infancy results in retarded growth and cretinism.
2. T_3 and T_4 are required for myelinisation of nerves.
3. Thyroid hormones stimulate heart, skeletal muscles, liver and kidney.
4. Body temperature is maintained by thyroxine and triiodothyronine.
5. Hormones of thyroid increase the number of beta-adrenergic receptors. They also increase sensitivity of beta receptors to catecholamines.
6. Stimulate metabolism of the body and increase oxygen consumption (increases basal metabolic rate).
7. Increase blood glucose by increasing breakdown of glycogen.
8. Reduce cholesterol in the blood.
9. Exert diuretic effect.
10. Important in menstrual flow and regulation of fertility.

Severe deficiency of thyroxine (due to drugs or disease) produces myxoedema (hypothyroidism). These patients

 (a) Do not tolerate cold weather.
 (b) Are usually constipated, lethargic.
 (c) Have thick coarse skin.
 (d) Mental activity is reduced.
 (e) Body weight is increased.

Role of iodine in thyroid diseases

Iodine in small quantities is needed for the production of thyroxine but in large amounts it blocks synthesis of thyroxine. This knowledge is employed clinically to treat patients of hyperthyroidism.

Present status of iodine in thyroid diseases

Deficiency of iodine as occurs in certain geographical areas is rectified by adding small quantities of iodine to table salt. This prevents endemic goiter and the problems associated with it.

Iodine in large doses is used these days only in the **preoperative management** of thyrotoxicosis. The action of iodine here is to render the hyperactive thyroid gland **less vascular with reduction of the size of the gland** with reduced thyroxine release of $T_3 + T_4$.

Uses of thyroxine

1. As substitution therapy when the gland is not functioning optimally, e.g. myxoedema and thyroxine cretinism. Therapy should be started with small doses and gradually increased.
2. In cretinism, therapy must be started as early as possible.
3. Simple goiter responds to thyroxine. The size of the gland is reduced.
4. It is given in thyroiditis.
5. D-thyroxine is used for lowering serum cholesterol.

Preparations of thyroid

(i) Dried thyroid powder — contains 0.2% hormonal iodine. It is available as 30 and 60 mg tablets.
(ii) Sodium L-thyroxine is available as tablet each containing 0.05 or 0.1 mg of this compound.

Following drugs should not be administered along with thyroid preparations as these drugs interact with thyroid hormone.
1. Tricyclic antidepressants.
2. Oral anticoagulants.
3. Cholestyramine.

Adverse reactions

1. Palpitations.
2. Precipitates angina and myocardial infarction.
3. Cardiac arrhythmias (auricular fibrillation) may occur.
4. Exophthalamus may develop.

Nursing care

1. Increase in pulse rate beyond 100/min should be reported and further dose of thyroid withheld.
2. If patient on thyroxine complains of tightness in chest or complains of being unwell this should be immediately reported to senior sister and further treatment stopped. This necessitates reduction of dosage. **Patients have died due to cardiac complications produced by thyroxine.**

ANTITHYROID DRUGS

If thyroid hormone is secreted in excess (hyperthyroidism) patient complains of irritability, nervousness, palpitations and loss of body weight (inspite of increase in appetite). Heat is not tolerated but cold weather is appreciated. Skin is sweaty and thin. Systolic blood pressure is raised without much change in diastolic pressure. **Menstrual functions are disturbed in hypo as well as hyperthyroidism.**

Antithyroid drugs specifically suppress the synthesis or release of thyroid hormones and are employed in thyrotoxicosis.

(a) Inhibitors of iodine trapping — thiocyanates and perchlorates

(b) Drugs which inhibit organification of iodine

   (i) Thiouracils — methyl thiouracil and propyl thiouracil

   (ii) Imidazoles — methimazole and carbimazole

(c) Radioactive iodine

(d) Inhibitor of iodine release — iodides.

Thiouracils

Propylthiouracil is the most commonly used drug in this group. It acts by:

(a) Inhibiting oxidation of iodide to iodine

(b) Inhibiting combination of iodine with tyrosine

(c) Inhibit coupling of tyrosine molecules to form $T_3 + T_4$.

Disadvantages

1. Takes at least 2–3 weeks for the action of these drugs to manifest.
2. Size of the thyroid gland is increased hence these agents are called goitrogens.
3. Vascularity of the thyroid gland is increased thereby making surgery more difficult.
4. Relapse rate is high.
5. All are toxic drugs.

Uses

1. Are given preoperatively to control symptoms of thyrotoxicosis.
2. To treat thyrotoxicosis in inoperable cases.

Adverse reactions

1. Nausea, vomiting and skin rashes.
2. Leucopenia and agranulocytosis.
3. Joint pain and lymphadenopathy are occasionally produced **methimizole** is preferred.

Nursing care

1. Reduction in pulse rate indicates the efficacy of this treatment.
2. Increase in body weight is a clear indication that drugs are effective.
3. WBC count should be done at least once a week.
4. Patient should be instructed to consult his physician immediately in case of any sore throat or any febrile condition. If patient receiving these drugs complaints of sore throat, matter should be reported to senior sister or the treating physician. Further administration of drug should be stopped.
5. In-door patient, any rise in body temperature should be immediately reported to sister. For this the body temperature should be taken thrice daily.

Thiocyanates and Perchlorates: These drugs by inhibiting the iodine uptake inhibit the synthesis of thyroid.

Adverse reactions

(i) Aplastic anaemia.

(ii) Drug rashes.

Because of their toxicity and availability of better drugs, they are rarely used now

Iodine and Iodides: Large doses of iodine inhibit release of T_3 and T_4 from thyroid.

Advantages

1. Quickest acting drug (action seen within 23 hours).
2. Decreases the size of the gland and makes surgery more manageable.
3. Decreases vascularity of the gland therefore reduces bleeding during surgery.

Disadvantages

1. Action is short lasting and self limiting. Hence its use is restricted to **preoperative period**.
2. Toxicity due to iodine is produced.

Uses

1. In preoperative stage of thyrotoxicosis.
2. In severe cardiac disease to counter overactivity of thyroid.

Adverse reactions

1. Allergic reactions.
2. On chronic use it produces increased salivation, lacrimation, swelling of lids and symptoms associated with gut.

Dose: Lugol's iodine 0.3 ml solution is given three times a day (consists of 5% iodine in 10% potassium iodide). Tablets of potassium iodide (60 mg three times daily) can also be used for the same purpose.

Radioactive Iodine: Sodium iodide (I^{131}) is used in diagnosis and treatment of thyrotoxicosis. The beta rays emitted by radioactive iodine destroy thyroid tissue to a limited extent. Gamma rays emitted by iodine are used for diagnosis.

Uses

1. Thyrotoxicosis for treatment.
   (a) It is specially useful in elderly patients or in patients of heart disease.
   (b) In patients where surgery is contraindicated.
   (c) For recurrent hyperthyroidism after antithyroid drug therapy has failed.
2. It is also used for making diagnosis of diseases associated with thyroid.

Advantages

1. No surgery is required
2. Gives permanent cure
3. It is convenient

Disadvantages

1. Onset of action is delayed.
2. Calculation of exact dose is difficult and may lead to permanent damage of the gland necessitating thyroxine administration.
3. Cannot be given to patients under 40 years.
4. Should not be given in pregnant patients.

Propranolol: It is used in thyrotoxicosis for the following effects:

(a) It inhibits the conversion of thyroxine (T_4) to triiodothyronine (T_3) the more active compound.

(b) It counters the symptoms of thyroid on heart and blood pressure. The effects are immediate.

Uses

1. Control peripheral manifestations, e.g. palpitations, sweating and tremors.
2. Drug of choice in thyroid storm.
3. Used for rapid effect before antithyroid drugs take effect.

Management of Thyroid Crisis: Thyroid crisis is a sudden acute condition of thyrotoxicosis. It is seen during surgery on thyroid. Drugs to be given—propranolol and hydrocortisone.

IV glucose and oxygen inhalation are given along with antithyroid drugs.

If heart is failing/failed add digitalis to this treatment (use caution).

50

Hormones of Pancreas

Pancreas releases various hormones. The important being

(a) Insulin from β cells.

(b) Glucagon from α cells. This hormone is released when there is hypoglycemia.

(c) Somatostatin from β cells.

1. INSULIN

Insulin is protein in nature and is secreted directly into bloodstream from beta cells of Langerhans. Normal pancreas secretes about 50 units of insulin per day.

Islet cells are not under the control of anterior pituitary. The secretion of insulin is regulated by blood glucose level, high glucose causing increase and low glucose causing reduction in insulin release.

Diabetes mellitus is a condition in which beta cells of islet fail to secrete enough insulin to meet the requirements of the body. There are two types of patients of this disease. The first are typically thin who tend to develop diabetes at an early age and have aberrant gene in chromosome 6. Plasma insulin is either low or absent. **These patients do not respond to sulfonylureas.** They are called insulin dependent diabetics (IDDM) and is now called **type I diabetes**.

In contrast, second **Type II diabetes** is noninsulin dependent diabetics (NIDDM). Patients of this type are over 40 years, obese and respond to both insulin and sulfonylureas. This group is less likely to develop ketoacidosis (diabetic coma) but suffer from **complications such as cataract, neuropathy, nephropathy and hypocholesteremia.**

Following substances stimulate release of insulin:

(a) Hormones from gut, e.g. glucagon, secretin, gastrin.

(b) Glucose, amino acids, fatty acids and ketone bodies.

(c) Growth hormone, steroids and thyroxine.

(d) β_2 receptor agonists.

(e) Cholinomimetics.

Following inhibit release of insulin:

1. α_2 receptor stimulants.

2. Somatostatin.

3. PGE.

Actions of insulin

1. Increases entry of glucose and potassium into cells of the body. All cells of the body except those of brain, heart, RBCs and kidney are dependent on insulin for glucose influx.
2. Increases peripheral utilisation of glucose.
3. Increases synthesis of glycogen in the liver and other tissues.
4. Reduces breakdown of fats and proteins (inhibits lipase).
5. Suppresses ketogenesis (increases entry of amino acids into cells).
6. On the contrary it promotes anabolism.

Through all these actions it lowers serum glucose.

Perparations of Insulin:

Soluble crystalline insulin: It is a clear solution can be given intravenously. Onset of action is quick (10–20 minutes) and duration is short (6–8 hours). It is used in diabetic coma and emergency management of diabetes mellitus.

Disadvantages

(i) It cannot be used for day to day treatment as at least 4 injections per day are required at regular intervals.
(ii) Solution of this preparation is slightly acidic and causes local irritation. Neutral solution is also available.

Insulin Zinc Suspension:

Zinc when added to insulin forms crystals has long duration of action. Zinc delays the release of insulin at the site of injection. Depending on the amount of zinc added to insulin, two kinds of suspensions are obtained.

(i) **Insulin ultralente** which has a duration of action of about **36 hours**
(ii) **Semilente** has quick onset of action (30 minutes) and its action lasts for **12 hours.**

Insulin lente is prepared by combining seven parts of insulin ultralente with 3 parts of semilente.

It controls the blood glucose for **18–24 hours** after single injection. It is given subcutaneously.

Advantages

1. One injection needs to be given a day to control blood glucose.
2. Unlike protamine zinc insulin it does not cause skin rashes.

Disadvantages

1. It can produce hypoglycemia at night.
2. It does not give good moment to moment control of blood glucose.

Globin Zinc Insulin:

This too is available as clear solution with globin and zinc containing 40 to 80 units of insulin per ml.

It is given subcutaneously, is long acting (effect lasts for 24 hours peak occurs a round 12 hours) and it takes 12 hours for the action to set in.

Use: It is used mainly for mild diabetic cases who can be controlled by a single dose.

Nursing care

If your diabetic patient being treated on this drug complains of severe headache on awakening in the morning this should be reported to your senior. Such a patient needs either readjustment of doses of the same drug or changing over to new drug.

Protamine Zinc Insulin: It is suspension of insulin with zinc and protamine. It is given subcutaneously. It is available in the concentrations of 40 and 80 units per ml. The onset of action is late (4–6 hours), peak occurs in 14–18 hours and duration 24–36 hours.

Advantage: It is long acting therefore single daily dose is sufficient to treat the patient.

Disadvantages

1. Does not provide smooth control of blood glucose. It cannot suit the circumstances of the moment.
2. Allergy is commonly encountered.
3. Skin rash is seen frequently.

NEWER INSULINS

These are more purified porcine insulins.

They are of two types:

1. Single peak insulins
   (a) Actrapid: Highly purified porcine and Lentard chromatographed insulin.
   (b) Insulatard: Highly purified isophane insulin (40 IU/ml).
   (c) Monosulin: Mixtard — good for elderly.

2. Monocomponent insulins
   (a) Actrapid MC.
   (b) Monotard MC.

Advantages

(a) Are neutral preparations and less often cause atrophy of the subcutaneous fat.
(b) Are less antigenic.
(c) Can be mixed with other preparations.
(d) Are more stable
(e) Lesser chances of developing resistance.

HUMAN INSULINS

Are produced by recombinant DNA technique.
   Available as regular, NPH, lente or ultralente preparation.

Advantages

(a) Are less immunogenic.
(b) Are absorbed more rapidly.
(c) Used in patients with insulin resistance due to A/B.
(d) Preferred during pregnancy.
(e) Dose needed is 10% less.

Disadvantages

(a) Have slightly shorter duration of action than conventional insulins.

(b) Are expensive.

(c) Hypoglycemia is more common.

Uses of insulin

1. Diabetes mellitus.

   (a) In IDDM patients.

   (b) In NIDDM patients undergoing surgery, stress or infection.

   (c) During pregnancy.

2. It is sometimes employed to stimulate appetite, e.g. anorexia nervosa.

3. In burns for anabolic effect.

4. To treat hyperkalemia as it pushes K^+ into cells.

5. It was used to produce convulsions in schizophrenic patients.

Precautions

Overdose with insulin can produce hypoglycemia, which is characterised by anxiety, sweating, tremors, convulsions and coma. This condition can be treated by giving glucose orally or intravenously according to the severity of the condition.

1. Repeated injection of insulin at the same site produce atrophy of the subcutaneous tissue. It is therefore advised to change the site of injection.

2. Allergic reactions are often seen as the above mentioned insulin is obtained from sheep, cows or pigs. The remedy lies in changing type of insulin.

Instructions for insulin

(a) Store vials in refrigerator.

(b) Remove vial from refrigerator before injection and let it stand for 5–10 minutes at room temperature. **Do not heat vials.**

Insulin Syringes: These are special syringes that — red contains 40 units in 1 ml and green has 80 units in 1 ml are calibrated in insulin units, hence patient can take exact dose.

Nursing care of hypoglycemia

1. Patient to be educated on symptoms of hypoglycemia and its management.

2. Nurse should be familiar with clinical picture of hypoglycemia.

   (a) Palpitation or sweating and mental confusion.

   (b) Injection site to be regularly changed.

   (c) Plane/regular insulin alone can be given IV.

   (d) Body temperature tends to fall.

   (e) Nausea and headache may occur.

ORAL HYPOGLYCEMIC AGENTS

Insulin cannot be given orally as it is destroyed by the enzymes of the gut. Drugs which can be given orally and produce lowering of blood sugar are called oral hypoglycemic agents. They are of three types.

1. **Sulfonylureas**
   (a) *First generation*
   Chlorpropamide
   Tolbutamide
   Acetohexamide
   Tolazamide
   (b) *Second generation drugs*
   Glibenclamide
   Glipizide
   Glimpride
2. **Biguanides**
   Phenformin
   Metformin
3. **Meglitinides**
   Repaglinide
   Nateglinide
4. **Thiazolidenediones (glitazones)**
   Rosiglitazone
   Troglitazone
   Pioglitazone
5. **Miscellaneous**
   Glymidine
   Acarbose
   Ciglitazone

SULFONYLUREAS

These drugs act by increasing the release of insulin. Hence, they are ineffective in those patients in whom functional tissue (beta cells of islet of Langerhans) are completely destroyed.

They also probably increase the sensitivity of the tissue to insulin by increasing insulin receptors thus enhance insulin mediated glucose metabolism. In addition they inhibit gluconeogenesis in liver.

Tolbutamide: Action of this drug lasts for 6–12 hrs. Two to three doses are required per day. It is given in 500–3000 mg/day in divided doses. It is safer in elderly patients.

Chlorpropamide: It is long acting and it accumulates in the body. Severe hypoglycemia (specially in elderly patients) may develop. Sudden change in mood or mental confusion in a patient on chlorpropamide should raise the suspicion of hypoglycemia. Dose 250–500 mg once daily.

Adverse reactions

1. Jaundice is produced by chlorpropamide.
2. Agranulocytosis and hepatic changes have been reported with acetohexamide and tolazamide.
3. All these drugs interact with alcohol and produce symptoms like disulfiram.
4. Sulphonamides and phenylbutazone potentiate the action of these drugs.

Tolazamide has slow onset.

Disadvantages of first generation sulphonyl ureas: Result in **several drug interactions**.

Second Generation Sulphonyl Ureas

Advantages

1. Are more potent.
2. Have fewer side effects.
3. Less drug interactions.

Disadvantages

1. Can cause hypoglycemia.
2. Cause kidney and liver damage.

Glibenclamide

(a) 200 times more potent than tolbutamide.
(b) Action lasts for 24 hours.
(c) On long-term treatment it accumulates.

Dose: 2.5–20.0 mg once a day.

Disadvantages

1. Should not be given in patients with liver and kidney damage.
2. Causes hypoglycemia in postprandial period.

Glipizide: In addition to antihyperglycemia it has antiplatelet aggregating activity. It has short half-life. Food delays absorption.

Biguanides: Metformin and phenformin

1. These are antihyperglycemic agents and do not cause hypoglycemia.
2. These drugs reduce absorption of glucose from intestine.
3. In liver suppress glucogenesis.
4. Increase influx of glucose into skeletal muscles.
5. Reduce low density lipoproteins and VLDL.
6. **Reduce body weight**.

Uses: Are used along with insulin and sulfonyl ureas in type 2 diabetes. When combined with these drugs, biguanides produce a better control of the blood sugar. They help in reducing the body weight. Reduce insulin resistance.

Adverse drug reactions: Metallic taste, abdominal discomfort.

Muscular weakness, loss of body weight and lactic acidemia are some of the common adverse reactions.

Dose: Phenformin 75–150 mg/day

Metformin 1.5–3.0 g/day

THIAZOLIDINEDIONE DERIVATIVES

Ciglitazone, pioglitazone, englitazone and troglitazone are effective in increasing sensitivity of tissues to insulin.

(a) Reduce peripheral insulin resistance.

(b) Increase peripheral glucose utilisation. Maximum effect comes in 14 weeks.

(c) Reduce hyperinsulinemia.

(d) Reduce blood glucose as well as glycosylated haemoglobin.

(e) Decrease plasma triglycerides.

(f) Increase HDL by about 10–15%.

Adverse reactions

1. Elevate hepatic enzymes.
2. Cause oedema and weight gain.
3. Increase tendency to CCF.

Disadvantages

1. Not recommended in pregrnancy.
2. Cause pill failure.

ACARBOSE AND MIGLITOL

(a) Inhibit α-glucosidase, glucoamylase and sucrase.

(b) Block digestion of starch, sucrose and maltose.

(c) Do not affect absorption of glucose do not cause weight reduction.

ADRs

Flatulence, abdominal bloating and diarrhea.

Use: Along with other hypoglycemic agent, are given to treat diabetes mellitus.

Drug therapy of diabetes mellitus

1. Treatment of maturity onset diabetes or noninsulin dependent diabetes.
   Drug treatment of these patients is started only after the diet and exercises have failed to control blood sugar. Reduction in body weight reduces the requirement of drugs.
   Tolbutamide (0.5 g twice a day) is given and dose is adjusted according to response of urinary sugar. In mild cases a single dose may also help.
   Chlorpropamide, acetohexamide and tolazamide are given once a day.

Insulin is given to few of these patients when they are not effectively controlled by these drugs or during condition of stress such as **fever, infection and surgery**.

2. Treatment of insulin dependent diabetes is initiated by giving 10 units of regular insulin, 20 minutes before meals at least 4 times a day. Subsequent doses are determined by response of urinary sugar. After control is achieved a single dose of long acting insulin may be substituted for regular insulin. The injection of long acting insulin is given before breakfast. Depending on the response of the patient and his/her food habits changes in the timings of the injection are made.

Intermediate acting insulin is sometimes added to long acting insulin for better control of blood sugar.

Following conditions increase the requirement of insulin:

(a) Infections.

(b) When excess food is consumed.

(c) During pregnancy.

(d) During treatment with corticosteroids.

(e) During treatment with oral contraceptives.

(f) During surgery.

TREATMENT OF DIABETES DURING PREGNANCY

1. Oral hypoglycemics should be stopped once the patient becomes pregnant and insulin must be started.

2. In the IDDM patients the dose of insulin needs to be increased.

TREATMENT OF DIABETIC COMA

Diabetic coma is also known as **diabetic ketoacidosis**. It is one of the medical emergencies frequently seen in casualty.

Diabetic coma must be clinically differentiated from hypoglycemic coma as the treatment must start before the laboratory report on blood sugar is received.

		Diabetic coma	Hypoglycemic coma
1.	History of diabetes	+	–/+
2.	History of taking insulin	+	–/+
3.	Smell of the breath	**Fruity**	None
4.	Skin	**Dry and wrinkled**	Cold and sweaty
5.	Administration of glucose	Does not help	Patient recovers
6.	Blood sugar	High	Low

1. Regular insulin is the mainstay of diabetic coma. It is given in the dose of 0.2–0.3 units/kg initially (half intravenously and the other half subcutaneously), followed by 0.1 unit/kg/hr.
   Intravenous infusion of insulin achieves better results. 2–10 units/ hour of insulin may be given through infusion. Hypoglycemia and hypokalemia are not seen with continuous infusion.

2. In diabetic patients there is deficiency of fluids — dehydration due to polyuria is a common feature of diabetic coma. Three to six liters of fluid may often be necessary before dehydration improves. Maintenance of input and output chart is therefore essential.

Treatment of fluid correction is initiated by giving 0.9% sodium chloride. Two bottles may be given to an adult. Subsequently 0.45% sodium chloride is administered if serum Na^+ is more than 150 mEq/liter. In severe dehydration fluids may be given at the rate of 20 ml or more per minute.

3. There **is deficiency of alkali** and pH of blood tends to be low. To obtain energy body fats are broken down into acids (p-hydroxybutyric acid and acetoacetic acid). These two compounds are termed as ketones (hence ketoacidosis). The breath and urine smell of acetone. Deficiency of alkali is corrected by giving **sodium bicarbonate** (50 mEq of sodium bicarbonate is added to 0.45% solution of sodium chloride).

4. After insulin therapy serum potassium tends to fall. If serum K^+ is low, it is given either in the form of **Ringer lactate solution** or orally through Ryle's tube. **Potassium should not be given if the urinary output is poor**. Serum potassium should be estimated at regular intervals.

5. **Deficiency of phosphate** is also noticed during diabetic coma. This can be corrected by administering phosphate of potassium instead of its chloride.

   Hyperosmolar coma is seen in noninsulin dependent diabetics. In this condition there is severe dehydration which is corrected by giving **sodium chloride (0.45%) potassium and insulin**. Glucose levels are monitored.

Nursing care of patient of diabetic coma

1. Chart must be maintained to record insulin administration its dose, route and time of administration.
2. Input and output chart is a must. Future course of treatment is guided by this chart.
3. Urine should be checked for glucose and ketone bodies regularly.
4. Respiratory rate and the character of respiration should be checked and recorded.
5. Temperature should be taken 4 hourly. In the event of increase in temperature, antibiotics must be started. Pulse should be counted regularly.
6. Record blood pressure regularly.

Insulin resistance: Patients requiring more than 200 units of regular insulin are said to be resistant to insulin. Resistance can be acute or chronic. Acute resistance to insulin is seen in infections due to Staphylococci or during stress. Treatment of this condition lies in treating the cause.

Biguanides reduce insulin resistance.

HYPERGLYCEMIC AGENTS

Glucagon: It is secreted by the alpha cells of the islets of Langerhans. The release of this hormone occurs during acute starvation and muscular exercise. It regulates release of insulin. It raises blood sugar and was employed to treat hypoglycemia in patients who could not swallow glucose, hypoglycemic coma or when it is not possible to give glucose intravenously. 0.9% sodium chloride is started intravenously and glucagon is added to it. It has positive inotropic and chronotropic effect on heart. It relaxes intestine.

Uses

1. Correction of hypoglycemia.
2. It is used to antagonise effects of beta-blockers on the heart.
3. For X-ray of intestine to relax intestine.

4. In diagnosis of insulinoma and pheochromocytoma.
5. In treatment of beta-blocker poisoning.

Adverse drug reactions

(a) Nausea and vomiting.
(b) Cardiac arrhythmias.

Somatostatin: It is released from α and δ cells of pancreas. Glucagon stimulates its release.

Actions: Inhibits release of insulin as well as glucagon.

Uses: It is given to inhibit release of insulin in insulinomas and carcinoid tumours.

Sandostatin: It is longer acting stomatostatin. It is used to treat:

(a) Esophageal varices.
(b) Peptic ulcer.
(c) Postprandial orthostatic hypotension.

Adverse drug reactions

1. Stones in bile duct or gallbladder.
2. Cardiac arrhythmias.
3. Hypoglycemia/hyperglycemia.

Diazoxide

1. It inhibits insulin release.
2. Increases adrenaline release and hepatic glucose output.
3. It is a direct vasodilator.

Uses

1. Hypertensive emergencies.
2. Treatment of resistant hypoglycemia.

51

Adrenal Cortical Hormones

Adrenal cortex has three zones that produce three types of hormones

(a) **Zona glomerulosa** produces mineralocorticoids (aldosterone, corticosterone and deoxy-corticosterone).

(b) **Zona fasciculata** releases glucocorticoids (hydrocortisone and corticosterone).

(c) **Zona reticularis** releases androgenic steroids (dehydroepiandrosterone and androstenedione).

Zona reticularis and fasciculata are under pituitary control. **Zona glomerulosa is not regulated by the pituitary**. Glucocorticoids are also referred to as corticosteroids which include both the natural and synthetic preparations.

All glucocorticoids have some degree of mineralocorticoid activity.

Actions of glucocorticoids

1. They increase blood sugar because:
   (a) they increase glucose formation from glycogen and proteins.
   (b) they reduce peripheral utilisation of glucose.
   They are capable of precipitating diabetes mellitus that may persist.
2. They reduce synthesis of proteins from amino acids and at the same time increase their breakdown **(catabolic effect)**. This results in:
   (a) reduction in growth rate in children.
   (b) osteoporosis in adults which can produce spontaneous collapse of a vertebral body or fractures of rib.
3. These drugs produce increased deposition of fat on shoulders and abdomen, swelling of the face partly due to retention of Na$^+$ and water. Face resembles full moon. Acneform rashes appear on the cheeks and because of the atrophic skin and increase in capillary fragility, spontaneous bruising develops.
4. Red blood cells are increased while the **number of lymphoid cells are reduced**. **Reduction in eosinophils** is most predominant. Thrombocytes increase in blood.
5. **Inflammatory response of body is suppressed** by these drugs. For this effect, corticosteroids are commonly used in medicine, e.g. rheumatoid arthritis. They do not remove disease process but symptomatology is suppressed.
6. **Immune responses are also suppressed.** Immunity is lowered. They suppress the abnormal production of antibodies which characterises various diseases namely autoimmune diseases, e.g. acquired autoimmune hemolytic anaemia, thrombocytopenia myasthenia gravis, etc. These drugs

are therefore **used in skin disorders, bronchial asthma and tissue transplant**. Heavy doses of these drugs are required for this purpose. As these drugs suppress antibody production they **increase liability to infection**. Commonest infections that usually prove fatal in these patients are tuberculosis and septicaemia.

7. Miscellaneous actions:

(a) Corticosteroid increase uric acid excretion in urine these are therefore used in gout.

(b) Peptic ulcers and gastric ulcers are precipitated because these drugs **interfere with healing process** and also increase acidity of stomach.

(c) **Cause retention of Na$^+$ and H$_2$O** therefore produce hypertension, increase in body weight and precipitate congestive cardiac failure. **Blood pressure should routinely be checked in these patients**. These drugs can be used even in hypertensive patients — only extra care is required.

(d) On chronic administration the size of the adrenal glands is reduced.

(e) Cause **increase in urinary excretion of calcium**. These drugs can therefore, **produce osteomalacia and osteoporosis**.

Adverse reactions of glucocorticoids

1. These drugs lower glucose tolerance **diabetes** may be precipitated in borderline cases and known diabetic may worsen.

2. Long-term and high dose therapy produces **wasting of muscles** and spontaneous fractures of bones.

3. **Hypertension and congestive cardiac failure** may occur.

4. Have tendency to **aggravate peptic ulcer**. Perforation of peptic ulcer may take place without its characteristic symptoms.

5. **Psychosis** may be precipitated. Euphoria is commonly encountered in patients. These symptoms disappear once these drugs are withdrawn.

6. Corticosteroids impair the resistance to infection. Aggravation of tuberculosis or any other chronic infection usually occurs.

7. Glucocorticoids with considerable mineralocorticoid activity produce considerable **K$^+$ loss** leading to muscle weakness and hypokalemic alkalosis. These are corrected by administering potassium chloride.

8. **Hypercoagulability of blood** is produced by these drugs.

9. These drugs lower resistance to stress such as infection, anaesthesia or injury.

10. The size of the adrenal glands is reduced by corticosteroids. To prevent this:

(a) These drugs should be given early morning.

(b) Smallest effective dose should be given.

(c) Corticosteroids can be given on alternate days.

(d) In between ACTH can be given to stimulate the gland.

11. **Sudden withdrawal of these drug results in acute adrenal failure.**

12. Cataract and glaucoma.

13. Delayed wound heating.

Preparations

Oral preparations

1. Cortisone	–25 mg
2. Hydrocortisone (**cortisol**)	–20 mg
3. Prednisolone	–5 mg
4. Triamcinolone	–4 mg
5. Dexamethasone	–0.5 mg
6. Betamethasone	–0.5 mg

Last four preparations cause less Na^+ retention

Injectable preparations

1. Prednisolone phosphate	–25 mg
2. Triamcinolone diacetate suspension	–25 mg/ml
3. Dexamethasone phosphate solution	–4 mg/ml
4. Betamethasone phosphate solution	–4 mg/ml
5. Cortisol acetate suspension	–50 mg/ml

Suspensions are meant for long-term effects. Solutions can be given intravenously as well as intramuscularly.

Locally used steroids — hydrocortisone, triamcinolone, dexamethasone, betamethasone, beclomethasone and clobetasol.

Uses

1. Replacement therapy in acute adrenal insufficiency and in Addison's disease. Small doses are used in these conditions. In hypopituitarism, in addition thyroxine and sex hormones have also to be given.
2. Rheumatoid arthritis (not responding to other drugs).
3. **Bronchial asthma** not controlled by other drugs.

   Steroids used in asthma for inhalation.
   (a) Beclomethasone dipropionate.
   (b) Triamcinolone acetonide.
   (c) Budesonide.
   (d) Flunisolide.
4. Locally applied in skin diseases.
5. Eye diseases such as allergic conjunctivitis, interstitial keratitis and iridocyclitis are treated by glucocorticoids given as eye drops during day and ointment at night.
6. **Acute lymphatic leukemia** responds very well to these drugs. Other drugs (6-mercaptopurine, etc.) are also given along with steroids.
7. Blood diseases such as acute hemolytic anaemia and thrombocytopenic purpura show a good response to these drugs.
8. In ulcerative colitis these drugs are given through retention enema.
9. Systemic lupus erythematosis and other collagen diseases.
10. Severe allergic conditions such as anaphylactic reaction.

11. In tuberculosis **meningitis and TB joints** these drugs prevent fibrosis and development of hydrocephalus, blindness and stiffness of joints.
12. In severe infections (typhoid or miliary tuberculosis), these drugs are helpful in everting shock and sustaining the patient while chemotherapeutic agents are taking effect.
13. **In shock**.

Nursing care of patients on long-term glucocorticoids

1. To prevent or reduce osteoporosis patient should be given diet rich in protein and calcium
2. Watch should be kept on his blood pressure, signs of impending cardiac failure may be specially looked for. To prevent this glucocorticoids with less Na^+ retention activity should be used or a diuretic added to therapy.
3. Patients with history of peptic ulcer and taking steroids should be given antacids routinely.
4. Before starting long-term treatment with these drugs X-ray chest should be taken to rule out tuberculosis. Signs of infection should be carefully looked for during treatment with corticosteroids. If infection develops, appropriate therapy should be started immediately.
5. K^+ blood level should be monitored. In case of its deficiency potassium chloride can be added to treatment.
6. In patient with history of thromboembolic disease and receiving these drugs, bleeding and clotting time should be routinely done and oral anticoagulants can be added to drug regimen.
7. During stress the dose of corticosteroids should be increased.
8. Urine should be routinely examined for glucose. It is important to detect glycosuria at the earliest and treat it accordingly.
9. Patient should be weighed weekly. Excessive increase in body weight demands reduction in dosage of these drugs.
10. Patients on steroids often develop septicaemia, pneumonia, peritonitis or internal haemorrhage without characteristic symptoms.

It is often the dealing nurse who detects that her patient is unwell. Patient looks toxic without complaints. This feature should be reported to treating physician immediately.

MINERALOCORTICOIDS

Aldosterone and desoxycortisone are mineralocorticoids.

Actions

1. Increase reabsorption of Na^+ in the renal tubules.
2. Increase K^+ and H^+ loss in urine.

Retention of Na^+ increases water retention resulting in increase in body weight and hypertension.

Most glucocorticoids have some degree of mineralocorticoid activity. Glucocorticoids with minimum mineralocorticoid activity are considered better.

Other mineralocorticoids

18-hydroxycorticosterone
17-oxocortisole
19-nor desoxycorticosterone

Uses: Replacement therapy in acute adrenal insufficiency.

Drugs blocking synthesis of steroids

Mitotane

Amphenone B

Metyrapone

Ketoconazole

Aminoglutethimide

These drugs are used to treat Cushing's syndrome and carcinoma of adrenal glands.

Sex Hormones: Sex hormones released from adrenals are the same as those released from gonads (refer pages 251–254).

52

Male Sex Hormones

These hormones are concerned with growth and function of the sex organs.

They are:

(i) Gonadotropins (covered under pituitary).

(ii) Male sex hormones (androgens).

(iii) Female sex hormones.

The release of these hormones is under the influence of gonadotropins that have been dealt with under pituitary.

ANDROGENS

Testosterone is the natural androgen, which is secreted by Leydig cells of the testes. 8–10 mg of testosterone is produced daily.

Actions: The external genitalia grow under its influence.

It is responsible for development of secondary sexual characteristics in male. This hormone is responsible for the development of pubic and axillary hair both in males and females and also for the appearance of moustache and the beard in male. In immature animal testosterone produces enlargement of prostate and seminal vesicles.

Skeletal muscles develop and the bones grow under its influence. The voice becomes low pitched and heavy. There is increase in libido and skin becomes oily.

Under the influence of this hormone, body retains:

(a) Na^+,

(b) K^+,

(c) PO_4 and Ca^{++}.

In adults testosterone is needed for:

(a) Normal spermatogenesis.

(b) Erythropoiesis.

(c) Maintenance of libido and physical well-being.

(d) Physical and mental aggressiveness in males and penile erections are also due to this hormone.

Adverse reactions

1. In females it produces:
   - (a) Masculinization
   - (b) Hoarseness of voice
   - (c) Development of facial hair.
2. Increase in body weight due to retention of water.
3. Predisposes to prostatic carcinoma.
4. If given to young children it may cause early closure of the epiphysis resulting in short height.
5. **Large doses can cause testicular atrophy.**
6. Cholestatic jaundice.

Preparations: Natural testosterone cannot be given orally. Testosterone propionate (25 and 50 mg/ml) is given intramuscularly. Testosterone cypionate and enanthate are available as depot preparations.

Uses

1. In castrated males or in patients of hypopituitarism it is used for restoring secondary sexual characteristics.
2. They are of value in cases of inoperable breast cancer (before menopause).
3. It is given in female patients to prevent osteoporosis.

ANABOLIC STEROIDS

These are derivatives of testosterone but possess greater anabolic than masculanisation effect.
Ratio of anabolic to androgenic is 1:6.

Action

(i) Increase conversion of amino acids to proteins and increase muscle development.

(ii) Cause retention of Na^+, K^+, and PO_4^-.

(iii) Exert weak androgenic activity which manifests after a long period in children and females.

Uses

1. Chronic debilitating illness resulting in catabolic state because these agents increase appetite and nitrogen retention.
2. Aplastic anaemia.
3. Osteoporosis at late age.
4. To promote growth in delayed puberty.
5. In chronic renal failure they reduce nitrogen load on kidneys to improve Hb in refractory anaemia.
6. **These drugs are abused by athletes.**

Preparations

Mesterolene and nandrolone phenylpropionate.

Contraindications

1. Pregnancy,
2. Carcinoma prostate
3. Infants and children
4. Renal, cardiac and liver diseases.

MALE CONTRACEPTIVES

GnRW agonists and antagonists are being tried as they inhibit gonadotropin secretion.
Various compounds have been tried but failed to completely suppress spermatogenesis.

Gossypol: Cotton seed derivative decreases sperm count and impair sperm motility but is not used as it can cause hypokalemia.

DRUGS USED IN MALE SEXUAL IMPOTENCY

Impotency is in ability of man to maintain penile erection.

Sildenafil (Viagra): It is effective orally, is given one hour before intercourse.

Adverse reactions: Headache, dizziness and nasal stuffiness. If taken with nitrates causes severe hypotension.

ANTIANDROGENS

Cyproterone, Flutamide, Danazol, Bicalulamide and Finasteride: These drugs oppose the action of androgens.

Uses

1. To decrease sexual drive in **precocious puberty.**
2. Prostatic cancer.
3. Hirsutism in females given along with estrogen.
4. In acne.
5. Virilizing syndrome.

Alpha Reductase Inhibitors: **Finasteride** decreases benign prostatic hypertrophy but does not decrease libido.

Nilutamide and casodex are being tried for treating male baldness.

53

Female Sex Hormones

These are:
1. Estrogens
2. Progestogens.

Estrogens (estrone, oestradiol and estriol) are substances which produce estrus in female animals (spayed) and are responsible for development of secondary female sexual characteristics in immature animals.

Estradiol is secreted by the graafian follicle in ovary and is converted to estrone and estriol in liver. Placenta also produces estrogens and in small amounts it is produced by adrenal glands.

Actions

1. Estrogens produce cornification of the vaginal epithelium making the vagina resistant to most infections. The cervical mucus becomes thin and copious under its influence. This forms basis of Spinnbarkeit phenomenon.
2. The size of the uterus is increased. Endometrium proliferates under its influence before ovulation.
3. Estrogens sensities the uterus to the effect of oxytocin.
4. Estrogens increase breast size because they increase the ductal tissue and the stroma of breasts.
5. Large doses of these agents produce inhibition of lactation and ovulation.
6. Serum lipoproteins and cholesterol are reduced while alpha-lipoproteins increase (they exert protective effect).
7. **Coagulability of the blood is increased.**
8. Secretion of FSH from pituitary is inhibited while release of LH is initiated by this hormone.
9. Inhibit bone resorption and maintain bone mass. The long bones grow rapidly initially and then estrogens cause closure of epiphysis.
10. Effects on lipids
    (a) HDL is increased.
    (b) LDL receptors are increased but serum level is reduced.
    (c) PGD_2 is increased and **Thromboxane** is reduced.

Adverse reactions

1. Nausea and vomiting.
2. Retention of sodium and water.

3. Gain in body weight.
4. **Precipitate migraine and epilepsy.**
5. **Promote venous thrombosis.**
6. **Promote carcinoma of breast.**

Uses

1. For treatment of postmenopausal symptoms such as flushing and anxiety and these symptoms are produced due to deprivation of estrogens.
2. Senile vaginitis.
3. Senile osteoporosis — estrogen needs to be given for long time.
4. In dysmenorrhoea and dysfunctional uterine bleeding estrogens are given in combination with progesterone.
5. Carcinoma of the prostate.
6. For inhibiting lactation large doses of estrogen have to be employed.
7. Turner's syndrome (hypogonadism).
8. It is used as contraceptive because it suppresses ovulation.
9. Carcinoma of the breast of postmenopausal origin.
10. Diagnosis of pregnancy.
11. In primary hypogonadism.

SYNTHETIC ESTROGENS

Ethenyl Estradiol and Mestranol

Non-steroidal

Diethyl stilbestrol is used for systemic effects and **hexestrol, dienestrol** for local effects.

Clomiphene is a partial agonist of estrogen receptor. It increases release of gonadotropins. In males it improves gametogenesis. In females promotes ovulation.

Adverse reactions

Hot flushes
Headache
Constipation
Multiple pregnancies.

ESTROGEN MODULATORS

Tamoxifen: It is partial estrogen agonist, it is used in advanced estrogen dependent breast carcinoma.

Raloxifene and toremifene have effects similar to tamoxifen.

(a) On **bone, lipid metabolism, brain and liver** they have **effects like estrogen.**
(b) At **breast, pituitary and on endometrium** these drugs **antagonise** the effects of estrogen.
(c) On genitourinary epithelium, bone modelling and cholesterol metabolism they have effects like estrogen but effect is less marked.

Tamoxifen and toremifene inhibit proliferation of tumor cells in breast, reduce bone resorption and decrease total cholesterol and are used in treatment of breast cancer.

Adverse reactions

Nausea, vomiting and hot flushes.

Aminoglutethimide inhibits synthesis of steroids and used in prostatic cancer.

PROGESTOGENS

Progesterone is secreted by the corpus luteum and during pregnancy by placenta. It is also synthesised in ovaries, testes and adrenals. **Progesterone is a precursor of estrogens, androgens and adrenocortical steroids.**

Progesterone Derivatives

Drugs like progesterone: Hydroxyprogesterone, medroxyprogesterone acetate, chlormadinone acetate.

Drugs resembling 19 testosterone: Norethindrone, norgestrel, norethyindrone. and levonorgestrel.

Synthetic: Megestrol acetate and norgestimate.

Actions

1. Vaginal secretions are made thick and scanty. This effect of progesterone contributes to its contraceptive action.
2. On uterus—prepares the endometrium for implantation of the fertilised ovum. Endometrium becomes secretory. It reduces the sensitivity of the uterus to oxytocin. It maintains pregnancy and keeps the uterus in a sedentary state.
3. Progesterone promotes development of glandular part of the breast. It prepares breasts for secretion of milk.
4. It has thermogenic action.

Uses

1. Used as contraceptive.
2. It is given in threatened or habitual abortion.
3. Endometrial carcinoma.
4. Carcinoma of breast and prostate.
5. Hormone replacement therapy (HRT).
6. In combination with estrogen is given to treat dysfunctional uterine bleeding, dysmenorrhoea and endometriosis.

Adverse drug reactions

(a) 19-nortestosterone derivatives lower HDL thus **increasing chances of atherosclerosis.**
(b) Breast engorgement.
(c) Increase in body temperature.
(d) Changes in mood.

ORAL CONTRACEPTIVES

These are of three types:
1. Combination of estrogen and progesterone.

2. Continuous use of progesterone.

3. Sequential administration of estrogen and progesterone.

Actions

1. These agents suppress pituitary gonadotropins and **inhibit ovulation and its maturation**.

2. Make endometrium unfavourable for implantation.

Combination of Estrogen and Progesterone:
It contains low doses of estrogen (ethinylestradiol or mestranol) and a progestin (desofestrel and norgestimate). Pill is started on day 5 of menstrual cycle, taken each day for 21 days followed by gap of 7 days during which menstruation occurs.

If woman misses a pill she should take 2 pills the next day and continue the courses. If more than 2 pills are missed then course should be withdrawn and should follow alternate method of contraception for that cycle and restart course on 5th day of menestruation.

If pregnancy occurs it should be terminated as these hormones are teratogenic.

Minipill: A low dose progestin is given daily without gap.

Advantage: Adverse effects of estrogen are avoided.

Disadvantage: Efficacy is low.

Postcoital Contraceptives: Combination of estrogen and progesterone is given within 72 hours of intercourse. Efficacy is 90–98%. 2 tablets immediately and 2 tablets are repeated after 12 hours. If failure occurs intrauterine device should be used within 5 days of coitus to prevent pregnancy.

Depot preparations: Depot medroxyprogesterone acetate (150–400 mg) or norethisterone enanthate (NETEN) 200 mg are given IM at 3–6 months interval.

Implants: Norplant capsule is implanted in subcutaneous tissue — works **for 5 years.**

Disadvantages

1. Amenorrhoea is frequent.

2. Permanent sterility may occur.

Transdermal Patches: Estradiol patches are applied 3–4 days for 3 weeks. Progesterone is to be taken orally during last 10–12 days of cycle.

Advantage: It has better acceptance but is expensive.

Vaginal Rings: Levonorgestrel containing rings are placed in vagina for 3 weeks and removed.

Uses

(a) As contraceptive.

(b) To treat endometriosis.

(c) To treat habitual abortion.

(d) Dysmenorrhea.

(e) Premenstrual tension.

Not to be used in patients

(a) Suffering from cancer breast/uterus.

(b) During pregnancy.

(c) 7 days after menstruation.

Adverse drug reactions

1. Nausea
2. Hypertension
3. Thrombosis
4. Precipitates diabetes.

Centchroman (SAHELI): It is non-steroidal contraceptive. It has both antiestrogenic and antiprogestogenic activity. 30 mg is given twice a week for 3 months followed by once a week till contraception is wanted.

Advantages

1. Success rate is 97–99%.
2. It is devoid of adverse effects of hormones.
3. It has no teratogenic or carcinogenic effects.

Adverse reactions

1. Causes enlargement of ovaries.
2. Causes prolongation of menstrual cycle in about 10% women.
3. Should be avoided in renal and hepatic insufficiency.

54

Pharmacology of Calcium Metabolism

Calcium is required for:
1. Excitation — contraction coupling in nerve, muscle and for tissue excitability.
2. Myocardial contractability.
3. Coagulation of blood.
4. As cementing substance of the bones.
5. Secretions from glands.

Normal serum calcium ranges between 9–11 mg% and 6–6.5 mg% exists in ionised form which is the active form. The average daily requirement of calcium varies between 0.5 and 0.75 g. During pregnancy and lactation the requirement is increased. Calcium is absorbed from small intestine by active transport. Absorption is increased during deficiency and by vitamin D.

Uses

1. To prevent and treat calcium deficiency.
2. Tetany — calcium is given slowly by 1V.
3. Vitamin D deficiency.

Preparations: 10% solution of calcium gluconate is used for intravenous administration during emergency. Oral calcium is used as supplement during pregnancy and lactation or when the dietary calcium is low.

In cases of osteomalacia and osteoporosis oral calcium is administered along with vitamin D_3.

In deficiency of parathyroid hormone oral calcium is given instead of the hormone.

PARATHYROID HORMONE

It is secreted by the parathyroid glands which are four in number and are situated close to thyroid gland. Occasionally during surgery on thyroid these glands get removed.

Parathyroid hormone maintains serum calcium between 9 and 11 mg%. It raises serum calcium by:
 (i) Increasing reabsorption of calcium at the proximal convoluted tubule in the kidney.
 (ii) Increasing mobilisation of calcium from the bone to the blood.
(iii) Increasing absorption of calcium from the intestine.
(iv) Increasing excretion of phosphates in the urine.
 (v) By stimulating synthesis of vitamin D which in turn increases Ca^{++} absorption from gut.

Uses: It is available as solution for injection (100 units/ml). It is given subcutaneously for diagnosing pseudohypoparathyroidism.

For treating chronic hypoparathyroidism vitamin D and calcium are quite effective.

CALCITONIN

This hormone is secreted by C cells of the thyroid gland. Secretion is regulated by plasma Ca^{++} concentration. It performs following functions:

(i) It **inhibits osteoclastic activity** and **promotes deposition of calcium** in the bones.

(ii) It lowers calcium phosphate in serum (high serum calcium triggers its release) by reducing absorption of calcium and phosphate.

It is available as solution for subcutaneous or intramuscular injections.

Dose: 100 units/day.

Uses

(i) To treat hyperclacemia.

(ii) To promote healing of bones.

(iii) To treat Paget's disease.

Adverse reactions

(i) Nausea and vomiting.

(ii) Swelling and tenderness of hands.

Sodium etidronate is a new compound. It has effects like calcitonin and can be given orally.

VITAMIN D

This is a fat soluble vitamin and is a **prohormone**. It is of two types D_3 (7-dehydrocholesterol) is of animal origin and is formed by sun rays in the skin. D_2 is termed calciferol and is of plant origin. D_2 and D_3 have similar pharmacological actions.

Adults do not require vitamin D normally. Children and adult females during pregnancy and lactation require 400–800 units of this vitamin daily. It is absorbed in presence of bile. Vitamin D (D_2 and D_3) performs following functions:

(i) It increases absorption of calcium and phosphate from the intestine.

(ii) It deposists calcium into bone (unlike parathyroid which removes calcium from the bones).

(iii) It raises plasma calcium and increases phosphate reabsorption from kidney.

(iv) It increases excretion of magnesium in the urine.

(v) **Improves muscle contraction.**

Adverse reactions: This vitamin accumulates in the body, hence on long-term treatment produces toxicity.

(i) It causes overcalcification of bone ends and calcification of soft tissues.

(ii) Hypercalcemia is produced which produces symptoms of weakness, fatigue, headache, nausea and renal failure.

Uses

1. Rickets and osteomalacia.
2. Pregnancy and lactation.
3. Hypothyroidism.

Hypercalcemia: Following conditions can produce this condition, e.g.

- Hyperparathyroidism.
- Excess vitamin D.
- Sarcoidosis.
- Adrenal insufficiency.

Symptoms: Recurrent attacks of renal colic and stones.

Treatment

1. High salt diet with high fluid intake.
2. Frusemide.
3. Drugs lowering serum calcium—**mithramycin, calcitonin, edetate disodium**.
4. Phosphates given orally.
5. **Etidronate** and **pamidronate.**

Hypocalcemia: Following conditions produce hypocalcemia:

- Malabsorption.
- Hypoparathyroidism.
- Deficiency of vitamin D.
- Renal failure.
- Pancreatitis.
- Excessive citrated blood transfusion.

Signs and symptoms: Increase in neuromuscular excitability resulting in muscle cramps (carpopedal spasms).

Tetany.

Treatment: 20% solution of calcium gluceptate slowly.

10% solution of calcium gluconate IV.

Calcium lactate and **calcium carbonate** are meant for oral administration.

Adverse reactions

1. Feeling of warmth over the body.
2. Tachycardia.

Digestive System

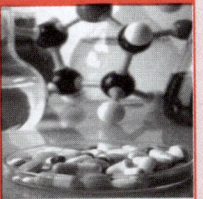

55

Pharmacology of Digestive System

PHYSIOLOGY OF SALIVARY GLANDS

Parasympathetic nerve stimulation causes vasodilatation and increased secretion (watery saliva). Stimulation of sympathetic nervous system causes vasoconstriction with scanty flow of thick and viscid saliva.

Dryness of mouth can be produced by all of the following drugs:
(a) Atropine, probanthine.
(b) Imipramine.
(c) Chlorpromazine.
(d) Levodopa.

Patients may be advised to chew bubble gum, chicklets and anisi which will reduce dryness of mouth.

APPETISERS

These are substances which are used to stimulate appetite in patients of anorexia. **Alcohol is the most popular appetiser.**

All bitters are appetisers.
Examples of bitters: Tincture of Nux vomica, Chirata. Tincture of orange peel, tincture of lemon.

CARMINATIVES

Dilute solutions of volatile aromatic substances like **peppermint water, cardamom, chloroform water,** etc. when taken orally cause mild irritation of gastric mucosa which produces a pleasant sensation of warmth and well-being. This sensation in often followed by eructation. These agents are given after meals.

DIGESTANTS

These are agents that promote the process of digestion. Agents usually employed are **hydrochloric acid, pepsin, pancreatin and bile salts.**

Hydrochloric Acid: 10% solution of this acid is given to patients of achlorhydria. It has to be diluted before taking (4 ml of acid in full glass of water).

It is sipped through a straw (so as to protect enamel of the teeth) during meals and also in between meals.

Pepsin: It is a natural enzyme of the stomach. It is obtained from stomach but is not very essential.

Pancreatin: This contains amylopsin, trypsin and strepsin which are destroyed by acidity. They are therefore, given in the form of enteric coated capsules in patients of chronic pancreatitis.

It is to be given before meals.

EMETICS

Drugs which produce vomiting are called emetics. They can produce vomiting either by acting on CTZ in the brain or by irritation of the gastric mucosa (local irritants).

Receptors involved in vomiting: Histamine (H_1) — in motion sickness.

M_1 cholinergic — motion sickness and disease such as dyspepsia.

Radiation and chemotherapy produces vomiting due to stimulation of 5-HT_3 receptors. Levodopa like drugs cause emesis due to stimulation of D_2 receptors.

Mechanical stimulation of fauces produces vomiting

1. **Local irritants are mustard, ipecac, tartar, hypertonic saline, copper sulphate and salicylates.**
2. Acting through higher centers in the brain — offensive visual and olfactory stimuli, motion sickness **apomorphine and ipecac.**

Sodium chloride is most harmless and can be used for emetic action (table spoonful of salt in a glass of water).

Drugs that produce vomiting as an unwanted effect

1. Most anticancer drugs.
2. Morphine and other opiates.
3. Aminoglycoside antimicrobials.
4. Ergot alkaloids.
5. Levodopa and theophylline.

Use of emetics: For treatment of poisoning where gastric lavage is not feasible.

Disadvantages

1. Should not be used in unconscious or semiconscious patients because there is a danger of vomitus being aspirated into the lungs.
2. Should not be used in corrosive poisoning.
3. In poisoning by CNS stimulants — as convulsions may be precipitated.
4. In poisoning due to petroleum products — as these can cause pneumonitis.

ANTIEMETICS

Vomiting as a symptom is associated with many diseases. The removal of primary cause (if can be recognised) is the best way to treat vomiting. However, for symptomatic relief antiemetics are given. Repeated vomiting can lead to imbalance of **electrolytes, dehydration, exhaustion, aspiration of vomitus into lungs and gastric hemorrhage**.

Drugs usually employed for their antiemetic effect are:

1. Anticholinergic drugs: Atropine, hyoscine, dicyclomine, benztropine and trihexyphenidyl.

Hyoscine is beneficial in motion sickness. Dose is 0.3 mg. It produces sedation therefore is not fit for pilots or drivers.

2. **Antihistaminics:** Promethazine, cyclizine, meclizine, diphenhydramine and cinnarizine. These are not better than hyoscine. They are not effective against apomorphine induced emesis. Most of these agents produce sedation.

3. **Nonspecific blockers of $D_1 + D_2$ — receptors phenothiazines:** Chlorpromazine.

These drugs are not useful in motion sickness but effectively control vomiting due to **uremia, radiation sickness, and carcinomatosis**. These drugs **are ineffective in morphine poisoning**.

Commonly used agents are prochlorperazine (stemetil) 5–10 mg.

Perphenazine — 2.5 to 5 mg.

Trimethobenzamide this is long acting drug which has no teratogenic action and does not produce sedation.

Metoclopramide is specific D_2 blocker. It is powerful antiemetic. It speeds the rate of transit through the bowel and prevents gastroesophageal reflux by increasing tone of esophageal sphincter. It produces less adverse reactions.

Adverse reactions: Drowsiness, diarrhea and sodium retention.

Domperidone: Does not cross BBB to a large extent. It blocks D_2 receptors in CTZ.

Cisapride, itopride and mesopride.

Advantages

1. Highly effective.
2. Do not cause sedation.
3. Do not produce Parkinsonism.

Disadvantages

1. Cisapride — cardiac arrest/arrhythmia appear on IV administration. Hence, not to be given IV.
2. Diarrhea and dry mouth.
3. 5-HT antagonists.

   Ondansetron and granisetron used mostly to control vomiting. They block 5-HT receptors in nucleus tractus solitarius and peripherally 5-HT$_3$ receptors in gut.

   (a) Vomiting due to cancer chemotherapy and radiotherapy.

   (b) Postoperative nausea.

   Act at both peripheral and central levels: Ondansetron is drug of choice. It is **ineffective in morphine posioning**.

   Granisetron is 10 times more potent that ondansetron.

   Are ineffective in motion sickness. May produce headache and gut problems.

4. **Miscellaneous**

   (a) **Cannabinoids** not often used as they produce too many unwanted effects.

   (b) **Pyridoxine** is a mixture of pyridixine, pyridoxal and pyridixamine, is soluble in water, is heat stable, is light sensitive, is useful in morning sickness and hyperemesis gravidum.

Actions

(a) Gets converted to pyridoxical phosphate which acts as a cofactor for enzymes involved in amino acid metabolism, e.g. conversion of tryptophan to 5-HT and methionine to cysteine.

(b) It is required for:

(i) Activity of glycogen phosphorylase.

(ii) For formation of antibodies.

(iii) For synthesis of 5-aminolevulinic acid.

Uses of pyridoxine

1. In patients of chronic anemia who have hyperferremia and abnormal tryptophan metabolism

2. To prevent as well as to treat neurological symptoms due to INH, cycloserine and hydralazine.

3. Morning sickness and hyperemesis gravidum.

4. Infantile convulsions:

(a) **Steroids:** dexamethasone and methyl prednisolone are found to be effective in controlling vomiting due to anticancer drugs.

(b) Cisapride rushes the gut content (by blocking 5-HT$_4$ receptors) and stops vomiting. It is banned because of its toxicity.

Nursing care in patient who is vomiting

(a) In a conscious patient, the cause of vomiting should be elicited through history.

(b) In medicolegal cases vomitus must be preserved.

(c) In unconscious state the patient should be tilted to one side so as to prevent aspiration of the vomitus.

Nursing care in vomiting due to pregnancy

(i) Patient is advised to take frequent small meals and excess of fluids.

(ii) Reassurance helps.

(iii) In pregnancy dry biscuits in the morning prevent vomiting.

(iv) If vomiting is severe, patient should be administered drugs which do not have teratogenic effect, e.g. pyridoxine is given and is found to be effective.

56

Drugs used in Treatment of Peptic Ulcers

Ulcer is discontinuity in the epithelial lining of gastrointestinal tract.

Factors increasing ulcers—cholinergic stimulation (M_1, M_2 and M_3), H_2 receptors stimulation and spicy foods, alcohol. Peptic ulcers occur at sites exposed to hydrochloric acid and pepsin. Healthy mucosa is resistant to these two offending agents but due to imbalance between acid pepesin secretion and mucosal defence factors ulcers are formed and their healing is prevented by the constant presence of irritant action of the above substances.

Drugs used for treatment of peptic ulcers

Classification

1. Drugs neutralising acidity—antacids
   (a) *Systemic antacids:* Sodium bicarbonate
   (b) *Non-systemic antacids:* Bismuth subnitrate, aluminium hydroxide, aluminium phosphate, magnesium hydroxide and magnesium trisilicate.

2. Drugs reducing gastric acid secretion
   (a) Anticholinergic agents—pirenzepine, propantheline
   (b) *H_2 receptor antagonists:* Cimetidine, ranitidine, famotidine, nizatidine, loxatidine
   (c) *Proton pump inhibitors:* Omeprazole, lansoprazole, pantoprazole, rabeprazole, esomeprazole
   (d) *Antigastrin agents:* Proglumide
   (e) *Prostaglandins:* Misoprostol, enprostil and esomeprazole

3. *Ulcer protectors:* Sucralfate and colloidal bismuth

4. *Drugs promoting healing of ulcers:* Carbenoxolone Na^+

5. *Anti H. Pylori:* Amoxycillin, metronidazole/tinidazole and tetracycline.

ANTACIDS

Systemic Antacids: Sodium bicarbonate

Advantages: It is very potent and has quick onset of action—stomach pH may be raised above 7. Does not reduce acid production. Taken on empty stomach, effect lasts for one hour but taken with meal it lasts for 2–3 hours.

Disadvantages

(a) Action is short lived.

(b) Has no adsorbent or demulcent action.

(c) Causes rebound acidity which increases chances of perforation of ulcer.

(d) **If kidney function is not proper — after absorption it produces alkalosis.**

(e) Worsens congestive cardiac failure.

Dose: 1–4 g.

Patient should be advised to keep this drug as a standby for emergency treatment of acute pain, but should not use this routinely.

Non-systemic Antacids

Magnesium hydroxide (milk of magnesia)

Advantage: Rapidly neutralises gastric acid and action is sustained

Highly potent
No systemic alkalosis

Disadvantage: Produces diarrhea — therefore it is given in combination with aluminium hydroxide (a constipating agent).

Aluminium hydroxide

(a) Delays gastric emptying.

(b) Raises gastric pH.

(c) Causes constipation and may cause intestinal obstruction.

(d) It binds and prevents absorption of phosphate in gut.

(e) It is slow acting.

Uses

(a) As antacid.

(b) In treatment of hyperphosphatemia in chronic renal failure and in treating phosphate stones.

ANTISECRETORY AGENTS

Anticholinergics

Disadvantages: Produce dryness of mouth as atropine inhibits secretions of salivary glands.

Increase heart rate and produce blurring of vision and therefore should be given only at night (bed time).

Reduce volume but do not raise pH have narrow therapeutic index.

Propantheline: It can be given in tablet form and has lesser side effects than atropine. It has shorter duration of action therefore the dose can be easily monitored.

Antispasmodic drugs are given in combination with antacids as they increase the stay of antacids in stomach which makes it more effective.

Pirenzepine: It is specific M_1 blocker

Advantages

1. Lacks CNS adverse reactions.
2. Does not cause:
   - (a) Tachycardia.
   - (b) Blurred vision.
   - (c) Delirium and confusion.

Disadvantages

1. It is less effective—causes 40–50% reduction in acid secretion.
2. Bioavailability is affected by food.
3. Adverse reactions such as thrombocytopenia and agranulocytosis are possible.

H_2 RECEPTOR BLOCKERS

Cimetidine: It blocks H_2 receptors and reduces secretion of HCl. However, it is not used now as it produces serious adverse reactions such as:

- (a) Antiandrogenic effect and causes **gynaecomastia** in males.
- (b) Confusion, restlessness, delirium, convulsions and coma.
- (c) Diarrhea and nausea.
- (d) Skin rash, itching
- (e) Blood—**thrombocytopenia and agranulocytosis.**
- (f) Drug interactions—it inhibits hepatic microsomal enzymes thereby inhibiting metabolism of certain drugs (theophylline, benzodiazepines, propranolol, digitoxin, warfarin and phenytoin). It increases half life of all these drugs.

Ranitidine

Advantages

- (a) It is more potent than cimetidine.
- (b) It does not inhibit microsomal enzymes in liver and therefore drug interactions are limited.
- (c) It has no anti-androgenic activity.
- (d) It is more potent and longer acting.

Dose: 150 mg b.d.

Adverse reactions

- (a) CNS—headache and mental confusion.
- (b) GIT—diarrhoea and nausea.

Nizatidine: It is as effective as ranitidine and has highest oral bioavailability (98%).

Adverse effects

Urticaria
Rhinitis, pharyngitis, cough
Headache

Roxatidine, Famotidine and Sufotidine: All have effects like ranitidine. Famotidine is more potent than ranitidine.

Uses of H₂ blockers

1. Gastric and duodenal ulcers.
2. Gastritis and dyspepsia.
3. Zollinger-Ellison syndrome.
4. Reflux esophagitis.

Ebrotidine in addition to antisecretory activity it exerts protective effect on the mucosa.

PROTON PUMP INHIBITORS

Omeprazole, Pentaprazole and Lansoprazole: $H^+ K^+$ ATPase (proton pump) is responsible for secretion of H^+ ions by parietal cells of gastric mucosa. These drugs bind to this enzyme and inhibit it thus blocking formation of HCl. These drugs **are as effective as H₂ blockers**. Inhibit both resting and stimulated HCl secretion.

Uses

1. Peptic ulcer.
2. Zollinger-Ellison syndrome.
3. Gastroesophageal reflex disease.

ANALOGUES OF PROSTAGLANDINS

Misoprostol: It is orally available preparation of PGE_1

Actions

(a) It is cytoprotective.
(b) Reduces secretion of HCl.
(c) Heals gastric as well as duodenal ulcers in 4–6 weeks.
(d) **Does not relieve gastric pain.**

Adverse drug reactions

(a) Diarrhoea
(b) Abdominal cramps, nausea, anorexia
(c) Headache
(d) Induces abortion.

Enprostil is more potent than misoprostal but has same actions and ADRs. It is useful in smokers.

ULCER PROTECTIVES

Sucralfate: It is combination of sucrose octasulfate and polyaluminium hydroxide.

Actions

1. As gel it adheres to gastric mucosa for 6 hours and thereby protects it against HCl.
2. More effective against duodenal than gastric ulcers.
3. Antacids reduce its efficacy.

4. Proteins enhance its efficacy.
5. It is not absorbed.
6. It is good for smokers.

Adverse drug reactions

(a) Constipation/diarrhoea.
(b) Interferes with absorption of tetracyclines, phenytoin and digoxin.

Colloidal Bismuth

Actions

(a) Inhibits pepsin activity and increases PGE_2 secretion.
(b) Increases mucus secretion.
(c) Acts with proteins in the necrotic area and form a barrier thus protecting ulcer from effect of acid.
(d) Causes lysis of *H. pylori*.
(e) It also neutralises acidity.

It has lower relapse rate.

Adverse drug reactions

(a) Staining of oral mucosa
(b) Osteodystrophy
(c) Encephalopathy can occur on long-term treatment

Gefarnate is safer but less effective than carbenoxolone.
Oestrogens are helpful in duodenal ulcers in men.

ANTIGASTRIN AGENTS

Proglumide, Oxethazine, Somatostatin, Octreotide

Proglumide: Chemically resembles gastrin. Blocks the effect of gastrin by occupying these receptors. It is as effective as cimetidine.

Oxethazine: Inhibits release of gastrin

Uses of gastrin inhibitors:
(a) Reflux esophagitis.
(b) Hiatus hernia.
(c) Gastritis.

Somatostatin, Octreotide (long acting somatostatin analogues) are under trial as these drugs reduce the H^+ secretion.

DRUGS PROMOTING ULCER HEALING

Carbenoxolone: It is extracted from liquorice root. It promotes healing of gastric ulcers but does not have much effect on duodenal ulcers. Onset of action is slow.

Disadvantages

Adverse reactions are common and occur in the form of:
(a) Fluid retention (especially in the elderly) producing increase in body weight and heart failure.
(b) It causes excessive potassium loss that leads to extreme muscle weakness.

Nursing care in patients on carbenoxolone

1. Serum potassium should be done routinely.
2. Patient should be asked to report any muscle weakness.
3. Patient should be weighed weekly. If there is sudden increase in weight doctor should prescribe diuretics.

Deglycyrrhinized liquorice preparations do not cause fluid retention but retain ulcer healing effect.

ANTI-*H. PYLORI*

H. pylori (an infective organism) is implicated in the causation as well as recurrence of peptic ulcers.

This infection is treated by giving combination of antimicrobials

Metronidazole with colloidal bismuth subcitrate

Tetracyclines and bismuth

Amoxacillin, clarithromycin, tetracycline and metronidazole.

Nursing care

Bland diet, devoid of spices is recommended. Excess tea or coffee are bad, spirits and smoking worsens ulcers.

Small frequent meals are better than large infrequent meals. Day's diet can be arranged in such a way that patient gets something to eat at two hourly intervals.

Advice given to the patient:

1. Reduce anxiety and conflict in life.
2. Smoking should be completely stopped.
3. Drinking should be reduced.
4. Bed rest and sedation help.
5. Eat short meals frequently.

57

Purgatives

These drugs promote passage of stools. Various nomenclatures are used; namely **cathartic (powerful) and (weaker) laxative** and aperient depending upon the degree of action.

With continued use of purgatives the muscles of the bowel become flabby and dependency on purgatives develops.

Classification of Purgatives

1. Bulk purgatives
   (a) *Saline purgatives:* Magnesium sulphate, magnesium hydroxide, sorbitol, lactulose, etc.
   (b) *Hydrophilic fibers:* Bran, isapgulla, agar and carboxymethyl cellulose
2. Lubricant or emollient purgatives or fecal softeners—liquid paraffin and dioctyl sodium sulphosuccinate (docusate)
3. Stimulant purgatives: Phenolphthalein, biscodyl, cascara, castor oil and senna.

Ideal purgative should be:
(a) Dependable.
(b) Devoid of systemic effects.
(c) Not produce any griping pain.
(d) Not be habit forming.
(e) Not cause after constipation.

BULK PURGATIVES

(a) **Saline purgatives:** Magnesium sulphate, milk of magnesia and magnesium citrate are commonly employed as purgatives. They exert an osmotic effect by holding considerable amount of water and increase bulk in small and large intestine. They produce a watery evacuation within 3 to 6 hrs. Due to their quick onset of action they are given early in the morning before breakfast.

These agents may cause dehydration and magnesium toxicity.

(b) **Natural or semisynthetic polysaccharides or cellulose, hemi-cellulose, pectin or gums** that are neither digested nor absorbed but adsorb water and increase the bulk of feces in lumen of bowel. In so doing they stimulate the small and large bowel to evacuate their contents.

   (i) The bulk so formed has emollient action and is sometimes used for relief of acute diarrhoea.
   (ii) They are also useful in obesity as they act as filling agents without caloric value.

Bran, isapgulla, agar and carboxymethyl cellulose are commonly used preparations.

LUBRICANT PURGATIVES

(a) Liquid Paraffin: It is mineral oil obtained from petroleum. It softens the stool and by interfering with absorption of water it increases the bulk. Acts both on small as well as large intestine.

Disadvantages

1. Unpalatable taste.
2. Leaks through anus and spoils the clothes.
3. Regular usage produces deficiency of vitamins A, D and K.

(b) Dioctyl Sodium Sulphosuccinate (Docusate): Surface active, emulsifying and wetting agent. It softens stools by lowering surface tension.

Advantages

1. It is safe
2. It is effective
3. It is useful in treatment of painful fissures or after surgery for removal of piles.

Should not be given with other drugs such as liquid paraffin.

IRRITANT PURGATIVES

The use of most of these purgatives has decreased. Only the following are used:

Senna, bisacodyl, phenolphthalein and castor oil these drugs act locally on the large bowel and stimulate evacuation of its contents. **Senna** is widely used. It contains anthraquinone which gets absorbed in intestine and is secreted in colon where it exerts its effect. It takes **6–8 hours to act**. It is available in tablet form. It is given at night.

Phenolphthalein: It is an active ingredient in many of the marketed preparations. It acts on large bowel and therefore takes 6–8 hours to act. It should be given at bed time.

A small portion of it gets absorbed and re-secreted into intestine. This is responsible for repeated purgation.

Adverse reactions

(i) Allergic skin rashes.
(ii) Prolonged effect.
(iii) Hepatic damage.

Bisacodyl (Dulcolax): It acts like phenolphthalein.

Needs to be given at bed time as it takes 6–8 hrs to produce effect. Also available as suppository it produces effect in 15–60 minutes.

Castor Oil: It is fixed oil obtained from seeds of Ricinus communis. It is hydrolysed in the intestine to yield ricinoleic acid that acts as an irritant purgative. It induces rapid peristalsis and produces fluid stools within 2–3 hrs. It is given early morning on an empty stomach. It is not effective in patients with bile duct obstruction. Emulsion of castor oil however will continue to exert its effects in these patients.

Disadvantages

1. Bad taste.
2. Chronic use produces intestinal damage.
3. Abdominal colic.

Uses: For purgation in pregnant woman **at term. This induces labour.**

Usually given as emulsion.

Uses of purgatives

1. They are required to be given before X-ray examination (bisacodyl).
2. Used for removal of unabsorbed poisons (castor oil or saline purgative is given).
3. In hepatic coma (magnesium sulphate).
4. Along with certain drugs which cause constipation, e.g. opioids.
5. After a few anthelmenthics
6. Before surgery on the large bowel.
7. To avoid straining at stools in piles or anal fissures or in cardiac conditions.

Purgative **should not be used in:**

1. Undiagnosed abdominal pain.
2. Intestinal obstruction.
3. Faecal impaction.
4. Magnesium salts should not be used in patients with renal impairment.
5. Emodin alkaloids should not be given to lactating mothers as they pass into breast milk and produce diarrhoea in the breastfed baby.

Adverse effects of purgatives

1. Constant use produces habituation.
2. Excess use can produce colicky pain in abdomen along with diarrhoea, dehydration and electrolyte imbalance.

SUPPOSITORIES (BISACODYL, GLYCERINE)

These agents produce an effect within one hour.

Suppositories containing anhydrous sodium acid phosphate and sodium bicarbonate produce carbon dioxide and stimulate gut by distention.

Suppositories with astringents or anti-inflammatory agent (indomethacin) or local anaesthetics (lignocaine) are also available for **non-purgative effects**.

ENEMA

Can be given for producing defecation (**evacuation enema**) or for absorption of a medicament for systemic effect (**retention enema**). These agents produce purgation by distending the bowel and increasing its motility. Plain water (at body temperature) or soap and water enema are usually given before conducting delivery.

Disadvantages

1. Psychologically patients do not prefer enema.
2. Are habit forming.
3. Requires time and equipment.

Uses

1. Enemas are used to remove impacted faecal matter from the rectum when suppositories have failed.
2. They are often used in bed ridden patients or in the elderly.
3. To empty large bowels prior to radiological examination.
4. Before surgery on the large bowels.
5. Before normal delivery.

Retention ememas are used in ulcerative colitis and may also be used to reduce intracranial tension (magnesium sulphate enema). They are also used to rehydrate the individual but it is not desirable.

DRUGS WHICH CONTROL DIARRHEA (ANTI-DIARRHEALS)

Diarrhea may be due to various diseases such as

  (a) Infection

  (b) Irritant food

  (c) Acute anxiety

  (d) Malabsorption.

Therapy against diarrhea is aimed at removing the cause, e.g. chemotherapeutic agents are indicated in infected diarrhea, e.g. tetracyclines for bacillary and metronidazole for amoebic dysentery.

Diarrhea may also be controlled by variety of drugs that have no effect on the cause but these drugs produce necessary symptomatic relief.

Uses of nonspecific antidiarrheals

  (i) In cases where there is no specific treatment.

  (ii) During the period when specific treatment is taking effect and taking time.

The nonspecific antidiarrheals are classified as follows:

  (i) Adsorbents

  (ii) Demulcents

  (iii) Opiates.

Adsorbents: These agents act by:

  (i) Providing a coating of the bowel mucosa.

  (ii) Adsorbing toxic substances (gases, toxins and microorganisms) generally they are used in combination with demulcents, or anticholinergic agents and opiates.

Kaolin: Chemically it is hydrated aluminium silicate. It is to be given several times a day. It is available as suspension containing 20% by weight of kaolin and 1% by weight of pectin.

Activated Charcoal: It is highly effective in **adsorbing gases and toxins** from the intestine. It is used in **alkaloidal poisoning** as alkaloids are adsorbed by this agent.

Aluminium hydroxide, magnesium trisilicate also possess adsorbent activity.

Demulcents: These agents have high molecular weight and form colloidal solutions exerting soothing effect on abraded skin and mucous membranes. These agents reduce irritation and produce soothing effect.

Opiates: Tinct, opium along with morphine and codeine have been in use as antidiarrheal. They reduce the propulsive activity of the large as well as small bowel. These are no more used for this purpose as they are addicting in nature and have serious adverse reactions (refer CNS).

Diphenoxylate: It is synthetic opioid and acts like morphine and codeine. This drug too produces euphoria and is liable to produce addiction. It is available in combination with atropine (lomotil) which contains 2.5 mg of diphenoxylate and 0.025 mg of atropine. **It is not safe for children.**

TRAVELLERS DIARRHOEA

This condition is probably due to contamination of food with Staphyloccocal or Enteroviruses or *E. coli*. Neomycin, tetracycline and the nonabsorbable sulphonamides were given for this condition. Due to their adverse reactions they are no more preferred. It is best controlled by one of the opiods which reduces gut movement, e.g. codeine phosphate tablets (30 mg) or lomotil, (diphenoxylate and atropine).

DRUG TREATMENT OF ULCERATIVE COLITIS

(i) Sulphasalazine should be given in maximally tolerated doses and the patient maintained on this drug.

(ii) Correction of electrolyte and fluid imbalance. Levels of serum potassium should be specifically corrected.

(iii) Glucocorticoids by enema are also indicated. If patient cannot retain enema give intrarectal drip of hydrocortisone (100 mg in 120 ml of water) twice a day.

(iv) Initiate therapy with prednisolone (60 mg/day) given in divided doses. In severe acute attacks intravenous route is adopted.

(v) **Broad spectrum antibiotics orally should never be given as they worsen the condition.**

DRUGS USED IN COLICKY PAIN (ANTISPASMODIC AGENTS)

Anticholinergic drugs (propantheline, atropine) reduce motility and tone of the gut. These agents are employed to relieve colicky pain.

DRUGS WHICH INCREASE BILE ACID EXCRETION FROM THE GUT

Cholestyramine: Bile acids if they accumulate in the blood (which they do in case of obstructive jaundice) produce severe itching. This drug combines with bile acids in the gut and prevents their absorption thus reducing their levels in blood. **This drug is effective only in partial blockade of bile duct.**

It is also useful in controlling diarrhea in patients of ileal resection.

Chenodeoxycholic Acid: It is used to dissolve gallstones.

Haemopoietic System

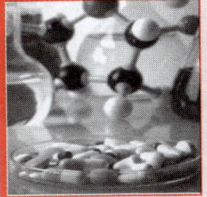

58

Haematinics

Haematinics are substances needed for synthesis of haemoglobin. This chapter describes drugs used in the treatment of anaemias.

ANAEMIA

It is defined as a deficiency of haemoglobin in red blood cells. Anaemia is measured in terms of haemoglobin (Hb) in blood. In men normal Hb concentration ranges between 13 and 14 gm per 100 ml. Hb values lower than these are indicative of anaemia.

Causes of Anaemia

1. Due to impaired blood formation. This condition is seen when there is deficiency of essential substances, e.g. iron, vitamin B_{12}, copper, etc. It is also seen in cases where bone marrow is depressed due to chronic infections, malignancy or drug therapy.
2. Anaemias also result from blood loss. Acute blood loss is seen in accidents or after major surgery. Chronic blood loss occurs in hookworm infestations or in diseases such as piles and peptic ulcer. In women excessive menstrual loss also produces anaemia.
3. Anaemias can also be produced in diseases where there is excessive breakdown of RBC, e.g. malaria.

Anaemia due to deficiency of iron is microcytic hypochromic type.

Iron: Total iron content of body is 4 g out of which 2.5 gm are present in haemoglobin.

Daily requirement of iron is 1 mg in men and 1.5 to 2.0 mg in women. Loss of iron (e.g. during pregnancy and lactation 600 mg) is more in women. Iron is naturally present in meat and leafy vegetables. In the bone marrow iron is used for synthesis of haemoglobin. In the skeletal muscles it gets incorporated in myohaemoglobin (protein found in muscle).

Iron administered orally is absorbed from the small intestine. The absorbed iron is transferred through plasma to reticuloendothelial cells of bone marrow, liver and spleen in combination with carrier protein.

Ferric form of the iron is converted to ferrous form by the action of hydrochloric acid before absorption. Only 10% of the dietary iron is normally absorbed by the body. The percentage of iron absorption increases in anaemia.

Absorption of iron is increased by the anemic state, gastric acid, ascorbic acid and succinate.

Phytates and phosphates reduce its absorption.

Route of elimination of iron
(a) Stools
(b) Urine
(c) Sweat.

Preparations of iron: Iron can be given to patients orally, intramuscularly or intravenously.

Ferrous Sulphate

Advantages

1. It is least expensive
2. It is well absorbed
3. It is well tolerated

It is available as tablet containing 200 mg of this salt.

Dose: One tablet three times a day.

Disadvantages: It produces gastric irritation. This can be avoided if the tablet is taken after meals. Dose of ferrous sulphate may be reduced to avoid this reaction. A tablet a day may be sufficient in many such cases.

Ferrous Gluconate and Ferrous Fumarate: Claimed to be better tolerated than the above preparation. Dose is 300 mg given three times a day.

Uses: In patients who cannot tolerate ferrous sulphate.

Disadvantages

1. Are expensive.
2. Produce nausea and vomiting
3. Liquid preparations stain teeth.

Ferric Ammonium Citrate: Absorption of iron from these tablets is poor. This preparation is more expensive than ferrous sulphate.

Precautions

(a) Chronic use of iron can lead to iron overload—this should be avoided.
(b) These preparations can cause gastric irritation, hence should be taken with meals.

Spansules of iron are available (FEFOL). Iron from spansules is released only in the duodenum or jejunum.

Preparations of iron for parenteral administration: Iron can be given intramuscularly as well as intravenously.

Following are the reasons for giving iron intramuscularly:
(a) When the patient is not tolerating oral iron.
(b) When the patient is suffering from malabsorption.

(c) In cases of severe anaemia when an early correction of anaemia is required, e.g. elective surgery in an anaemic patient.

Preparations of iron available for intramuscular injection:

1. Iron dextran injection.
2. Iron sorbitol citric acid complex injection.

Iron Dextran: This contains 50 mg per ml of elemental iron. 0.5–1.0 ml can be given on alternate day.

Disadvantages

1. It stains the site of injection. This can be avoided by giving injection in Z form.
2. It is painful.
3. Malignancy may be produced at the site of injection.

Iron Sorbitol Citric Acid Complex: This injection contains 50 mg/ml of iron.

Advantages: Allergic reactions to this preparation are less common.

(i) This preparation does not produce malignant change at the site of injection.
(ii) It does not stain skin.

Intravenous preparations

Saccharated iron oxide can be given intravenously.

Uses of iron therapy

1. In anaemias due to nutritional deficiency of iron.
2. Anaemia of pregnancy and infancy. Supplemental iron is given to pregnant and lactating mothers to avoid development of anaemia.
3. In patients suffering from diseases associated with chronic blood loss.

Adverse reactions of parenteral iron

1. Pain at the site of injection.
2. Staining of the skin at the site of injection, lymphadenopathy.
3. Headache, fever, arthralgia, backache and tachycardia.
4. Haemolysis and circulatory collapse.

IRON TOXICITY

Acute Toxicity of Iron: This condition is seen in children who consume large number of iron tablets mistakenly. These tablets produce:

1. Severe gastrointestinal irritation leading to nausea and vomiting followed by colicky pain and diarrhea. Shock may be precipitated. Death may occur in 6 to 8 hrs.
2. If the patient recovers:
   (a) He may still die in 12–24 hrs.
   (b) But if he survives a few months later he shows symptoms of stenosis of bowel.

Treatment of acute iron toxicity

1. Gastric lavage is done using **sodium bicarbonate and albumin**.
2. Fluid loss and electrolyte imbalance is corrected.
3. Specific chelating agent **desferrioxamine** is given to trap the free iron. This helps in:
   (i) Inactivating free iron which is responsible for toxicity.
   (ii) Removal of the iron through kidneys.

Chronic Toxicity: Chronic toxicity of iron is produced by either taking iron treatment for too long or consuming heavy doses in short span resulting in haemosiderosis.

It is treated by:
(a) Repeated bleeding (500 ml at a time).
(b) By giving 1–3 g of desferrioxamine intravenously to achieve rapid iron excretion.

Adjuvants to Iron Therapy: **Vitamin C, cobalt and copper** are added to iron to help its absorption and better utilisation. These agents **are of help only if they are deficient**.

Disadvantages of adjuvants

1. Many preparations available in the market have vitamin C, folic acid, vitamin B_{12} and cobalt. Cobalt and copper may produce toxicity.
2. Folic acid and B_{12} may mask megaloblastic anaemia that gets only partially treated. It hampers in making correct diagnosis.
3. Addition of these substances adds to the cost of the product making it difficult for the poor man.
4. Addition of these agents is both harmful and wasteful.

Nursing care in anaemia

Nurse has a major role to play in these cases, both in the out-door and in-door patients.

1. Unhygienic conditions breed infections. Most of our population lives below poverty line and lacks the knowledge about personal hygiene. Nurses can play the role of health educationists and help in eradication of these diseases. Patient of anaemia is prone to infections and is likely to suffer greater morbidity. Cliping the finger nails prevents development of helminthic infections.
2. Patient must be educated on good dietary habits. Explain the utility of eating green vegetables.
3. Warn the patient against self medication of these drugs and abuse of tonic.
4. Guide patient regarding storage of these drugs so as to prevent accidental acute toxicity in children.
5. While injecting iron intramuscularly exercise care that the drug does not leak into subcutaneous tissue as this produces discolouration of the skin.

Folic Acid: Folic acid—as the name suggests is present in leafy vegetables, e.g. spinach. It is also synthesised by the intestinal bacteria. When given orally two thirds gets absorbed from the upper part of small intestine. In body it is converted to folinic acid before use.

It is needed for synthesis of purines and also for conversion of serine to glycine, homocysteine to methionine and deoxyuridylate to thymidylate.

Deficiency of folic acid occasionally develops in pregnancy (because of the increased demand of the foetus), in malabsorption and during treatment with certain drugs (phenytoin, and primidone). Deficiency of this agent produces **macrocytic anaemia, glossitis, chelosis, dyspepsia and diarrhea.**

Folic acid deficiency responds favourably to treatment with oral folic acid (except in malabsorption).

Dose: 5 mg tablet given two to three times a day. In malabsorption — injections containing 15 mg/ml of folic acid are given IM.

Uses

1. Megaloblastic anaemia due to nutritional deficiency of folic acid.
2. In pregnancy and lactation.
3. Malabsorption syndrome.
4. Megaloblastic anaemia in alcoholics and scurvy.

Precautions: Folic acid alone should not be given in undiagnosed, megaloblastic anaemia. It should be given along with vit B_{12}. Folic acid given alone in B_{12} deficiency (pernicious anaemia) improves the haematological picture by diverting B_{12} from the nervous tissue to the bone marrow. Neurological signs are therefore aggravated.

Anaemia due to vitamin B_{12} deficiency is produced in:
  (i) Pernicious anaemia.
 (ii) Gastrectomy.
(iii) Malabsorption syndrome.
 (iv) In blind loops of bowel.

Folinic Acid: In the body folic acid needs conversion to folinic acid before it can produce effects. Folinic acid is available in 1 ml ampoules containing 3 mg of this vitamin.

Uses

1. In treatment of methotrexate toxicity.
2. In treatment of methyl alcohol toxicity. Liver preparations containing B_{12} and folic acid are available. These can be used in conditions where there is deficiency of these agents.

Disadvantages

1. All these preparations have short shelf life.
2. Injections of liver are painful.
3. These can produce allergic reactions.

Pyridoxine

(a) It is useful in patients of hereditary or acquired sideroblastic anemia.
(b) Anemia that is associated with use of isoniazid and pyrazinamide. Routine use is not advocated.

Copper: Deficiency of Cu^{++} occurs in malabsorption. It is present in food in quantities sufficient for daily requirements.

(a) 1–2 mg/day may be given to patients on parenteral nutrition.
(b) 0.1 mg/kg of cupric sulphate is given orally in patients of multiple nutritional deficiencies.

Cobalt: It stimulates erythropoiesis. Improves Hb value and RBC counts in sickle cell anaemia, thalassemia and anemia associated with renal disease, neoplasias and chronic infections.

Adverse drug reactions

(a) Large amounts depress RBC production.
(b) Cutaneous flushing.

(c) Retrosternal chest pain
(d) Nausea and vomiting
(e) Myxedema

Cyanocobalamine (B$_{12}$):

Cyanocobalamine (B$_{12}$): Vitamin B$_{12}$ is produced by microbes and colonies of the fungus — *Streptomyces griseus*. This vitamin (except legumes) is totally absent in plant kingdom. Commercially it is obtained from *Streptomyces griseus* which also yields streptomycin. It is a red coloured compound.

It is needed for the maturation of RBCs and plays a role in lipid metabolism of neural tissue.

Daily requirement of this vitamin is about one microgram.

Given orally (dietary) it is absorbed from ileum. It needs intrinsic factor for its absorption. Intrinsic factor is secreted by gastric mucosa. In very large doses, a small part of the vitamin B$_{12}$ gets absorbed even in the absence of intrinsic factor. Vitamin B$_{12}$ is stored in the liver.

Deficiency of this vitamin produces atrophic glossitis, megaloblastic anaemia and subacute combined degeneration of the spinal cord. In all the above conditions Vitamin B$_{12}$ is given parenterally

Preparations: Cyanocobalamine injection 100 µg/ml.

Hydroxycobalamin injection 100, 500 and 1000 µg/ml.

Oral preparation containing B$_{12}$ along with intrinsic factor is also available.

Adverse reactions: Allergic reactions have been reported.

Uses

1. Nutritional megaloblastic anaemia.
2. Peripheral neuropathies.

59

Coagulants and Anticoagulants

Mechanism of Normal Blood Coagulation

Body has a mechanism to maintain blood in a liquid form in the vessels. If you sustain injury (cut your finger) bleeding starts which generates events which automatically stop bleeding through vasoconstriction as well as clot formation.

There are certain clotting factors which participate in the formation of a clot. There are two mechanisms which result in clot formation.

Clotting Factors

   (i) Fibrinogen: A protein produced by the liver.

  (ii) Prothrombin: A glycoprotein produced by the liver. This needs vitamin K for its synthesis and release.

 (iii) Tissue thromboplastin produced by injured tissues.

 (iv) Calcium.

  (v) Accelerator globulin which is a plasma protein.

 (vi) **No such factor.**

 (vii) Prothrombinogen is produced in liver and is present in plasma.

(viii) Anti-haemophilic factor—deficiency of this factor produces haemophilia.

 (ix) Christmas factor: It is produced by liver. Deficiency of this factor is responsible for Christmas disease and haemophilia B. It is vitamin K dependent factor.

  (x) Stuart factor: It is produced by liver, it requires vitamin K for its synthesis.

 (xi) Plasma thromboplastin antecedent.

 (xii) Hageman factor: It initiates clotting *in vitro*.

(xiii) Fibrin stabilizing factor.

Intrinsic System

All the factors which participate in this system are present in blood. It is slow and takes several minutes.

Antihaemophilic factor (VIII) combines with Christmas factor (IX) + Ca^{++} + factor (X) + factor (V) and the platelet factor (released from the damaged platelets) to form thromboplastin.

Extrinsic System

In the extrinsic system **thromboplastin** is formed from **tissue extract** of the damaged tissue. This converts factor X to Xa in presence of Ca^{++}, factor VII acid V. It is rapid but needs tissue factor.

Clot formed from the blood is composed of a vast number of extremely tiny strands of fibrin (protein). Blood cells get enmeshed among these fibres. Fibrin is not normally present in the body. Its precursor—fibrinogen is soluble in water and circulates in the blood. Fibrinogen gets converted to fibrin by the combined action of thrombin and calcium.

Unless thrombin is present in the blood, fibrinogen will not be converted to fibrin.

Thrombin too does not exist in blood in the active form. It is generated by the action of thromboplastin (in presence of calcium) on prothrombin. Thromboplastin for its generation need either damaged platelets or tissue extract (damaged tissue). Thus, injury (either of platelets or tissue) is required to initiate the process of clotting.

PHYSIOLOGICAL ANTAGONISTS OF COAGULATION

(A) Inhibitors of Clotting Factors: Antithrombin III—inhibits conversion of prothrombin to thrombin

(a) inactivates factors XIIa, XIa, IXa and Xa
(b) Inactivates thrombin
(c) Inhibits factors VII, IXa, Xa , XIIa. Factors IIa and Xa being most sensitive

(B) Fibrinolytic Agents: Kinase—converts plasminogen to plasmin-a proteolytic enzyme—that dissolves fibrin.

ANTICOAGULANTS

Anticoagulants are drugs that interfere with the clotting properties of the blood. Anticoagulants are of two types.

1. Injectable—heparin and warfarin Na.
2. Oral anticoagulants.
   (a) Coumarins
   (b) Indandione.

Heparin: It is released from mast cells, liver and lungs and exerts anticoagulant effect both in vitro and in vivo. It prevents conversion of prothrombin to thrombin. In high doses, it also prevents platelet cohesion and formation of fibrin monomer. It is of three types:

(a) Low molecualr weight.
(b) High molecular weight.
(c) Physiological heparin.

Other actions

(i) It activates lipoprotein lipase and it reduces lipids in blood after meal.
(ii) It increases excretion of sodium chloride and water.
(iii) It has weak anti-inflammatory activity.

Adverse reactions

1. Allergic and anaphylactoid reaction.
2. It produces transient alopecia.
3. On chronic use results in osteoporosis and spontaneous fractures of ribs and vertebrae.

Advantages

1. It is effective both in vitro and in vivo.
2. It has immediate effect, therefore, it can be given in conditions where there is an urgent need for anticoagulant action, e.g. in myocardial infarction or deep vein thrombosis.
3. It has no effect on the foetus and can be used in pregnancy.
4. Toxicity is easily managed.
5. Inhibits spontaneous metastasis from malignant neoplasms.

Disadvantages

1. Action is short lived and therefore repeated injections have to be given. **Low molecular wieght heparin is long acting.**
2. It produces pain at the site of injection.
3. Allergic reactions are commonly encountered.
4. It is expensive
5. May delay healing
It is available as 1000, 5000, 10,000 and 20,000 units in vials.

Dose: 20,000 to 30,000 units of heparin are added to 1 liter of 5% dextrose or 0.9% saline solution and administered as infusion in 24 hrs.

Bolus of 5,000 units may be given before the infusion.
It should not be given IM.

Low Molecular Weight Heparin

Advantages

(a) It is rapidly absorbed.
(b) Haemorrhage occurs less frequently.
(c) It is long acting and given once a day.
(d) Has low antiplatelet effect.

Nursing care

1. Sensitivity testing should be done before administering heparin.
2. Clotting time of the patient should be done on alternate days. Drug should be withdrawn if clotting time is prolonged beyond 1.5 times.
3. Appearance of symptoms of toxicity of heparin (bleeding, etc.) should be closely observed by the nurse and heparin withdrawn at the earliest.
4. Monitor PTT or clotting time.

Treatment of toxicity of heparin

1. Stop heparin
2. Give fresh blood

3. **Protamine sulphate** is given to neutralise its effect. It is administered as 1% solution intravenously (50 mg over a 10 minute period).

Precaution in use of protamine sulphate high dose of this drug exerts anticoagulant effect, therefore limit the dose.

ORAL ANTICOAGULANTS

Coumarin Derivatives: Bishydroxycoumarin (dicumarol) and warfarin are the preparations commonly used. These drugs antagonise the effects of vitamin K resulting in inhibition of synthesis of prothrombin and factors VII, IX and X as these require vitamin K for their synthesis and release.

Dose of these drugs is adjusted by **monitoring prothrombin time**.

Advantages

1. These drugs can be given orally.
2. These are inexpensive.
3. Can be given to out patients.
4. Vitamin K acts as antidote.

Disadvantages

1. These drugs exert anticoagulant effect only in vivo.
2. Onset of action is delayed.
3. Monitoring of dose is more difficult than of heparin.
4. Toxicity of these drugs is difficult to treat.
5. Action is influenced by diet and other drugs.
6. **Cross placenta and cause foetal defects if taken in pregnancy.**

Adverse reactions

1. Haemorrhagic tendencies.
2. Urticaria, anorexia, vomiting and diarrhoea may occur in few patients.

Dicumarol and Bishydroxycoumarin: Long acting drugs (4–14 days). Action sets in 12–24 hours. Initial dose varies between 200–300 mg while the maintenance dose is 25–150 mg per day.

Ethyl Biscoumacetate: It is less potent than Bishydroxycoumarin. Peak effect is obtained in 18 to 30 hours. The effect lasts for 2 to 3 days.

Disadvantage: It is difficult to achieve steady state with this drug.

Warfarin Sodium: It is completely absorbed from the gut. Peak levels are reached in 2–12 hours. Action starts in 36 hours and lasts for 3 days. Dosage is individualised. It is not effective in vitro. It crosses placenta therefore should not be given in pregnancy.

Adverse reactions

1. Haemorrhage.
2. Alopecia (hair loss from scalp).

3. Urticaria and dermatitis.

4. Allergic reactions are common.

Advantages

1. It is completely absorbed.

2. It can also be given orally as well as parenterally.

3. Adverse reactions are less as compared to other drugs in this group.

Indandione Derivatives: **Phenindiones, diphenindione and chlorphenindione.** These drugs are toxic and therefore usually not used.

Uses of Anticoagulant Therapy

1. Venous thrombosis and pulmonary embolism.

2. Myocardial infarction: These drugs do not dissolve the clot responsible for myocardial infarction but are helpful in preventing the spread of clot. However, they are not found to be very useful in this condition. Drugs which inhibit platelet aggregation (low dose of salicylates) are highly effective.

3. These drugs prevent deep vein thrombosis in patients when they are bed ridden.

4. In rheumatic heart disease these drugs prevent emboli.

5. Disseminated intravascular coagulation: Heparin is found to be useful.

Following are the conditions in which these drugs should not be given:

1. Haemorrhagic tendencies.

2. In gastric ulcers.

3. In subacute bacterial endocarditis.

4. Threatened abortion.

5. In regional and lumbar block anesthesia.

6. Renal damage.

7. Hypertension.

Nursing care of the patient receiving oral anticoagulants

1. Prothrombin time is done before administration of these drugs and is then done repeatedly. The aim of the therapy is to depress the prothrombin content of the blood. Prothrombin time is maintained at two and a half times the normal.

2. Patients on long-term therapy are advised to attend hospital regularly and prothrombin time should be done on every visit.

3. Patients are informed about the dangers of these drugs (bleeding tendencies) and are instructed to approach hospital at the earliest in the event of bleeding (bleeding from gums, epistaxis, and haemoptysis, blood in stools).

4. Blood grouping of the patient should be done before starting therapy.

5. In the event of toxicity fresh blood should be immediately administered and drug completely withdrawn. Vitamin K oxide is injected.

6. Patient should be informed about drugs, which interact with anticoagulants and these should be avoided.

TREATMENT OF TOXICITY DUE TO ORAL ANTICOAGULANTS

1. Stop anticoagulant.
2. Give fresh blood.
3. Administer **vitamin K₃**.

ANTICOAGULANTS USED IN VITRO TO MAINTAIN BLOOD FLUIDITY

1. Oxalates and citrates. Citrate is used as anticoagulant for blood used for transfusion (0.38%).
2. Ethylenediaminetetra-acetic acid.
3. Hirudin
4. Heparin

DRUGS AFFECTING PLATELET AGGREGATION

1. Aspirin.
2. Dextran (both 40 and 70).
3. Sulfinpyrazone.
4. Dipyridamole

Aspirin

1. It irreversibly blocks ADP and PG mediated aggregation of the platelets.
2. Small doses (75 mg) are required.
3. It should be taken at the same time each day.

Uses

1. In arteriosclerosis
2. In all conditions associated with thrombus formation, e.g. prevention of coronary thrombosis, mitral stenosis and deep vein thrombosis.

Dipyridamole: Inhibits platelet and is used in coronary bypass surgery. It is used along with aspirin.

Sulfinpyrazone, Ticlopidine and Tranexamic Acid: Have similar effects like aspirin but are costly.

Uses of antiplatelet drugs

(a) Myocardial infarction—aspirin reduces reinfarction.
(b) Angina pectoris.
(c) Prosthetic heart valves.
(d) Cerebral thrombosis.

Adverse reactions

(a) Nausea, vomiting, diarrhea and giddiness.
(b) Thrombophlebitis at the site of injection.

Snake Venoms: Venoms of Russell Viper and Copperhead snakes decrease coagulability.

AGENTS USED TO CONTROL BLEEDING

Locally acting substances

1. **Thrombin powder** is used for skin grafts.

2. **Thromboplastin** is used in surgery

3. **Fibrin** — available as strips that can be cut according to size and used. Strip is dipped in thrombin and placed at bleeding area.

4. **Gelfoam:** It is applied on the surgical wound. It gets absorbed in 4–6 weeks. It is left in place after suturing of wound.

5. **Oxidised cellulose:** It is treated with nitrogen oxide before application. It gets absorbed in 2–10 days. It should not be applied on bony tissue as it interferes with regeneration of the bone.

6. **Adrenaline** (110000) is used in tooth sockets and nasal packs for treating bleeding from gums and epistaxis.

Fibrinogen: It is present in human plasma. On addition of thrombin it is converted to fibrin. It is combined with thrombin and applied locally. **For systemic effects it is given to patients of afibrinogenemia.**

Uses

(a) Applied to control bleeding when there is deficiency of fibrinogen.

(b) Disseminated intravascular coagulation.

AGENTS GIVEN SYSTEMATICALLY

1. Fibrinogen

2. Epsilon Aminocaproic Acid:
It reduces fibrinolytic activity. It inhibits activation of plasminogen. It is used in treatment of overdose of streptokinase or urokinase and in menorrhagias.

3. Antihemophilic Globulin (AHG):
It is freeze dried powder containing factor VIII. This is used in cases of patients of haemophilia A (this condition is associated with deficiency or absence of factor VIII). It is given intravenously. It produces allergy and is very expensive.

4. Human Factor IX Complex:
Contains coagulation factors II, VII, IX and X. It is useful in treating Christmas disease (haemophilia B) characterised by deficiency of factor IX. It is sometimes used to treat hemorrhagic disease of the newborn.

5. Plasma or Fresh Blood
These are given in:

(i) Toxicity due to oral anticoagulants.

(ii) In treating Christmas disease.

(iii) It is advisable to use concentrated solution of factors (isolated from blood) rather than whole blood as the latter increases blood volume and results in precipitation of congestive cardiac failure.

6. Vitamin K:
This is a fat soluble vitamin. It is of three types. K_1 is present in plants. K_2 is produced in intestine. Vitamin K_3 (menadione) is a synthetic preparation of this vitamin.

Vitamin K is required for the synthesis and release of certain coagulation factors (II, VII, IX and X). Deficiency of this vitamin results in deficiency of these factors. Deficiency of vitamin K is produced:

(i) During malabsorption syndrome.

(ii) By use of oral anticoagulants.

(iii) Bile duct obstruction and cirrhosis of liver.

Disadvantages

1. Onset of action is late (K_1 = 12 hrs; K_3 = 24 hrs) and in extensive bowel resection fresh blood or the coagulation factors must be administered to the patient to cover the duration before vitamin K_3 becomes effective.

2. Adverse reactions are manifested in the form of jaundice.

Uses

1. Vitamin K is indicated whenever bleeding is suspected because of its deficiency.

2. Hypoprothrombinemia in premature infants.

3. Hemolytic anemia.

4. Kernicterus in newborn.

7. Platelets are Transfused in Dengue

FIBRINOLYTIC AGENTS

Fibrinolysis is a process which is responsible for the dissolution of the clot in the body. Agents used to produce fibrinolysis are called fibrinolytic agents. These are used in coronary artery disease.

Fibrinolysin (Plasmin): It is obtained from human plasma.

Disadvantages

1. Can produce febrile attacks.

2. Can produce haemorrhages.

3. The action of the drug being nonspecific it can destroy other proteins also.

Streptokinase and Urokinase: These enzymes are obtained from beta haemolytic Streptococci and human urine respectively. These agents can lyse clots in human veins.

Adverse reactions

1. Allergic reactions.

2. Febrile reaction.

3. Haemorrhage from sutured wounds.

4. They have self-limiting effect as antibodies develop.

Venom of the Malaysian Pit Viper: It removes fibrinogen from blood.

Platelets are not affected. In 2–3 weeks the fibrinogen level returns to normal.

Advantage: It does not produce haemorrhagic tendencies.

Drugs Acting on Urinary Tract

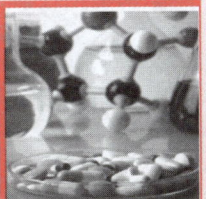

60

Drugs Acting on Urinary Tract

This chapter describes the mode of action and uses of **diuretics** and also deals with treatment of **urinary tract infections**.

DIURETICS

Diuretic is defined as a drug which brings about loss of sodium and water. These agents are used in diseases causing sodium and water retention leading to hypertension and oedema. Certain agents in common use such as tea and coffee produce diuresis.

Physiology of Urine Formation: Urine is an ultrafiltrate of plasma which is concentrated and modified by the renal tubule.

Fluid filters from the blood in the glomeruli across **Bowmen's capsule** into the lumen of the **proximal convoluted tubule**. This fluid contains the electrolytes of the plasma but is devoid of proteins and blood cells. Drugs increasing glomerular filtration rate (GFR) such as **digitalis, caffeine and aminophylline** increase urinary output.

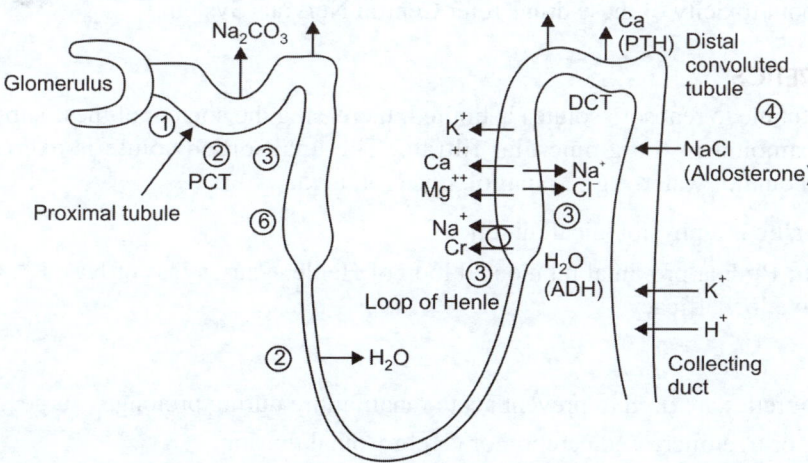

Diuretics: 1. Acetazolamide (C.A.I.), 2. Osmotic diuretics, 3. Loop diuretics (high ceiling), 4. Aldosterone antagonist, 5. ADH antagonist and 6. Thiazide.

In the proximal tubule large amount of water (80%) is reabsorbed along with active reabsorption of sodium, potassium chloride and bicarbonate. Uric acid and urea are partly reabsorbed while the reabsorption of glucose and amino acids is complete.

In the loop of Henle, sodium chloride and water are reabsorbed but hyperosmolarity of the tubular fluid is retained by counter current multiplier system in this area.

(a) **Descending limb:** Water is reabsorbed and fluid becomes hypertonic.

(b) **Ascending limb:** 25% of filtered Na^+ is reabsorbed due to active Na^+ K^+ Cl^- co-transport.

In the **distal tubule** sodium is reabsorbed actively and water absorption is facultative. K^+ is lost in the tubular fluid while absorbing Na^+. (Na^+ exchanges for K^+). Acidification of urine takes place here.

In **collecting tubule**, water is further reabsorbed under the influence of antidiuretic hormone and urine gets concentrated.

Diuretics: Diuretic drugs can produce their effect by one of the following mechanisms.

1. By increasing glomerular filtration rate, e.g. xanthines and digitalis.
2. By reducing reabsorption of water through osmotic action — osmotic diuretics, e.g. sodium chloride, glucose, mannitol, urea and glycerol.
3. By reducing absorption of sodium at the level of loop of Henle, e.g. furosemide, thiazides, ethacrynic acid and triamterene.
4. Drugs which antagonise the effect of aldosterone, e.g. spironolactone.
5. Miscellaneous — organic mercurials and carbonic anhydrase inhibitors.

Xanthines (caffeine, theophylline and theobromine) produce diuresis by:

(a) Increasing glomerular filtrate

(b) Inhibiting tubular reabsorption of sodium. Aminophylline is given intravenously for this purpose.

For details about toxicity of these drugs refer Central Nervous System.

OSMOTIC DIURETICS

Capacity of the tubule to reabsorb solutes is limited. Increasing the content of these substances in blood increases their amount in the glomerular filtrate. The unabsorbed solute is excreted along with proportionate amount of water, e.g.: Mannitol, glycerol, urea.

Sodium chloride is a physiological diuretic.

Site of action: Both at proximal tubule and loop of Henle. Causes loss of Na^+, K^+, Ca^{++}, Mg^{++}, Cl^- HCO_3^- PO_4^{2-}. Have low efficacy.

Uses

1. Osmotic diuretics are used to prevent acute renal failure during prolonged surgery or trauma.
2. To prevent or treat increased cerebral or cerebrospinal tension.
3. To treat glaucoma.

Glycerol is given by mouth just before eye surgery to decrease intraocular tension.

Advantages

1. It is very effective.
2. It is not metabolised in the body and acts on the tubule as well as loop of Henle.

Disadvantages

1. To be effective it has to be given in large doses.
2. It cannot be given in congestive cardiac failure or in conditions associated with sodium retention as it does not cause sodium loss.
3. It increases workload on the heart.

Uses

1. It is used in shock specially of hypovolemic type.
2. It is used in cases of barbiturate or other poisonings so as to increase the rate of excretion of these poisons.

Dose: 100 to 400 mg of 25% solution is given by slow intravenous infusion.

Urea: It has following disadvantages

1. It is less effective.
2. Has a bad odour and taste.

Uses: Intravenous infusion of 100–200 ml of 30% solution is used in cerebral oedema.

Glycerol and glucose are used for the same purposes.

Mannitol: It is administered intravenously.

Uses

1. For prevention or treatment of oliguric phase of acute renal failure.
2. For treating increased intracranial pressure in brain and spinal cord.
3. For reducing refractory intraocular hypertension.

Adverse reactions

1. It increases circulatory load and may precipitate congestive cardiac failure.
2. It may cause electrolyte imbalance.

THIAZIDES

Benzthiazide, chlorothiazide, hydrochlorothiazide, polythiazide, chlorthalidone. These act on ascending limb of loop of Henle. These are drugs which are chemically and pharmacologically related (benzothiadiazines) cause loss of Na^+, Cl^- and K^+ in urine.

Advantages

1. They are highly effective. Action begins in 2 hours.
2. They can be given orally as well as parenterally (for quick action).
3. Various drugs are available in this category with difference in their duration of action and dosage, therefore, selection of the appropriate drug is easier.
4. **On chronic use these agents lower blood pressure.**

These act on multiple sites on the renal tubule. They remain effective even in various kidney diseases.

Disadvantages

1. These drugs cause hyperglycemia and glycosuria (i.e. they precipitate diabetes mellitus).
2. Thiazides reduce excretion of uric acid and precipitate gout.
3. **These agents produce severe loss of K^+.**

Adverse reactions

1. Allergic reactions, e.g. thrombocytopenic purpura, dermatitis.
2. In renal or hepatic insufficiency these agents can produce renal as well as hepatic failure.
3. Loss of K^+ caused by thiazides can precipitate cardiac arrhythmias specially if given with digitalis.

Uses

1. In oedema due to:
   (a) Cardiac failure.
   (b) Nephrotic syndrome.
   (c) Liver cirrhosis.
   Chlorothiazide and hydrochlorothiazide are given twice a day in these conditions.
2. Hypertension—in mild cases these agents may be used alone while in moderate and severe hypertension these are added to other antihypertensive agents.
3. Premenstrual tension.
4. Nephrogenic diabetes insipidus.
5. In treatment of calcium stones in kidney.
6. Management of bromide toxicity.

Following drugs should not be given along with thiazides as they interact, e.g. allopurinol, ibuprofen, calcium carbonate and indomethacin.

Thiazides are not given in pre-eclampsia as they cause decrease in blood volume and compromise placental circulation.

Chlorthalidone: This drug has effects like thiazides but has longer duration of action and hypotensive effect is more marked.

Doses

Chlorothiazides	250–500 mg (1 g/day)
Hydrochlorothiazide	25–200 mg/day
Hydroflumethiazide	25–200 mg/day
Bendroflumethiazide	10 mg

All of the above drugs exert effect for 12 hours

Chlorthalidone	100 mg
Polythiazide	1 mg

These agents have long half-life should be given early morning

LOOP DIURETICS

Furosemide, bumetamide, ethacrymic acid and torsemide. These drugs inhibit absorption of Na^+, K^+, Cl^-, Ca^{++}, Mg^{++} and H_2O.

Furosemide (Frusemide): Chemically it resembles thiazides but it differs from them in the following respects.

(a) Has more rapid onset of action.
(b) Efficacy is more.
(c) **Continues to be effective in renal failure.**

After oral administration the action starts in 30 minutes, reaches a peak in 2 hours and is over in 6–8 hours. Intravenous injection of this drug produces immediate effect which lasts for about 2 hours.

Uses: This drug is employed in all the conditions in which thiazides are used and in addition it is used when:

(a) Thiazides have failed to show good effects.
(b) Immediate action is desired, e.g. in left ventricular failure, hepatic failure, nephrotic syndrome and renal failure.
(c) Hypercalcemia.
(d) Poisoning due to barbiturates, salicylates and other NSAIDS.
(e) Cerebral oedema.
(f) Hypertension.

Dose: 40 mg daily orally. In renal failure higher doses are used.

Adverse reactions

(a) Hyperuricemia
(b) Hypokalemia
(c) Hypocalcemia
(d) Hypomagnesemia.

Ethacrynic Acid: It has actions similar to frusemide but has even quicker onset of action.

Uses

1. In severe and refractory cardiac, hepatic or renal oedema.
2. Management of bromide toxicity.

Adverse reactions

1. Gastrointestinal symptoms such as anorexia, nausea and vomiting are produced.
2. Increases serum uric acid which can precipitate gout.
3. Produces K^+ loss.
4. All the reactions seen with thiazides are also seen with this drug.
5. On chronic use it can cause tinnitus and deafness.

Signs and symptoms of hypokalemia

1. **General effects:** muscle weakness (flabby muscles), speech changes, reflexes are reduced, breathing is shallow.
2. **Abdominal:** anorexia, vomiting and distension. Paralytic ileus may develop.

3. **Cardiovascular:** Cardiac arrhythmias, decreased intensity of heart sounds, weak pulse and decreased blood pressure, heart block and ventricular fibrillation in systole may develop. ECG shows — prolonged PR interval, depressed ST segment, flat or inverted T waves.

4. Hearing loss — sometimes permanent may occur with frusemide.

5. **Frusemide should be withdrawn in patient complaining of difficulty in hearing.**

Nursing care (thiazides and loop diuretics)

1. All diuretics should be given early morning. If given at night it will inconvenience the patient.

2. Brisk diuresis in the elderly (particularly in males with enlarged prostate) is associated with risk of precipitating urinary retention. This should be avoided.

3. Before giving lasix or thiazides parenterally, sensitivity test should be done as allergy is known to occur with these agents.

4. Body weight of the patient be checked. If drugs are effective there will be reduction in body weight.

5. Potassium depletion is common among patients using these drugs.

6. Diabetes is known to worsen. Blood sugar and urinary sugar should be done routinely.

7. Provide dietary potassium supplement with these drugs. Potassium chloride (0.6 g twice daily) in form of effervescent drink maybe given.

8. In in-door patients nurse should maintain input-output chart. This helps in regulating the dose and judging efficacy of therapy.

Pulse of these patients must be taken carefully. Increase in K^+ supplementation or withdrawal of frusemide maybe indicated if the nurse notices ectopic beats.

CARBONIC ANHYDRASE INHIBITORS

Acetazolamide and Ethoxazolamide:
Carbonic anhydrase enzyme is responsible for the formation of H ions in the renal tubule and $NaHCO_3^-$ reabsorption.

This drug inhibits carbonic anhydrase in kidney, eye and the central nervous system. It seems to be less effective against carbonic anhydrase of stomach and the pancreas. Acetazolamide by inhibiting this enzyme produces **loss of sodium, potassium, bicarbonate and water** in urine. It **reduces intraocular tension** and is useful in epilepsy.

Disadvantages

1. It is only a mild diuretic.

2. Action of this drug is self-limiting. This drug should therefore be used intermittently.

3. It causes metabolic acidosis, CNS depression and fatigue.

Advantages:
Lowers intraocular tension in glaucoma. Reduces cerebral congestion. It has antiepileptic effect.

Uses:
It is not preferred as a diuretic as better and safer drugs are available.

1. It can be used along with mercurial diuretics.

2. In glaucoma 0.5 g may be given as injection for immediate action.

3. In petitmal epilepsy 0.25 g of this drug is given twice or thrice daily.

Precautions: As it increases K$^+$ loss, serum K$^+$ level must be routinely done in these patients (specially in renal failure).

Dose: 100 mg twice daily.

Use: Same as for thiazides.

POTASSIUM SPARING DIURETICS

Spironolactone: It chemically resembles aldosterone (steroid).

Actions: It **antagonises the action of aldosterone** at the level of renal tubule. It increases sodium loss in the urine (diuretic effect) but reduces potassium loss. It **causes retention of K$^+$.**

Uses

1. It is used in cases of hyperaldosteronism (hepatic cirrhosis or ascites).
2. It is combined with frusemide, thiazide or ethacrynic acid to reduce potassium loss produced by these agents.

Adverse reactions

1. Skin rash.
2. Gastrointestinal symptoms.
3. Gynaecomastia (enlargement of breasts in male), menstrual irregularities.
4. Hyperkalemia.

Dose: 50–100 mg daily.

Triamterene: It has effects similar to spironolactone but it does not antagonise the effects of aldosterone.

Lowers glucose tolerance. Produces hyperkalemia and megaloblastic anemia.

Amiloride: Acts at the distal tubule causes excretion of Na$^+$, retention of K$^+$ and has long duration of action. It is given once a day. At higher doses it blocks Na$^+$ and Na$^+$ –Ca^{++} antiport and Na$^+$ pump.

Uses: It is given along with more potent diuretics that cause K$^+$ loss.

Adverse reactions

(a) Hyperkalemia
(b) Glucose intolerance in diabetic patients.

OTHER DRUGS PRODUCING DIURESIS

1. **Digitalis** produces diuresis by:
   (i) Improving cardiac output.
   (ii) Increasing kidney perfusion thereby kidney function is improved.
2. **Glucocorticoids** induce diuresis in patients of glomerulonephritis because anti-inflammatory activity of these agents improves glomerular functions.

Clinical conditions and diuretic agent of choice

1. Congestive cardiac failure   Loop diuretics, **thiazides can worsen cardiac conditions due to hypokalemia**. This should be prevented

2. Kidney diseases   Loop diuretics can be given cautiously. Avoid K^+ sparing diuretics and acetazolamide.

3. Cirrhosis   Spironolactone or loop diuretic with K^+ sparing diuretic are prefered.

DRUGS USED IN DIABETES INSIPIDUS

1. **Antidiuretic hormone** (for details please refer Endocrinology).
2. **Benzthiazides.**These drugs are known to produce diuresis, but in cases of diabetes insipidus they tend to produce anti-diuretic action. This is probably achieved through lowering of glomerular filtration rate.

Chlorpropamide: It is orally acting hypoglycemic agent. It is useful in diabetes insipidus (but not of renal origin). 250 mg is given once a day.

Uses

1. Idiopathic diabetes insipidus.
2. Nephrogenic diabetes insipidus.

DRUGS PRODUCING RENAL TOXICITY

(a) Antibiotics: Tetracyclines, aminoglycosides and long acting sulphonamides.
(b) Heavy metals: Arsenic, bismuth, gold and iodides.
(c) Miscellaneous: Phenacetin, phenylbutazone, methysergide, antineoplastic drugs and corticosteroids.

URINARY TRACT INFECTIONS AND THEIR TREATMENT

Urinary tract infections are common in all age groups. **Females are more prone** to these infections than males. Congenital anomalies of the urinary tract and obstructive lesions (stones) predispose to repeated infections in this area. Acute infection of lower part of urinary tract — urethra and bladder produces:

(a) increased frequency of urination

(b) urgency of micturition

(c) painful urination

(d) pain in the perineum.

Urine in this condition is full of pus cells. Chronic urinary tract infections produce:

(a) Loss of body weight

(b) Generalized ill health, fever

(c) Hypertension

(d) Renal failure may occur.

Urine is full of bacteria as well as pus cells. Following organisms are usually responsible for urinary tract infections.

(a) *E. coli* (commonest)

(b) *Proteus mirabilis* (second commonest)

   (c) *Klebsiella*

   (d) *Aerobacter*

   (e) *Pseudomonas aeruginosa*

   (f) *Enterococci*

   (g) *Streptococci* and *Staphylococci*.

In chronic cases infection is caused by more than one organism and **mixed infections are difficult to treat.**

Nursing care

1. Collection of urine for investigations: Urine for microbiological investigation is collected either by midstream technique or through suprapubic bladder puncture. For midstream technique patient is instructed to void off initial urine, then pass the midstream urine into a sterile bottle and the remaining urine can be voided.
2. Urine sample should be sent for culture as well as sensitivity. In practice it is seen that most of the bacteria responsible for causing urinary tract infections are resistant to various drugs. It is therefore, essential to get sensitivity of the bacteria done.

   It is equally important to remember that sensitivity of the bacteria (done in vitro) may not correlate with in vivo response.
3. Catheterisation should be avoided as it helps in spread of infections.
4. Urine normally contains bacteria and therefore a value of over 1,00,000 organisms per ml of urine alone is termed significant.
5. Sample of urine should be sent for pH estimation.

DRUG TREATMENT OF URINARY TRACT INFECTIONS

Sulphonamides: Sulphasomidine (elkosin) and sulphamethazine are usually used.

Advantages

1. These drugs are effective against most of the organisms in urinary tract infections specially— *E. coli* and *Proteus* and these are present in high concentrations in urine.
2. Are cheap and can be given orally.
3. They are safe.
4. Sodium bicarbonate is given along with sulphonamides. This increases efficacy as well as safety of sulphonamides.
5. Fluids should be given in excess. This reduces crystal formation and also dilutes infectious organisms in urine.

Disadvantages

1. Not effective in mixed and chronic infections.
2. Dose: 2.0 g initially followed by 1.0 g every 6 hours for 10–14 days.

Cotrimoxazole: It is effective against ***E. coli* and *Proteus***, but not against *Pseudomonas*.

Adverse reactions

1. Chills, fever, cough and chest pain.
2. Pulmonary infiltration, pleural effusion with eosinophilia.

These are completely reversible if treatment is of short duration. Long-term treatment produces permanent interstitial pneumonitis and pulmonary fibrosis.

3. Peripheral neuropathy in patients with impaired renal function.

Ampicillin: This is a very useful drug as it is effective against many bacteria, e.g. *E. coli*, *Aerobacter* and *Proteus*. It is not effective against *Pseudomonas*. It can be used to treat UTI in pregnancy.

E. coli has gradually become resistant to this drug and there is greater relapse rate. (for details please refer to Chemotherapy.)

Cloxacillin and Methicillin: Used when infection is due to penicillinase producing Staphylococci.

Carbenecillin; piperacillin or ticarcillin are used in *Pseudomonas* infections.

Tetracyclines: These drugs are effective against most of the bacteria invading urinary tract. They are ineffective against *Proteus* and *Pseudomonas*. These drugs should not be given to patients with imparied renal functions or during pregnancy.

Not preferred as many organisms have developed resistance. These drugs can be combined in sequential order with sulfonamides or nitrofurantoin.

Fluoroquinolones: **Are highly effective.** Are useful even if renal function is subnormal.

Norfloxacin and **ciprofloxacin** are often used.

Use should be restricted to non-responders to other drugs as resistance develops.

Nitrofurantoin

1. It is used in cases resistant to other drugs.
2. Useful in cases of mixed infections.
3. It is effective in UTI but not in systemic infections. It is urinary antiseptic. It is used prophylactically as well as for long-term suppressive therapy.

Precautions

1. It should not be given if kidney function is poor (creatinine clearance below 20 ml per minute).
2. It should not be given along either with nalidixic acid or oxolinic acid.

Aminoglycoside Antibiotics (Streptomycin, Kanamycin and Gentamicin): These drugs are effective against **gram-negative bacilli,** *E. coli* and *Proteus*. **Gentamicin** is the drug of choice for *Pseudomonas* infection.

Precautions

1. Care should be exercised in giving these drugs in renal failure. They cause kidney damage.
2. Urine should be made alkaline as it enhances its antibacterial activity.
3. Few of the adverse reactions are irreversible (hearing loss and renal damage), these should be prevented by early detection.

Hence used in complicated cases only.

Methenamine Mandelate: It is highly effective against gram-negative organisms and *C. albicans*. Formaldehyde is released in acidic urine which exerts antiseptic effect. The efficacy is improved by maintaining the urine on the acidic side (pH less than 5). It is effective against most common pathogens except *Proteus* and *Pseudomonas*.

Advantages

1. Adverse reactions are not common.
2. Bacteria do not develop resistance to it.
3. It is useful in chronic infections.

Disadvantages

1. It is not effective in treating infections of the upper part of urinary tract.
2. Gastric upsets are common.

Precautions

1. It should not be given along with sulfamethiazole (forms insoluble precipitate with formaldehyde).
2. Urine must be made acidic by giving ammonium chloride or other acidifying salts.

Nalidixic Acid: It is a toxic drug and is used only in patients not responding to commonly employed drugs and the microbes infecting urinary tract are sensitive to this drug.

Dose: 1 g 4 times a day for 10–14 days.

Cycloserine: It is highly effective against *E. coli* infections. Its action does not depend on pH of urine.

Dose: 50 mg/day.

Precaution: This drug should not be used in patients with poor renal function.

Cephalosporins: These agents are of special value in cases of infections with penicillin resistant *Staphylococci*, *E. coli*, and *Proteus* resistant to other antibiotics.

They are given in septicemia due to urinary tract infections.

Polymyxin B: It is given to treat resistant strains of *Pseudomonas* infection. Cycloserine is effective against coliforms and *Proteus*.

ANTIMICROBIAL ACTIVITY AND URINARY pH

The activity of certain antimicrobial agents is affected by urinary pH. A few antimicrobials act better in **acidic medium,** e.g. **nitrofurantoin, methicillin, tetracycline, methenamine**.

A few antimicrobials act better in **alkaline medium — sulphonamides, aminoglycosides, flouroquinolones, cephalosporins.**

Drugs used for alkalinisation of urine.

Potassium citrate, sodium citrate, sodium bicarbonate, sodium acetate and acetazolamide.

Mixture of potassium citrate and sodium bicarbonate (2 g of each) is given 3–4 times a day. This mixture has the advantage that it is simple effective and cheap but has a bad taste. Therefore, it should be given with fruit juice.

Advantage of alkalinisation

1. It prevents burning micturition.
2. It improves the antibacterial activity of certain drugs, e.g. sulphonamides and aminoglycosides.
3. It reduces the risk of crystal formation in patients receiving sulphonamides because sulphonamides completely dissolve in alkaline urine but tend to form crystals in acidic urine.

Drugs used for Acidification of Urine: Ascorbic acid, ammonium chloride, calcium chloride.

Phenazopyridine is given to relieve pain and reduce urgency, frequency and burning of micturition. **It changes the colour of the urine to red.** Patient should be informed about this feature of the drug.

Nursing care in patients of urinary tract infections

1. Nurse should watch for the appearance of adverse drug reactions. In case of nephrotoxic drugs (aminoglycosides) input output chart should be maintained. Renal functions tests should be done routinely.
2. Patient should be instructed to take large volumes of fluid as
   (a) Large urinary volume dilutes such drugs which otherwise can form crystals and form stones in the kidney and urinary tract, e.g. sulphonamides.
   (b) At least 3 liters of fluids/day must be given to these patients.
   (c) Dehydration usually occurs in febrile patients. Excess of fluids correct this dehydration.
3. Drugs must be used in proper dosage and for adequate period.
4. The last dose of the drug should be given after instructing the patient to empty his bladder.
5. Urinary pH should be adjusted to suit the antibiotic. Nurses should administer the acidifying and alkalinising salts accordingly.

Prevention of development of urinary tract infections

1. Catheterisation should be avoided as far as possible. If needed, it should be done under complete aseptic conditions.
2. Prophylactic antibiotics should be started in following conditions.
   (a) Following instrumentation of urinary tract.
   (b) With indwelling catheter.

61

Drugs Affecting Uterine Motility

The motility of uterus is important during pregnancy. Sedate uterus is needed during pregnancy but at the time of delivery increase in uterine tone and motility are desired.

DRUGS INCREASING UTERINE MOTILITY (OXYTOCIC OR ECBOLIC AGENTS)

Oxytocin
Ergometrine
Prostaglandins

Oxytocin: It is a natural hormone of the posterior pituitary. The release of this hormone is increased by coitus, suckling and at birth of the child.

Actions

(a) Stimulates both frequency and intensity of uterine contractions. As the gestation progresses sensitivity of uterus is increased to oxytocic effect.
(b) Contractions of myoepithelial cells in the breast result in ejection of milk.
(c) In doses that are used to induce labour it causes fall in blood pressure.
(d) Large doses produce retention of Na^+ and hypertension.
(e) Has anti-diuretic effect.

Uses

1. Induction of labour—5 units in 500 ml of 5% dextrose solution. Start with 0.1–0.2 ml of solution/min and increase to maximum of 2.0 ml/min.
2. Uterine inertia.
3. To control postpartum haemorrhage: 2–5 unit IM or SC **after placenta is delivered**.
4. Abortion during 2nd trimester.

Ergot Alkaloids: Are derived from fungus — *Claviceps purpurea*.

This fungus has several alkaloids:
(a) Ergotoxine (mixture of ergocristine, ergokryptine and ergocornine)
(b) Ergotamine (used in migraine)
(c) Ergometrine

311

Ergometrine: Though all the alkaloids stimulate uterus, **ergometrine** is preferred as it has greater specificity and is less toxic.

Actions

(a) Produces spasmodic contractions of the uterus without any in between relaxation.
(b) Unlike oxytocin it contracts cervical segment of the uterus. If given during pregnancy this can result in rupture of uterus and fetal death.

This is therefore **not used to induce labour** but is used to prevent and **control postpartum bleeding**. It is used in cases of incomplete abortion.

Methyl ergometine maleate, a semisynthetic preparation, is also used for same effects.

Uses

1. To control postpartum haemorrhage.
2. To cause uterine involution.

Prostaglandins: PGE_2, PGF_{2a} and semisynthetic derivative — 15-methyl PGF_{2a} (carboprost) are used in obstetric practice.

Actions: Stimulates uterine muscle causing contraction.

Sensitivity of uterus to prostaglandins increases as the gestation progresses.
Motility of the uterus is increased.
Local application on cervix causes ripening of cervix.

Adverse drug reactions

Vomiting
Fever
Diarrhoea
Should be used with caution in patients with increased intraocular pressure, hypertension, angina, epilepsy and diabetes mellitus.

Uses

(a) Carboprost (15-methyl PGF_{2a}) is used as abortifacient during second trimester.
(b) For induction of labour in patients not responding to oxytocin.
(c) Local application on cervix for producing ripening of cervix.

Not to be used in asthmatics.

Nursing care

1. Before using **oxytocin** — cephalopelvic disproportion should be ruled out.
2. Oxytocin should not be given to patients with placenta previa, malpresentation and those with uterine scars.
3. Doses should be regularised by monitoring fetal heart rate.
4. Smoking and alcohol should be avoided during use of **prostaglandin** and for 48 hours afterwards.
5. Carboprost should be stored at 2–4°C.
6. Signs of uterine hypertoxicity to foetal distress should be watched for.

UTERINE RELAXANTS (TOCOLYTICS)

1. CNS sedatives — diazepam and barbiturates are used to sedate uterus.
2. 20% **magnesium sulphate** IV is used to control fits and sedate uterus during eclampsia.
3. Calcium channel blockers such as **nifedipine** (sublingual).
4. Beta agonists — **ritodrine, salbutamol, nylindrine** and **isoxsuprine.**
5. Inhibitors of prostaglandin synthesis, e.g. **indomethacin**. It has the disadvantage of causing fluid retention and early closure of ductus arteriosus.
6. Antagonists of oxytocin — such as **atosiban**.
7. **Progesterone** — it can prevent preterm labour but is not effective if labour has already started.

Atosiban: Inhibits uncomplicated prematured labour and is used between 24 and 33 weeks of gestation. Dose is 6.75 mg given IV over 1 minute for 4–8 hours.

Ritodrine is used IV (50 mcg/min) and dose is increased every 20 minutes till uterine relaxation is obtained and then maintained for 60 minutes followed by reduction in dose.

Magnesium sulphate is given IV (4–6 gm loading dose) followed by 2–4 gm hourly by infusion for total period of 24 hours. It is used if adrenergic β_2 agonists are contraindicated.

Uses of tocolytics

1. To delay premature labour.
2. In threatened abortion.
3. Dysmenorrhoea.

Nursing care

1. Adrenergic β_2 **agonists** given IV can produce fatal pulmonary oedema, hence these should be administered in minimum fluid volume.
2. These are contraindicated in pre-eclampsia, intrauterine death and antepartum haemorrhage.

Uses of uterine relaxants

(a) Prevention of preterm labour and threatened abortion.
(b) To treat dysmenorrhea.

Section
XI

Chemotherapy

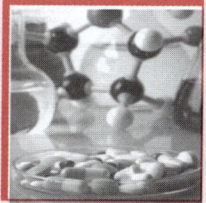

62

Chemotherapy

Chemotherapeutic agent is a chemically synthesised substance which either kills or inhibits the growth of microorgnisms (bacteria and viruses). An **antibiotic** is a substance which is derived from a living organism which antagonises the growth or life of other microorganims (bacteria or fungi).

Chemotherapy includes **anitbacterial, antiviral, antifungal and antihelmintic drugs**.

HISTORY

Use of cinchona bark in malaria was known even during 17th century. Ehrlich tried treating syphilis with certain chemicals. Introduction of penicillin (first antibiotic) however brought in a new era.

Some of the antibiotics which were originally obtained from microorganims are now synthesised, e.g. **chloramphenicol**.

Semisynthetic drugs are available which have more desirable qualities than the natural product, e.g. **ampicillin, cephaloridine,** etc.

A **bacteriocidal** agent kills bacteria, e.g. **penicillin** and **streptomycin**.

A **bacteriostatic** agent does not kill but stops further multiplication of bacteria, e.g. **sulphonamides** and **tetracyclines**. Once the bacteriostatic drugs have produced their effect these microorganisms get cleared by the defence—mechanisms of the body.

None of the antibiotics or chemotherapeutic agents is of value in the absence of polymorphs. That is why agranulocytosis is an extremely dangerous and often fatal condition.

Selection of the antimicrobial drug depends upon the

(a) Nature and type of the infecting organism.

(b) State of health or otherwise of the patient including his sensitivity (allergy) to these agents.

(c) Availability and cost of drug.

In theory, it may seem that bacteriocidal drugs are better but in practice there is not much difference except in severe acute infections.

Mode of action of antimicrobials

These drugs act in one of the following ways:

1. Interference with the **synthesis of cell wall of microbes,** e.g. pencillin, cephalosporins, bacitracin, vancomycin and cycloserine.

317

2. **Damage the membrane** inside the cell wall so that cell membrane no longer acts as an effcient barrier, e.g. **Polymyxins, colistin and polyene antibiotics**.

3. **Interference with protein synthesis** in the microbe, e.g. **aminoglycosides, tetracyclines, chloramphenicol, macrolide antibiotics and lincomycin**.

4. Interference with genetic information (on the ribsome), e.g. **rifampicin**.

5. Interference with metabolism of the microbe, e.g. sulfonamides, sulfones, para-aminosalicylic acid, ethambutol and trimethoprim.

6. Drugs acting by inhibiting gyrase, e.g. **quinolones**.

Advantages of combination of these drugs

1. To obtain greater efficacy, e.g. pencillin plus gentamicin in treatment of enterococcal endocarditis.
2. To delay the development of resistance, e.g. in treatment of tuberculosis, leprosy and HIV.
3. To enlarge the scope of their activity (that is to widen the spectrum), e.g. mixed infections.
4. To reduce severity and incidence of adverse reactions.

Duration of therapy

1. Too short a therapy fails to completely remove the infection. It may recur.
2. Too long a therapy produces adverse reactions and increases cost hence the **duration of therapy should be appropriate to degree of infections.**

Resistance: Experimentally the sensitivity of the microbe to a chemotherapeutic agent is expressed in terms of the minimum inhibitory concentration (MIC) determined in vitro in a test tube. Clinically however, this may be different. Organism is said to be resistant when it cannot be removed by the highest recommended doses of the drug.

Microbes can become resistant by one of the following means:

(i) Through mutation.

(ii) Microbes develop enzymes which destroy antibiotic, e.g. pencillinase which destroys pencillin, chloramphenicol acetyl transferase destroys chloramphenicol.

(iii) Microbes learn to grow in the presence of antibiotic, e.g. certain streptomycin dependent strains.

(iv) Microbes develop alternate path of metabolism.

(v) Bacteria may lose affinity for antimicrobial agent and penetration may be affected.

Cross resistance: An organism which has developed resistance to one chemotherapeutic agent automatically exhibits resistance towards chemically related other drugs, e.g. organisms resistant to erythromycin are often resistant to oleandomycin.

Precautions to be taken to inhibit development of resistance strains

1. Use proper agents in proper dosage for adequate duration.
2. Two or more agents can be combined, e.g. in tuberculosis.
3. Avoid indiscriminate use of these drugs.

CHEMOPROPHYLAXIS

This deals with use of agents for prevention of the disease. This is used in following conditions:

(a) Used before or after instrumentation of the urinary tract.

(b) Preoperatively in abdominal surgery.

(c) In suspected cases of rheumatic fever.

(d) In contacts of patients of tuberculosis and leprosy.

(e) In animal bites, e.g. rabies vaccination after dog bite, snake antivenom after snake bite.

(f) In malaria.

(g) After tooth extraction.

(h) For prevention of acute on chronic infection, e.g. bronchitis, cystic fibrosis, etc.

(i) During epidemics of dysentery, meningococcal meningitis.

(j) For syphilis and gonorrhoea after contact.

Precautions in the use of chemotherapeutic agents

No drug is without risk — chemotherapeutic agents are no exception. Following risks are inherent in their use.

(a) All antibiotics and chemotherapeutic agents can lead to **allergic reactions**.

(b) The misuse of these agents produces **resistant strains** of microbes that are difficult to treat.

(c) These drugs not only kill pathogenic microbes but also those which synthesise folic acid and vitamin K. Their use can therefore produce:

 (i) Deficiency of these vitamins.

 (ii) Lead to development of **superinfections.**

(d) Given during pregnancy many of these agents produce foetal damage.

(e) Few of them produce serious adverse reactions (aplastic anaemia, renal damage, hepatic damage, loss of hearing and vision) which may be irreversible in nature. Hence, their indiscriminate use can cure one illness and may produce another serious disease.

To avoid the above hazards, these drugs should be handled with great care.

1. Antimicrobial agent and its dose should be selected with great care.

 (a) Disease and the offending organism should be identified.

 (b) Severity of the disease should be taken in view.

 (c) General condition of the patient — status of health, function of kidneys and liver should all be considered.

 (d) Sensitivity of the offending microbe decides the selection of the drug.

 (e) In our country cost of the product and cost of total treatment should also be considered.

2. Dose of the antibiotic should be appropriate. This is determined by taking into account:

 (a) age of the patient,

 (b) functions of liver and kidney, and

 (c) severity of the disease.

3. **Dose schedule should be strictly adhered to**.

4. Combinations of antibiotics should not be encouraged except when the situation demands.

5. Chemotherapeutic agent should be given by **appropriate route**.

6. Fixed dose combinations should be discouraged except in cotrimoxazole.

The collection of samples for bacteriological examination. Collect the infected material (pus from wound, cerebrospinal fluid, sputum and urine) before starting the treatment and send it to the bacteriological laboratory. These samples are then used to culture the infecting organism. Offending organisms are identified.

Sensitivity test is done by growing these organisms in a culture plate in presence of antibiotic. Resistant microbes continue to grow, those bacteria which are sensitive fail to grow.

Nurse is responsible for collection of infected material

Following care has to be exercised:
- (a) Sterile container is not mishandled before use.
- (b) Samples should not get contaminated.
- (c) Sample for culture and sensitivity should reach the laboratory at the earliest. If the sample cannot be transported immediately it should be preserved at 37°C.

63

Sulphonamides

They were discovered while working on dyes for killing bacteria, and introduced in clinical practice in 1935. These dyes however were toxic. Hence, search was made for safer dyes. This search brought out *prontosil rubrum* into the forefront. This compound gave birth to sulphonamides.

These are bacteriostatic and are effective against bacteria that form folic acid.

There are many varieties of sulphonamides now available. They are classified as follows:

1. Those which are used for treating systemic infections (according to duration of action).
   (a) Long acting (half life 30–40 hrs): Well absorbed—sulfamethoxypyridazine, sulfadimethoxine and sulfamethopyrazine (given once a week), sulfadoxine (half life 8 days).
   (b) Intermediate acting (8–16 hrs): Sulfamethoxazole and sulfaphenazole.
   (c) Short acting (4–8 hrs): Well absorbed and rapidly excreted (most important group)— sulfadiazine, sulfadimidine, sulfamerazine, sulfanilamide, sulfasomidine, sulfamethiazole and sulfafurazole.
2. Sulphonamides used for their local action on GIT. These are poorly absorbed from gastrointestinal tract, e.g. sulfaguanidine, succinylsulfathiazole, phthalylsulfathiazole and sulfapyridine.
3. Locally acting on skin: Silver sulphadiazine and magenide (on burns).
5. Sulphonamides with special uses:
   (a) Sulfasalazine in ulcerative colitis.
   (b) Sulfapyridine in dermatitis herpetiformis.
   (c) Sulphacetamide as eye lotion.
   (d) Mefenide in burns.

Actions

These drugs act by inhibiting the conversion of para-aminobenzoic acid to folic acid that is needed for normal metabolism of the microbes.

Site of action of sulphonamides

$$PABA \longrightarrow Folic\ acid \longrightarrow Folinic\ acid$$

Sulphonamides inhibit the multiplication of following groups of microbes:

— Chlamydia
— *Streptococci, Staphylococci, Gonococci, Pneumococci. Meningococci, Bacillus anthracis, H. influenzae, Vibrio cholera, E. coli, C. diphtheriae, P. pestis, C. welchii.*

— *Actinomycetes*, *Toxoplasma* and *Nocardia*. Viruses of trachoma, Lymphogranualoma inguinale, Psittacosis and Ornithosis.

Microbes now resistant to sulphonamides are *Staphylococci*, *Streptococci*, *Pneumococci* and *E. coli*.

Action of sulphonamides is improved when combined with trimethoprim.

Factors reducing the efficacy of sulfonamides

1. Presence of para-aminobenzoic acid at site of action.
2. Presence of pus and necrotic material.
3. Drugs such as procaine, amethocaine and procainamide.

Sulphonamides are metabolised in the liver and excreted through the kidney. The metabolite of sulfonamides (acetylated compound) tends to form crystals in the acidic urine. Administration of alkali further increases absorption and reduces development of crystal formation.

Sulfisoxazole and sulfisomidine are soluble in alkaline urine hence used for treating urinary tract infections.

Adverse reactions

1. Allergic symptoms may be produced.
2. Anorexia, nausea and occasionally vomiting.
3. Crystalluria and haematuria.
4. **In patients who are deficient in G6PD enzyme, these drugs cause haemolysis.**

Drug interactions

In premature babies these agents produce kernicterus.

Sulfadiazine: It is less acetylated, 20% is excreted in urine as such. In meningococcal meningitis it can also be given intravenously.

Dose: 2 g initially, followed by 1 g 6 hourly.

IV dose 100 mg/kg in saline. Total dose is injected in 5 minutes.

Sulfasomidine

Advantages

1. This drug is excreted in urine in an active form.
2. Does not form crystals in urine
3. Action of this drug does not depend on pH of urine. Hence, it is preferred in urinary tract infections.

Sulfisoxazole

Advantages

It is tasteless and can be given to children. Dose of all the above drugs is same as sulfadiazine.

Sulfamethoxazole: It is combined with trimethoprim because the half-life of this drug is similar to half-life of trimethoprim.

Dose: 1–2 g initially followed by 1 g every 8–12 hourly.

Sulfacetamide: 20% solution of this drug does not irritate conjunctiva. It is used as eye drops.

Sulfamethoxypyridine and Sulfadimethoxine: Both these drugs are used for treating infections of urinary tract and for prophylaxis. Dose: 1 g initially and 0.5 g once a day.

Sulfadoxine: **It has half-life of 7 days.** It is therefore, employed for single dose treatment of urinary tract infections and prophylaxis.

Succinylsulfathiazole and Phthalylsulfathiazole: These are not absorbed when given orally, and are used to treat bacillary dysentery.

Dose of succinylsulfathiazole is 0.25 g/kg per day.
Dose of phthalylsulfathiazole is 125 mg/kg/day.

Sulfasalazine: It is used to treat ulcerative colitis. Relapses occur in 33% of cases. Also found effective in regional enteritis and granulomatous colitis.

Mafenide: To prevent bacterial growth it is applied locally on burns.

Silver sulfadiazine—1% cream is used in burns and is effective against many common bacteria.

Uses of sulfonamides

1. Meningococcal meningitis (sulfonamides are given intravenously in this condition).
2. Bacillary dysentery.
3. Urinary tract infections.
4. Trachoma—sulfacetamide eye drops are used during day and ointment at night. In severe infections tetracyclines can be combined with this drug.
5. Plague.
6. To treat certain venereal diseases, e.g. *H. ducreyi*.
7. These drugs are used for prophylaxis of:
   (i) Rheumatic fever in children who are sensitive to penicillin.
   (ii) Bacillary dysentery.
   (iii) Meningococcal infections during epidemic.

Precautions to be taken

1. Before giving these drugs find out whether patient is allergic to it or not. Stop the drug if allergy develops.
2. Whether the bacteria is sensitive to this drug or not. *E. coli* and Meningococci are usually sensitive.
3. **Should not be given during the last months of pregnancy.**
4. Advise your patient to take high fluid intake (3 litres per day).
5. Give sodium bicarbonate to make urine alkaline.
6. These drugs should be given after meals.

Adverse reactions

1. Allergy, drug fever, skin rash and eosinophilia. Conjunctivitis is common. In severe form of allergy serum sickness and leucopenia may occur.
2. Nausea and vomiting.

3. Renal toxicity: Crystalurea may occur.

4. Methemoglobinemia in patients with G6PD deficiency. Jaundice in newborn.

5. CNS: ataxia, tinnitus.

COTRIMOXAZOLE

This is a combination of sulfamethoxazole (400 mg) with trimethoprim (80 mg). Trimethoprim inhibits the conversion of folic acid to folinic acid.

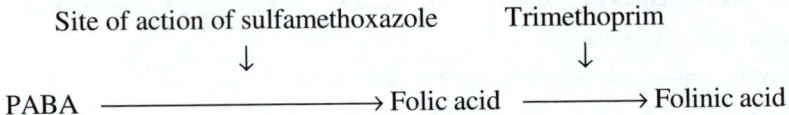

Sulphamethoxazole and trimethoprim have nearly same half-lives.

Advantages

1. The combination of these two drugs makes the product bactericidal and broad spectrum and relatively safe.

2. Microbes not sensitive to either sulfonamides or trimethoprim are killed by this combination.

3. It is cost effective.

5. Development of resistance is slow.

6. **Adequate concentrations reach CSF**.

Cotrimoxazole is effective against *Haemophilus*, *Proteus*, *E. coli*, *Neisseria*, *Salmonella*, *Shigella*, *Streptococcus and Staphylococcus*.

Pseudomonas however is resistant to this drug.

Adverse reactions: Same as with sulfonamides.

In addition megaloblastic anaemia is produced. This is treated by giving folinic acid.

Uses

1. For treatment of urinary tract infections due to *Shigella*, *E. coli* and *Proteus*.

2. For treatment of respiratory tract infections (bronchitis, sinusitis otitis media).

3. For treating gonorrhoea and typhoid.

4. Prostitis.

Dose: 2 tablets given every 12 hours.

Intravenous and intramuscular preparations are also available. Treatment should be continued for 14 days.

Other combinations available are:

(a) Trimethoprim 80 mg with 400 mg of sulfamethoxazole.

(b) 90 mg of trimethoprim with 410 mg of sulfadiazine, one tablet a day is sufficient in urinary tract infections.

Precautions: This drug should not be used in

(a) Infants under 2 months of age.

(b) During pregnancy.

(c) During nursing period.

Nursing care

1. IV route should not be employed in cardiac and renal patients.
2. Paediatric preparations (tablets and suspensions) contain 2 mg of trimethoprim and 100 mg of sulfamethoxazole and should be differentiated from adult preparations.
3. If creatinine clearance falls below 30 ml/min once a day treatment suffices. It should be avoided if creatinine clearance is less than 15 ml/min.

Uses of combination of sulphonamide with other antimicrobial agents.

Sulpha	Combination with	Use
Sulfadiazine	Chloramphenicol	*H. influenzae*
Sulfadiazine	Streptomycin	*H. influenzae*
Sulfadiazine	Penicillin	*Actinomycosis*
Sulfadiazine	Penicillin	*Anthrax*
Sulfadiazine	Trimethoprim	(a) *E. coli*, *Proteus* (in urinary tract infections)
		(b) Upper respiratory tract infections
		(c) GI infections — cholera, enteric fever and Shigellosis
		(d) *P. falciparum* and *P. vivax*
		(e) *H. influenzae*
		(f) Gonorrhoea

64

Penicillins

Penicillin is produced by *Penicillin notatum* and *P. chrysogenum.* It was introduced in clinical practice in 1941. In 1957 semisynthetic pencillins were developed. Penicillins available differ in bacterial activity.

Penicillins are classified as follow:

(a) **Narrow spectrum penicillins:** Benzylpenicillin, phenoxymethyl penicillin, phenothicillin and propicillin.

(b) **Broad specturm penicillins:** Ampicillin, amoxicillin, becampicillin, pivampicillin, hetacillin and carbenicillin.

(c) **Pencillinase resistant pencillins:** Methicillin, oxacillin, cloxacillin, dicloxacillin and naficillin.

These are used against organisms which are resistant to pencillin. Resistant microbes generate an enzyme (penicillinase) which destroys penicillin.

(d) **Anti Pseudomonas penicillins:** Carbenicillin, carbenicillin indanyl, ticarcillin, ureido penicillins (azlocillin, mezlocillin, piperacillin).

Penicillins act by interfering with synthesis of peptidoglycan layer of the cell wall which normally protects the bacteria from its environment. Due to differences in the osmotic pressure the bacterial cell swells and explodes.

Penicillin has **no action against resting organisms**.

Microbes sensitive to penicillins

Streptococcus beta haemolyticus, Pneumococci, Meningcocci, *C. diphtheriae, B. anthracis, Clostridium tetani, Clostridium welchii* and *T. pallidum. Actinomyces bovis* and *Nocardia.*

Less sensitive organisms: Gonococci, Streptococci alpha haemolyticus and strep viridans.

Benzylpenicillin (Penicillin G): Crystalline penicillin.

Actions

(a) Highly active against gram-positive organisms and gram-negative *Neisseria* and *Treponema pallidum* undergoing rapid multiplication.

(b) It is **acid labile** hence cannot be given orally.

(c) It is destroyed by organisms producing penicillinase (β-lactamase).

(d) Quick onset but short duration of action.

(e) It is widely distributed.

(f) Probenecid prolongs its duration of action.

Advantages: **Is best for quick results in cases suffering from penicillin sensitive microbial infections.**

Adverse reactions of penicillins

1. **Allergic reactions:** These are very common. Skin rash, drug fever, urticaria and even angioneurotic oedema may develop. **Sensitivity test should be done before administering penicillins.**

2. **Acute anaphylatic shock** is often noticed, which needs immediate attention. Intravenous adrenaline with steroids and antihistaminics have to be given immediately to save life of an individual.

3. **Local irritation at site of injection**

   (a) It produces pain at the site of injection.

   (b) When given intravenously it may produce thrombophlebitis.

   (c) When given intrathecally it may produce aseptic meningitis.

   (d) On oral administration it produces nausea and vomiting.

   (e) Jerish-Heximer reaction (occurs 12–72 hours. after injection)—fever, lymphadenopathy.

Development of resistance is due to

(a) Development of penicillinase, e.g. Staphylococci, *E. coli*, *H. influenzae*, Gonococci and *Bacillus subtilis*.

(b) Inability to penetrate bacteria.

(c) Altered protein binding sites by bacteria.

Uses

1. Respiratory tract infections, e.g.:

   (a) Acute phyaryngitis and tonsilitis.

   (b) Rheumatic fever.

   (c) Diphtheria.

   (d) Bronchitis.

   (e) Pneumonia.

2. Meningitis by Pneumococci or Meningococci.

3. Subacute bacterial endocarditis.

4. Venereal diseases, e.g. syphilis and gonorrhoea.

5. Cellulitis.

6. Gas gangrene and tetanus—penicillin is given in addition to antitoxic sera.

7. Rat bite fever.

Penicillin is excreted through kidneys hence dosage schedule needs to be changed in renal failure.

Procaine Penicillin: It is penicillin in combination with procaine moiety.

Advantages

1. Delayed onset but duration is prolonged.
2. Effect lasts 12 hrs hence two injections a day are sufficient.

Benzathine Penicillin G

(a) There is delayed absorption
(b) Has long duration of action. Blood levels are effective against established infection and **can prevent infection for 3 weeks**.
(c) Sufficiently high levels in blood are maintained for 10 days.

Penicillin as prophylactic agent

1. In rheumatic fever: Benzathine penicillin.
2. To prevent gonorrhoea: Procaine penicillin.
3. To prevent traumatic tetanus: Procaine penicillin.

Nursing care

All penicillins are cross sensitising and cross reacting.

Sensitivity to penicllin may be introduced by food or cosmetics:

1. Question the patient about history of reactions to penicillin.
2. An intradermal test (0.1 ml of a dilute solution of penicillin) may be carried out to detect allergy. However, **this test is not complete reliable**.
3. Be prepared to treat allergic reaction because **test dose itself may produce reactions**.
4. During intravenous infusion of penicillin the site of injection must be changed every 12 hourly.

Preparations: For injections

Benzyl penicillin injection is given IM every 6 hrs.
Procaine penicillin injection is given once or twice a day. Benzathine penicllin—1.2 mega units is given IM at 2–4 weeks intervals.

Preparations used locally

1. Penicillin lozenges—1000 units.
2. Penicillin eye ointment contains 2000 units of benzyl penicillin per gram.

Penicillin should not be applied on the skin as it causes allergic reactions

Doses

1. In gonorrhoea—4.8 million procaine penicillin with 1.0 g probenecid given once.
2. In Gonococcol arthrits, salpingitis or prostatitis 10 million units of procaine penicillin given for 4–14 days.

Preparations for Oral use

Phenoxymethyl penicillin tablets (Penicillin V)

(a) It is 1/5th as active as penicillin G. used for treating Streptococcal pharyngitis and tonsilitis.
(b) Can be destroyed by penicillinase.

Disadvantage: It is less effective against *H. influenzae* and Gonococci.

Phenethicillin: No advantage over penicillin V.

Given orally on empty stomach.

ANTISTAPHYLOCCAUS (PENICILLINASE RESISTANT) PENICILLINS

Cloxacillin

1. It can be given orally.
2. It is penicillinase resistant.
3. It is effective against benzylpenicillin resistant Staphylococci.

Precautions: Food interferes with its absorption. It **should be given on an empty stomach.**

Dose: 500 mg 6 hrly.

Oxacillin, dicloxacillin and nafcillin have similar qualities.

Actions

(a) Are acid resistant.
(b) Are penicillinase resistant.
(c) Can be given orally.

Hepatitis has been reported as adverse reaction with oxacillin.
Floxacillin (Fluxacillin): Actions same as oxacillin 250 mg orally or IM 6 hrly.

Methicillin

Advantage: It is active against penicillin resistant as well as sensitive strains.

Disadvantage: It has to be given by injection as it is destroyed by gastric acid.

Dose: 1 g intramuscularly at 4–6 hours intervals.

EXTENDED SPECTRUM PENICILLINS

Ampicillin, Amoxicillin, Carbencillin Indanyl, Ticarcillin, Bacmpicillin

Ampicillin

Advantages

1. It can be given orally.
2. It has broad spectrum of activity. It is active against both gram-positive and gram-negative bacteria (*H. influenzae, E. coli, Shigella* and *Salmonellae,* etc.)
3. It has no teratogenic effect.
4. It is bacteriolytic

Disadvantages

1. As compared to Penicillin G it is less effective against gram-positive organisms.
2. It is destroyed by penicillinase. It is therefore ineffective against *Staphylococci, Pseudomonas, Klebsella* and *Proteus.*

3. Food interferes with its absorption.

Uses

1. In mixed upper respiratory tract infections.
2. Urinary infections.
3. Meningitis due to *H. influenzae*.
4. Typhoid carriers.
5. Cholecystitis.
6. Subacute bacterial endocarditis.
7. Whooping cough.

Dose: 0.5 to 1 g orally every 6 hours.

Adverse reactions

1. Allergy rashes in AIDS and leukemia.
2. Nausea, anorexia and diarrhea.

Amoxicillin

Advantages over ampicillin

1. It is better absorbed from the gut than ampicillin.
2. Food does not interfere with absorption.
3. It is more effective against *Salmonella* and *Streptococcus faecalis*.
4. It is highly effective in chronic bronchitis.
5. It does not produce diarrhoea.
   It is preferred over ampicillin.

Disadvantage: Less effective against *H.influenzae* and *Shigella*.

Hetacillin, Talampicillin and Pivampicillin: All are prodrugs yield ampicillin in the body. Have no advantages over ampicillin.

Carbenicillin

Advantages

1. It is effective against Proteus and *E.coli*.
2. It is effective against ***Pseudomonas aeruginosa.***
3. It is used to **treat septicaemia.**

Disadvantages

1. As compared to ampicillin it is less effective against gram-positive organisms.
2. It is destroyed by penicillinase.
3. It is destroyed by gastric acid. It has to be injected.
4. Higher doses cause Na$^+$ retention.
5. Causes bleeding as it interferes with platelet functions.

Dose: 8–12 g/day in divided doses.

Uses
1. Urinary tract infections.
2. For treating infected burns.
3. Septicemia.

Nursing care
Do not mix carbenicillin with gentamicin in the same syringe.

Ticarcillin: Resembles carbenicillin but is more potent.

Advantage: More effective against *Pseudomonas* strains. **Some strains of *Pseudomonas* resistant to carbenicillin may respond to this drug.**

Disadvantage: Is inactivated by beta lactamases.

Action is better if given along with β-lactamase inhibitors (**clavulanic acid or sulbactam**).

Piperacillin: Effective against *Pseudomonas* is drug of choice for treating this infection.

Advantages
(a) Six to eight times more potent against *Pseudomonas* than carbenicillin.
(b) It is broad spectrum—**effective against *Klebsiella* and mixed infections due to aerobes and anaerobes.**

Uses
1. It is given along with gentamicin to treat *Pseudomonas* infections.
2. It is useful in treating immunocompromised patients.

PENICILLINS EFFECTIVE AGAINST *PSEUDOMONAS*
Carbenicillin, carbenecillin indanyl, ticarcillin, azlocillin, mezlocillin, piperacillin.

Points to remember about penicillins
1. Oganisms sensitive to penicillin show best response to penicillin G.
2. If a person sensitive to penicillin needs to be treated with this drug he should be desensitised under cover of corticosteroids and antihistaminics.
3. Cross-sensitivity is exhibited.
4. Cloxacillin, methicillin and flucloxacillin are used to treat severally ill patients with infections caused by penicillin resistant Staphylococci.
5. Carbenicillin is used as an adjuvant to treat resistant Staphylococci.
6. Ampicillin has no action against penicillin resistant Staphylococci but is active against gram-negative bacilli which are resistant to penicillin.

Penicillins are highly useful in treating tetanus, diphtheria and syphilis.

NON-PENICILLINS NON-CEPHALOSPORINS BETA-LACTAM ANTIBIOTICS

Carbapenems
Imipenem: Actions

Inhibits cell wall synthesis:

(a) It is **effective against aerobic as well as anaerobic organisms.**

(b) Not absorbed if given orally.

(c) It is effective against *Clostridium difficile* that is responsible for causing pseudomembranous colitis.

Disadvantages

(a) Needs to be given IV.

(b) Convulsions are produced.

Uses

(a) Urinary tract infections

(b) Respiratory infections

(c) Intra-abdominal and gynaecological infection

(d) Bone and joint infections

MONOBACTAMS AND CARBAPENEMS—AZTREONAM, TIGEMONAM AND MEROPENEM

Aztreonam

(a) Resistant to beta lactamases

(b) Active against *Pseudomonas aeruginosa, H. Influenzae,* Gonococci, *H. enterobacteriaceae.*

(c) Not effective against gram-positive bacteria and anaerobic organisms.

Can be given to patients allergic to penicillin and cephalosporins.

Can be given IV

Tigemonam: Can be given orally. It is active against gram-negative bacteria.

Carumonam: Injectable antibiotic with effects like aztreonam.

BETA LACTAMASE INHIBITORS

(a) Clavulanic Acid: Does not have anti-microbial activity.

Inhibits beta lactamases therefore prolongs the anti bacterial activity of penicillins. It is combined with amoxicillin and is used for the treatment of infections caused by beta lactamase producing strains of *H. influenzae, S. aureus, E. coli, Klebsiella* and *Enterobacters.*

(b) Sulbactam: It has very weak antimicrobial activity. Along with ampicillin it is used in treating intra-abdominal as well as pelvic infections.

(c) Tozabactam: Has actions similar to above and is combined with pipracillin.

CEPHALOSPORINS

First generation

(A) Parenteral—Cephalothin and cefazolin.

(B) Oral—Cephalexin, cephradine, cefadroxil and cephaloridine.

Disadvantages of first generation

1. Parenteral administration (cephalothin and cefazolin).
2. Are toxic.
3. Do not cross blood brain barrier.

Second generation: Cefamandole, cefaclor, cefuroxime, cefoxitin, cefonicid, cefotetan, cefprozol, loracarlef.

Advantages over first generation

(a) A few can be given orally (cefaclor and cefuroxime axetil).
(b) Are more resistant to beta lactamases.
(c) 10% of drug passes to CSF.

Third generation: Parenteral—ceftizoxime, ceftriaxone, ceftazidime, cefotaxime, cefitoxime, cefoperazone and Ceftazidime have antipseudomonal effect.

Oral—cefixine, cefpodoxime, cefdiner and cefoperazone.

Fourth generation

Cefepime

Ceffirone

These are semisynthetic bacteriolytic antimicrobials similar to penicillin in chemical structure and mode of action.

Cephazolin: It is drug of choice for surgical prophylaxis.

Cephlexin: It is used in oral infections, does not act upon bacteriodes and can be given orally.

Cephadroxil: It is better absorbed.

Cefoxtin: Used in anaerobic and mixed infections.

Cefuroxime axetil: Used in mixed infections (diabetic foot).

Ceftriaxone: Longest acting, is ineffective against anaerobes.

It is used in serious infections and in immunocompromised patients used in meningitis and typhoid fever.

Adverse reactions: Pain, thrombophlebitis. Ceftazidime produces neutropenia.

Actions: Are effective against gram-negative, anaerobic and pathogens resistant to I and II generations of cephalosporins.

(a) Are broad spectrum antibiotics.
(b) **Are more toxic than penicillins.**
(c) Are effective against Staphylococci resistant to penicillins.
(d) Are ineffective against Enterococci.

Advantages

(a) Wider spectrum of activity.
(b) Greater potency of action against gram-negative microbes.
(c) Can be used in patients allergic to penicillins.

Disadvantage: Activity against gram-positive organisms is less than those of first generation.

65

Broad Spectrum Antibiotics

Chloramphenicol and tetracyclines are referred to as broad spectrum antibiotics as they are effective against gram-negative as well as gram-positive organisms.

Group I: Tetracycline, chloretracycline, oxytetracycline.

Group II: Demeclocycline, methacycline and lymeclocycline.

Group III: Doxycycline and minocycline.

TETRACYCLINE

Actions

1. These drugs are **bacteriostatic**.
2. Are effective against gram-negative as well as gram-positive organisms. Tetracyclines affect the following microbes. ***Klebseilla pneumoniae,*** *Aerobacters*, ***Vibrio cholerae,*** Salmonella, ***T. pallidum, H. influenzae, E.coli, Shigella,*** *Listeria*, Propeonibacterium (causes acne), Mycoplasma, Spirochetes, malarial parasite, viruses of Lymphogranuloma, Psittacosis group, *Entamoeba histolytica*, Rickettsieae.
3. In addition they inhibit multiplication of Rickettsieae, Chlamydia and Actinomyces (fungi).
4. Act by inhibiting protein synthesis of the bacteria (305 ribosome)
5. Are concentrated by the sensitive strains of bacteria. Resistant strains do not concentrate these drugs.
6. They have chelation property also.
7. Bacteria develop resistance to these antibiotics due to defective concentrating mechanism.
8. **They cross placental barrier and adversely affect the foetus.**
9. Absorption is reduced by concurrent intake of milk, Ca^{2+}, Mg^{2+} and Fe^{3+}.

Resistance of tetracyclines

(a) It is plasmid mediated and therefore, bacteria develop resistance to many drugs simultaneously.

(b) **Staphylococci resistant to tetracycline may respond to minocycline.**

(c) Bacteroides resistant to tetracycline may remain sensitive to doxycycline.

Adverse reactions

1. Allergy is common.
2. Nausea, vomiting and loose stools.

3. Patients tend to develop superinfections with fungi.

4. Liver damage (oxytetracycline is safer).

5. Kidney damage (doxycycline is safer).

6. Produce weight loss.

7. They get deposited in teeth and bones.

8. Increase intracranial tension.

9. If given to pregnant women, they reduce growth of bones and stain teeth of foetus.

10. Reversible Fanconi syndrome occurs if **outdated tetracyclines** are used.

Uses

1. Patients sensitive to penicillin are treated with these drugs for following infections — syphilis, gonorrhoea, rat bite fever, Clostridial infection and Meningococcal infections.

2. Trachoma.

3. Plague.

4. Bacillary dysentery.

5. Cholera.

6. Primary atypical pneumonia.

7. Granuloma inguinale.

8. Rickettsial infections.

9. Acne vulgaris (minocycline).

10. Diagnostic use — for detection of certain cancers.

Semisynthetic Tetracyclines

Demethyl chlorteracycline (Demeclocycline)

1. It is more stable.

2. It is more effective.

3. Absorption from gut is 100%.

4. Dose of the drug is determined by severity of infection.

5. All other properties are like parent compound.

Dose: 300 mg/twice a day.

Adverse drug reactions

(a) Photosensitivity.

(b) Diabetes insipidus.

(c) Diarrhea.

Methacycline: Behaves like demethylchlortetracycline.

Adverse drug reactions

(a) Low incidence of phototoxicity.

(b) Diarrhea.

Doxycycline

1. It is long acting.
2. **Does not produce renal damage.** It can even be given in patients of renal failure.
3. Does not aggravate azotemia.
4. It is lipid soluble and well distributed.

Disadvantage: Not effective in urinary tract infections.

Dose: 100 mg/once a day.

Minocycline

Advantages

1. Better absorbed when given orally.
2. Effective even against organisms that are resistant to other tetracyclines, e.g. *Staphylococcus aureus, Streptococcus, pyogenes, Enterococci, Meningococci* and *E. coli.*
3. It is effective against *Mycobacterium tuberculosis.*

Disadvantages: In addition to all the adverse reactions produced by tetracyclines, it also produces vestibular damage (VIII nerve).

Nursing care

(a) Tetracyclines should be avoided during pregnancy and lactation.
(b) Should be avoided in patients of myasthenia gravis as it gets aggravated.
(c) Antagonises the effect of penicillins and other bacteriolytic agents. Hence, should not be combined.
(d) Tetracyclines should not be given with milk or along with antacids and salts of magnesium or calcium.

CHLORAMPHENICOL

It was obtained from *Streptomyces venezuelae,* but now for commercial use, it is synthetically prepared. It inhibits 50s ribosome.

Advantages

1. It is well absorbed when given orally.
2. It passes into tissues as well as CSF.

It is more effective against *S. typhi, E. coli, H. influenzae, Klebsiella pneumoniae* and *A. aerogenes.* Resistance occurs due to R factor.

Disadvantages

1. It is bacteriostatic.
2. It is very toxic.

Adverse reactions

1. Suppresses bone marrow which manifests as anemia, leucopenia and thrombocytopenia (aplastic anemia). May even produce aplastic anemia.

2. In premature children—produces gray baby syndrome (vomiting, unconsciousness, cyanosis and lactic acidosis).
3. Nausea, vomiting and diarrhea.
4. Allergic reactions
5. Superinfections may occur.

Dose: In typhoid fever—0.5 g every 6 hours for 10–14 days.

Uses

1. Typhoid fever (70–80% strains in India are resistant).
2. Bacillary dysentery.
3. For treating resistant strains of Staphylococci.
4. Urinary tract infections.
5. Anaerobic infections (*H. influenzae* meningitis).

Nursing care

1. Never use this drug if less toxic antibiotics are effective against microbes.
2. Complete dose should be given for specified period.
3. Blood counts should be done on alternate days.
4. Do not give this drug to either pregnant ladies or premature children.

66

Aminoglycosides and Miscellaneous Antibiotics

Following drugs belong to this group.

1. Streptomycin	2. Kanamycin
3. Gentamicin	4. Neomycin
5. Framycetin	6. Tobramycin
7. Amikacin	8. Netilmicin

The effect of these drugs is dose dependent. These are bacteriocidal but in lesser concentrations produce bacteriostatic effect.

These drugs interfere with transcription of amino acids on ribosomes and lead to formation of incorrect amino acid sequences in peptide chain resulting in formation of abnormal proteins that kill the bacteria.

They **act better in alkaline medium**. Aminoglycosides **show post antibiotic effect** — that is antibacterial activity persists even after drug has been completely elminated. Therefore despite the fact that their half life is 2–4 hours, they act longer. This effect is also seen with **fluroquinolone and β-lactamase antibiotics**.

Advantages of aminoglycosides

1. They are bacteriocidal in nature.
2. Streptomycin is effective against tuberculosis.
3. They are highly effective in infections caused by gram-negative bacteria.
4. They can be combined with penicillins and cephalosporins. Additive effect is produced.
5. Are more active in alkaline than acidic medium.

Disadvantages

1. None of these drugs is absorbed when give orally. **They have to be injected**.
2. Bacteria **develop resistance at a rapid rate**.
3. They are toxic to kidneys.
4. These drugs do not cross into CSF.
5. Antibacterial activity is reduced in blood, CSF and serum.
6. **Causes eighth cranial nerve damage** (get concentrated in endolymph and perilymph of inner ear). This is serious side effect of these antibiotics.

This nerve consists of two parts:

(i) Vestibular — the part that is responsible for the maintenance of balance.

(ii) Auditory — which is responsible for hearing activity. These drugs may either affect auditory or vestibular parts or both may get affected.

In the initial stages the damage is reversible but if severe it is likely to become irreversible.

Streptomycin: This drug is active against *M. tuberculosis, Shigella, E. coli, Proteus, Pseudomonas* and *Y. pestis.*

In tuberculosis, streptomycin has to be given for long duration. It is excreted through kidneys and in patients with impaired kidney functions, high blood levels of this drug are maintained for a long period. This is particularly liable to induce damage to the eighth cranial nerve. Dehydration aggravates this reaction. **Nurse must therefore, ensure that patients take fluids. It is specially important in older patients and those with high fever.**

Adverse reactions

1. Given intramuscularly it causes irritation.
2. Intrathecal injection can produce convulsions and death.
3. Allergic reactions can occur.
4. It **produces VIII nerve damage**. Hearing gets impaired. High frequencies are affected early and later lower frequency is affected— deafness can be permanent.
5. **All aminoglycosides produce skeletal muscle relaxation and worsen myasthenia gravis.** Therefore lesser dose of skeletal muscle relaxants is required during anesthesia.
6. **Kidneys get damaged if treatment with these drugs is prolonged.**

Uses

1. Tuberculosis.
2. Urinary tract infections caused by *E.coli, Proteus, A. aerogenes* and *Enterococci.*
3. In meningitis caused by *H.influenzae*, it is combined with sulfonamides and given in this condition.
4. Along with penicillin it is given to treat subacute bacterial endocarditis (caused by *Streptococci*) and bactremia due to *Pseudomonas* and other gram-negative aerobes.
5. Plague (acute phase).
6. Tularemia (drug of choice).
7. Brucellosis
8. It is given by oral route to clean bowels before surgery.
9. In the treatment of chancroid and granuloma inguinale.
10. In cases of empyema. it is injected into pleural cavity.

Dose: Streptomycin sulphate–1.0 g/day intramuscularly.

Kanamycin: It is second line treatment for TB.

Advantages over streptomycin

1. Resistance is slow to develop.
2. Organisms resistant to streptomycin continue to be sensitive to kanamycin but organisms resistant to kanamycin are also resistant to streptomycin.

Disadvantages

1. It is not effective against *Pseudomonas*.
2. It has narrow range of antimicrobial activity.

Adverse reactions

1. Same as with streptomycin
2. **Renal toxicity is more marked.**
3. **Respiratory and cardiac arrest may occur if this drug is injected intravenously.**

Dose: 1–1.5 gm per day in 2–3 divided doses.

Uses: It is used only in cases of severe infections

1. Septicaemia due to gram-negative bacteria.
2. Subacute bacterial endocarditis due to gram-negative bacteria.
3. Peritonitis.
4. Meningitis due to gram-negative bacteria.

Gentamicin: It is cheapest and most commonly used aminoglycoside.

It is more effective than kanamycin against Pseudomonas, *M. tuberculosis* and *Mycoplasma pneumoniae*. Effective against both gram-positive and gram-negative microbes.

Microbes which are highly sensitive to gentamycin include *Staph aureus, E.coli, Klebsiella, Aerobacter, Proteus* and *Pseudomonas*.

If given with carbenicillin it is highly effective against *Pseudomonas*.

Adverse reactions

1. Allergic reactions.
2. VIII nerve toxicity leading to deafness and problems involved in balancing.
3. Blood urea is increased.

Uses

1. Used locally on infected burns (*Pseudomonas*).
2. Used for cleaning bowels before abdominal surgery.
3. Though it is effective in various other infections it is not recommended when safer drugs are available.
4. Urinary tract infections, pneuomonia and meningitis caused by organisms resistant to other antibiotics.
5. Used in serious gram-negative infections with or without penicillin or cephalosporin or with piperacillin.

Dose: 1–3 mg/kg/day in divided doses.

Tobramycin

Advantages

1. It is more effective against *Pseudomonas aeruginosa* than gentamicin.
2. It is less toxic.

3. It has broadest antimicrobial range.
4. It is not destroyed by enzymes capable of destroying aminoglycosides.

Dose: 3–5 mg/kg is given every 6 hours.

Uses

1. In treatment of osteomyelitis.
2. Pneumonia.
3. Bacteremia.
4. Along with ticarcillin it is used to treat gram-negative sepsis.
5. Along with penicillin it is used to treat Enterococcal endocarditis.

Disadvantage: Needs to be given IM or IV.

Paromomycin: It resembles streptomycin in its actions. In addition it is effective against amoeba (*E. histolytica*).

Adverse reactions

1. Headache.
2. Vomiting and diarrhea.
3. Superinfections with fungus.

Uses

1. In hepatic coma.
2. In chronic bacillary dysentery.
3. For cleaning bowels before surgery.

Neomycin: It is active against Staphylococci, *C. diphtheriae, H. influenzae, Proteus, Vibrio cholera, Salmonella* and *Shigella*. It is used for local effects. It is not absorbed when given orally.

Uses

1. Locally used in skin and eye infections.
2. In hepatic failure it is given orally to kill intestinal bacteria.
3. For irrigation of the urinary bladder.
4. Drug of choice for wound preparation before surgery.

Adverse reactions

1. VIII nerve damage.
2. Kidney damage.
3. Respiratory paralysis.
4. When given orally it produces malabsorption.

Framycetin: Its actions are similar to neomycin, is used for local effects.

Uses

1. For local applicaion –0.5% ointment is used.
2. For cleaning gut it is given orally.

Amikacin: It is semisynthetic derivative. Most active against gram-negative organisms.

It has widest spectrum of activity.

It is used as reserve drug to treat septicaemia, infections of respiratory tract, bones and joints.

Sisomicin: More effective against *Pseudomonas* and beta haemolytic Streptococci.

Uses: **Local**

(a) Burns

(b) For treating ophthalmic infections.

Systemic: To treat bacteremia and septicemia.

Netilmicin: It is water soluble bactericidal amminoglycoside. It is used to treat **bacteraemia, septicaemia,** infections of bones, joints, burns, kidney and genitourinary tract. It is effective against microorganisms resistant to kanamycin, gentamicin, tobramycin, sisomicin and amikacin. Causes neurotoxicity and nephrotoxicity.

Sodium fusidate is a steroid antibiotic.

Advantages

(a) Penetrates all body tissues including bone except CSF.

(b) It is used for treating **severe Staphyloccocal infections** resistant to penicillins.

(c) It is used in **osteomyelitis**.

Adverse reactions: GI—nausea and vomiting.

Jaundice may appear.

POLYPEPTIDE ANTIBIOTICS

This group comprises following antibiotics:

(a) Polymyxin.

(b) Colistin (polymyxin E).

(c) Tyrothricin.

(d) Bacitracin.

(e) Cycloserine.

Advantage: **Polymyxin and colistin** are highly effective against *Pseudomonas aeruginosa.*

Tyrothricin and bacitracin are used only for local applications.

Polymyxin B: These are a group of antibiotics A, B, C, D and E. Polymyxin B is least toxic and is clinically used. Polymyxin B a mixture of polymyxin B1 and B2.

Used for treating gram-negative infections in skin, eyes, ear and for irrigation of urinary bladder.

Disadvantages

1. Not absorbed when given orally.

2. It is toxic compound. Toxicity manifests in the form of:

(a) Renal damage.

(b) Skeletal muscle paralysis—patient finds difficulty in speech and swallowing.

(c) Dyspnoea and respiratory paralysis are produced in higher doses.

Uses: In infections due to gram-negative organisms not responding to other antibiotics.

Colistin: It has same effects, toxicity and uses like polymyxin B.

Tyrothricin: It is a mixture of two antibiotics — **tryrocidine and gramicidin.**

It is mainly active against gram-negative microbes.
It is applied on ulcers and wounds in the form of ointment.

Bacitracin: It is mainly active against gram-positive organisms. It is used as ointment in ophthalmic and dermatological practice.

Uses

(a) Suppurative conjunctivitis.
(b) Infected corneal ulcer.

Disadvantage: It is nephrotoxic.

Gramicidin: Used locally in combination with tramycitin. Neomycin as cream ointment for treating skin sepsis.

Cycloserine

1. It is used as second line of treatment in tuberculosis.
2. It is used to treat *E.coli* infections of the urinary tract.

Precautions

1. All these drugs are **highly toxic**.
2. These drugs should be avoided as far as possible.
3. Their use should be restricted to conditions not responding to safer antibiotics.
4. Renal function tests should be done routinely.
5. Lesser dose should be given in patients with renal failure.

67

Macrolide Antibiotics

Following antibiotics belong to this group:

Erythromycin, oleandomycin, azithromycin, clarithromycin, roxithromycin, spiramycin, lincomycin, vancomycin and novobiocin.

All these antibiotics are obtained from the moulds of Streptomyces. **They are bacteriostatic in small doses but bacteriolytic in higher doses.**

Erythromycin acts by **inhibiting protein synthesis**.

1. Its bacterial spectrum resembles penicillin.
2. In addition it is effective against penicillin resistant Staphylococci.
3. Does not cross BBB but crosses placenta.
4. It is effective against *S. pyogenes, S. pneumoniae* and *Listeria*.

Resistance

(a) Cross resistance among members of macrolide antibiotics is complete.
(b) Cross resistance to lincomycin is present.

Uses

1. Upper respiratory tract infections.
2. In infections caused by Staphylococci.
3. Vaginitis due to Chlamydia.

Preparations: Erythromycin stearate and erythromycin estolate are available. Estolate is better absorbed but produces liver toxicity hence succinate is preferred.

Precautions: To be effective it should be strictly taken on 6 hourly schedule. It should be used with caution in liver disease.

Spiramycin

Advantages

1. It stays in tissues for a longer time.
2. Exerts lesser side effects.

Uses: Respiratory tract infections.

Dose: 500 mg 6 hourly.

Oleandomycin: Its salt triacetyloleandomycin is well absorbed. Not much used as it does not have any advantage over erythromycin.

Use: It is used in cases of endocarditis resistant to penicillin.

Dose: 500 mg 6 hourly.

Roxithromycin: Roxithromycin is used to treat pneumonia, acute bronchitis, sinusitis, tonsilitis, pharyngitis and genital infections.

Adverse reactions: Nausea, vomiting, rarely rashes and rise in liver enzymes.

Clarithromycin: Broad spectrum antibiotic.

Uses

1. Upper and lower respiratory tract infections.
2. Skin and soft tissue infections.
3. Sinusitis.

Teicoplanin: It is bactericidal both against aerobic and anaerobic gram-positive bacteria.

Uses

1. Prophylaxis against gram-positive endocarditis in dental surgery in high-risk heart patients.
2. Intraperitoneal administration to treat peritonitis in patients on peritoneal dialysis.

Azithromycin: Like erythromycin it is effective against gram-positive as well as gram-negative pathogens but has increased activity against many gram-negative and atypical microorganisms.

Uses

1. Upper and lower respiratory tract infections.
2. Skin and soft tissues infections.
3. Urogenital infections.

Precautions: Azithromycin should be taken 1 hour before or at least 2 hours after meal.

Not recommended in children below 3 years.

Adverse effects: Dizziness, headache, flatulence and vomiting.

Aztreonam: It is useful to treat sepsis and other gram-negative infections. It is highly effective against *Pseudomonas aeruginosa.*

Uses

1. Septicaemia/bacteremia.
2. Pyelonephritis and other complicated urinary tract infections.
3. Gynaecological infections caused by gram-negative organisms.
4. Adjunct to surgery in treatment of abscesses and hollow viscous perforations.

Adverse reactions: Pain at site of injection.

Roxithromycin

Advantages

(a) It has longer half-life.

(b) It is resistant to acid hydrolysis therefore better absorbed when given orally.

(c) It has better penetration into tissues.

Adverse reactions

1. Nausea and vomiting.
2. Flatulence and bulky stools.
3. Allergic reactions

Dose: 250–550 mg 4 times a day.

Novobiocin: It has same activity as erythromycin.

Adverse reactions

1. Nausea and vomiting.
2. Leucopenia.
3. Haemolytic anaemia.
4. Super infections with fungi.

Lincomycin: It has activity like erythromycin but is far less prone to produce adverse reactions.

Use: In treatment of acute and chronic osteomyelitis because it has better penetration into bone.

Adverse reactions

1. Nausea and vomiting.
2. In few patients it may produce dizziness, headache and vaginitis.
3. Diarrhoea.

Dose: 500 mg 3–4 times a day.

Clindamycin: Advantages over lincomycin

1. It is better absorbed.
2. Absorption is not affected by food.
3. Penetrates into bones better than other antimicrobials.

Uses: It is used for treating infections due to anaerobic organisms. For treating abdominal sepsis, bone and joint infections.

Disadvantage: Penetration into CSF and eyes is poor.

Adverse reactions: Same as with lincomycin.

Vancomycin: It is bactericidal against gram-positive cocci.

Disadvantages

1. It can not be given orally.

2. Intramuscular administration is painful.

3. Serious ADRs limit its uses.

Adverse reactions

1. Allergic reactions.
2. Local thrombophlebitis.
3. Loss of hearing.
4. Kidney damage.

Spectinomycin: Effective against gram-negative bacteria. Resistance develops due to mutation.

Uses

1. Given to patients allergic to penicillins and quinolones.
2. To treat penicillin resistant gonorrhoea.

68

Quinolones and Fluoroquinolones

QUINOLONES

Nalidixic acid is bactericidal against gram-negative organism (***E. coli, Shigella, Proteus and Klebsiella***). Like fluoroquinolones **inhibits DNA gyrase** required for DNA replication and transcription.

Nalidixic acid is well absorbed and circulates in blood. It is quickly excreted in urine, therefore, effective antibacterial concentrations are not reached in blood. **Concentration in urine is 20–50 times that of plasma and is effective for treatment of UTI.**

Uses

1. For treatment of urinary tract infection.
2. Diarrhoea due to *E. coli, Shigella* and *Proteus*.

Adverse reactions

Allergic reactions, headache and drowsiness.

FLUOROQUINOLONES

Fluoroquinolones include the following:

Ciprofloxacin, Ofloxacin, Norfloxacin, Pefloxacin, Rosoxacin, Cinoxacin, Enoxacin, Lomefloxacin, Sparfloxacin, Levofloxin and Acrosaxin

They are bactericidal and act by inhibiting enzyme called DNA gyrase that prevents normal formation of DNA helix.

They are effective against both gram-positive and gram-negative bacteria. Have better antimicrobial activity, achieve clinically useful concentrations in the body and have low toxicity.

Ciprofloxacin: It is effective against *Salmonella, Shigella* and *Campylobacter*. It has less activity against gram-positive organisms. It has high post-antibiotic effect.

Dose: 250–750 mg twice a day.

Uses

1. Urinary tract infections.
2. Typhoid (acute) and carriers.
3. Gonorrhoea.

4. Bone, soft tissue, gynaecological and wound infections.
5. Eye and ear infections.
6. Systemic gram-negative infections.
7. Anthrax.

Adverse effects

1. Nausea, vomiting and diarrhea.
2. Headache, dizziness and tremors.
3. Abnormal liver function or skin rash may develop.

Drug interactions

1. Ciprofloxacin raises serum level of theophylline.
2. Co-administration of antacids reduces the levels of fluoroquinolones.

Ofloxacin: Unlike ciprofloxacin, it is **active against Chlamydia and Mycoplasma. It is active against *M. tuberculosis, M. leprae,* and *M. Kansasii.***

Uses: For genitourinary, respiratory, gastrointestinal, skin and soft tissue infections. Peritonitis and for treating gonorrhoea.

Dose: 200–400 mg twice daily.

Exposure to sunlight and ultraviolet light should be avoided.

Norfloxacin: It is less potent than ciprofloxacin.

It is specially used for the treatment of urinary tract infection as it **concentrated in urine**.

It should not be administered to children or pregnant women.

Dose: 400 mg twice a day for 7 to 10 days.

Uses: Primarily for genital and urinary infections.

Gonorrhea: For complicated UTI, treatment is extended to 21 days.

Pefloxacin: It is effective against gram-negative as well as gram-positive bacteria. Advantage over ciprofloxacin is **its higher CNS penetrability.**

Dose: Initial loading dose of 800 mg followed by 400 mg twice daily.

Uses

1. Surgical, bone and joint infections.
2. Severe systemic infections.
3. Infections in mouth.
4. Gynaecological infections.

Precautions

Patients with hepatic disease require dose adjustment. Interval between the 2 doses should be increased up to 36 hrs.

It should **not be given to children, pregnant and lactating mothers** and those with G6PD deficiency.

Gatefloxacin: It is broad spectrum fluoroquinolone. It is effective against many gram-positive microbes as well as anaerobic organisms.

Uses

1. Acute bacterial exacerbation of chronic bronchitis.
2. Acute sinusitis.
3. Urinary tract infection.
4. Acute pyelonephritis.
5. Gonorrhoea.

Precautions: Renal impairment.

Adverse reactions

1. Convulsions.
2. Rapid heart beat.
3. Mental confusion, hallucination, and agitation.

Gemiofloxacin: It is fourth generation fluoroquinolone.

Uses: Treatment of mild to moderate community acquired pneumonia and acute exacerbation of chronic bronchitis.

Moxifloxacin: It is effective against β-lactam and macrolide resistant bacteria.

Uses

1. Treatment of acute bacterial sinusitis.
2. Acute bacterial exacerbation of chronic bronchitis.
3. Community acquired pneumonia in adult patients (over 18 years).

Adverse reactions

1. Allergy.
2. CNS — insomnia and agitation.

Special precautions

Not to be given to children, pregnant and lactating women.

Prulefloxacin

Uses

1. Treatment of urinary tract infections.
2. Respiratory tract infections.

Adverse reactions: Blood dyscrasias, CNS disorders and gastrointestinal disorders.

Lomefloxacin: It is not active against *M. leprae* is effective in need to moderate infections.

It does not interact with theophylline and ranitidine but may enhance the anticoagulant effect of warfarin.

Uses

1. For treatment of uncomplicated and complicated UTI.
2. Mild to moderate infection of the respiratory tract.

Dose: 400 mg once a day for 10 days for chronic bronchitis and for 14 days for UTI.

Sparfloxacin: Highly concentrated in nasal mucosa and sinus mucosa.

Advantages

1. Broader spectrum of activity.
2. Dose alteration not required in patients with compromised renal or hepatic functions.

Uses

1. Commonly acquired respiratory tract infections including *Streptococcus pneumoniae* and atypical pneumonia.
2. STD in males.

Adverse effects

1. Abdominal pain, nausea and vomiting.
2. In rare cases, headache, sleep disorders and moderate increase of transaminases.

Dose: 400 mg on the first followed by 200 mg tablet each day for 10 days.

69

Chemotherapy of Tuberculosis and Leprosy

Tuberculosis is a chronic granulomatous condition caused by *Mycobacterium tuberculosis*. It is highly prevalent in underdeveloped countries like ours. AIDS is increasing prevalence of TB.

It was one of the fatal diseases till 1944 as none of the antibiotics available then were effectice against this organism. **With the advent of streptomycin, isoniazid and rifampicin this disease is now curable.**

Problems associated with treatment of tuberculosis.

1. *M. tuberculosis* is an acid fast bacilli, and is not sensitive to common antibiotics.
2. *Mycobacterium tuberculosis* is an intracellular microbe. There are only a few antibiotics and chemotherapeutic agents (**INH, rifampicin and pyrizinamide**) which reach this organism.
3. *Mycobacterium* is **quick to develop resistance**.
4. The treatment needs to be continued for long time. Patients usually ignore this fact.
5. Caseation of the tissue blocks blood vessels in necrotic area and antitubercular drugs do not reach *Mycobacterium*.
6. Mycobateria remain alive in macrophages.

1. Standard drugs
   (a) Bactericidal: Isonicotinic acid hydrazide (H), rifampicin, streptomycin (S) and pyrizinamide (Z).
   (b) Bacteriostatic: Ethambutol (E) and thiacetazone (T).
2. Second line drugs
   (a) Bactericidal: Capreomycin (A), kanamycin (K), amikacin, fluoroquinilones (Q).
   (b) Bacteriostatic: Ethionamide (EE), cycloserine (C) and clofazimine.

New drugs: Rifabutin, ofloxacin and azithromycin and chlarithromycin.

Streptomycin

Disadvantages

1. It is not absorbed when given orally therefore it **has to be given by injection (intramuscularly)**.
2. It is less effective than INH.
3. It **does not reach brain**.
4. Resistance is quick to develop.
5. It produces damage of VIIIth nerve.

To overcome the above problems it is given in combination.

Advantages of combination

1. Development of resistance is delayed.
2. Efficacy is improved.

Dose of streptomycin is 1 gm/day for 3 months.

Isonicotinic Acid Hydrazide (INH): It is active only against *M. tuberculosis*. **It has no action against any other bacteria.**

Advantages

1. It is bactericidal.
2. It is well absorbed when given orally and can also be given intrathecally.
3. It penetrates cell membrane and enters CSF as well as caseous material.
4. It is well distributed.
5. Toxicity is less.
6. Absence of cross resistance to other anti-TB drugs.
7. It is effective against atypical mycobacteria.

Adverse reactions

1. Allergic reactions.
2. Peripheral neuritis due to deficiency of vitamin B_6.
3. It stimulates central nervous system. It produces euphoria. In a few it may cause convulsions.
4. Dryness of mouth and urinary retention (specially in elderly males) are produced.
5. Hepatotoxicity occurs specially in fast acetylators.

Dose: 300 mg daily orally.

Adverse reactions: Peripheral neuritis, hepatitis and psychotic behaviour.

Rifampicin: It is semisynthetic deriative of rifamycin B. It is active against *M. tuberculosis, M. leprae, Staphylococcus aureus, C. welchii, Strept viridans,* and *Strept haemolyticus*, Pneumococci and ***Bacillus anthracis***.

Advantages

1. It is bactericidal.
2. It is well absorbed when given orally.
3. It is well distributed.
4. It is effective against many bacteria.
5. Combination with INH is highly effective.
6. **It acts on persisters**.

Adverse reactions

1. Nausea, vomiting.
2. Leucopenia.
3. Serious liver damage, specially when given with INH and in the elderly.

4. It stains urine, stool and saliva.
5. Renal failure may be produced.
6. Chronic flu like syndorme.

Drug interactions: It interacts with certain drugs and reduces their effect, e.g. **contraceptive pill, Steroids, digoxin and dapsone**. It should not be combined with PAS as its absorption is reduced.

Refapentine: It is longer acting rifampicin. It is not given in initial phase but is used during continuous phase.

Uses

1. To treat tuberculosis.
2. To treat leprosy.
3. For treatment of severe Staphylococcal and Meningococcal infections (septicaemia).

Dose: 450–600 mg/day.

Precautions

1. It should not be used to treat simple infections as resistance is fast to develop.
2. It **causes pill failure**. Women on rifampicin must use other methods of contraception.
3. It should not be combined with PAS.

Rifabutin: It is derived from rifamycin. It is more effective than rifampicin.

It is active against atypical TB, has less drug interactions as compared to rifampicin.

ADRs

1. Allergic rash.
2. Nausea, vomiting and diarrhea.
3. Neutropenia.

Ethambutol

Advantages

1. It is effective against Mycobacteria that have developed resistance to INH, PAS and streptomycin.
2. It is also effective against atypical mycobacteria.
3. Mycobacteria develop resistance at a lower rate.
4. No cross resistance.

Disadvantages

1. It is bacteristatic and less effective than INH and rifampicin. Therefore, it has to be combined with bactericidal drug.
2. **It damages retina and reduces vision**.

Adverse reactions

1. Peripheral neuritis.
2. Reduction in visual acuity and red green colour blindness.

Dose: 25 mg/kg for 8–12 weeks. Dose is reduced gradually to 15 mg/kg/day. It is given for 12 months.

Para-aminosalicylic Acid (PAS): It inhibits the multiplication of Mycobacteria (bacteristatic).

Advantages

1. It improves INH levels in the blood.
2. It delays development of resistance.

Disadvantages

1. It is not very effective.
2. It produces many adverse reactions.
3. Patients do not like to take this drug as the dose is very heavy.

Adverse reactions

1. Allergic reactions.
2. Anorexia, nausea and vomiting.
3. Aggravates peptic ulcer.
4. Suppresses bone marrow.
5. It damages liver.
6. Renal stones may be formed.

Dose: 10–15 g/day.

Thiacetazone: This drug has properties like PAS, but it does not delay the development of resistance. Adverse reactions are similar to PAS, but it takes 2–3 months for these reactions to manifest. It should **not be used in HIV** patients as it can cause fatal skin reaction.

Dose: 150 mg/day.

Uses: In treatment of TB it is given along with INH.

Pyrazinamide: It is effective against *M. tuberculosis* that is resistant to INH and streptomycin. Combination of this drug with INH and streptomycin is highly effective. Can be given orally.

If given with INH and rifampicin in the initial period it sterilises the tuberculous area.

It produces liver damage and is considered more toxic than ethionamide or ethambutol.

Dose: 500 mg three times a day.

Morphazinamide: It is more potent than pyrazinamide. Adverse effects are same.

Ethionamide: Chemically it resembles INH and there is cross-resistance between these two drugs.

Advantages

1. It is effective against tubercle bacilli which have become resistant to other drugs.
2. It is effective against atypical Mycobacteria.

Disadvantage: Cross resistance shown with thiacetazone.

Dose: 250 mg twice a day.

Adverse reactions

1. Nausea, anorexia and vomiting.
2. Allergic reactions.
3. Hepatic damage is produced in diabetic patients.

Capreomycin: It is less effective than streptomycin. It is effective against bacteria resistant to streptomycin, INH and PAS.

Disadvantages

(a) If given alone resistance develops quickly.
(b) Does not penetrate cell wall.
(c) Cross resistance with kanamycin and viomycin is present.

   Adverse reactions are similar to streptomycin, e.g.:

(i) Renal damage.
(ii) VIII nerve damage.
(iii) Allergy.
(iv) In addition it causes loss of Ca^{++} Mg^{++} and K^+.

Dose: 1 g/day for 60 days.

Kanamycin and Amikacin

Advantages

1. Effective in severe or resistance cases.
2. Effective in multidrug resistant TB.

Disadvantages

1. To be injected intramuscularly everyday.
2. Produce kidney damage and deafness.

Viomycin: It is highly toxic to VIIIth nerve and kidneys.

Advantages

1. It is effective against streptomycin and INH resistant strains of mycobacteria.
2. It can be given twice a week.
3. Organisms resistant to viomycin are resistant to streptomycin and kanamycin.

   Rarely used.

Dose: 2 g/twice a week.

Cycloserine: It is broad spectrum antibiotic useful in TB and gram-negative infections. It is effective against MTBR atypical TB. CNS toxicity occurs that can be prevented by pyridoxine.

Advantages

1. It is active against streptomycin, INH and PAS resistant strains of mycobacteria.

2. Resistance is slow to develop.

3. It is freely distributed in body fluids. It reaches CSF.

Adverse reactions

1. Causes CNS toxicity: Insomnia, restlessness, twitching of muscles and convulsions.

2. Nausea, vomiting.

3. Peripheral neuritis.

4. Renal damage.

Dose: 250 mg two to three times a day.

Clarithromycin and Azithromycin: Clarithromycin is four times active against *M. tuberculosis* as compared to azithromycin but penetration into cells is poor. Also used to treat atypical tuberculosis.

Quinolones: Ciprofloxacin, ofloxacin and sparfloxacin are effective and are given as short term treatment in AIDS patient along with INH and rifampicin.

Useful in treating *M. tuberculosis* and *M. avium* complex resistant to standard drugs and relapse.

Nursing care

1. Caution the patient to take all drugs. Help patients to achieve compliance.

2. Patient or his relation be made aware of the adverse reactions that are likely to occur. Instruct him to report these to the physician.

3. Doses of most of these drugs depend upon the renal functions and need to be reduced in children and elderly.

4. Treatment should be continued for **6–18 months after the closure of the cavity in lungs**.

5. Pyridoxine given to patients who develop neuropathy.

6. Patient should be advised to come for frequent check ups to:

   (i) Evaluate the success or failure of treatment.

   (ii) For appearance of reactions.

7. All contacts should be traced and treated.

8. Outpatients should be checked at least once in two weeks.

10. Monitor laboratory data for adverse drug effects. Inform physician when these occur.

11. Maintain a slow infusion rate.

12. Reassure the patient for IV administration.

13. Advise him to improve nutrition.

Regimens used for Treating TB

1. H + R + Z + E daily two months followed by

   H + R daily (self administered) or H + R twice weekly (supervised) for 4 months.

2. If patient cannot be given Z then

   H + R + E daily for 2 months followed by

   H + R daily for 7 months.

3. Directly observed treatment short courses (DOTS): This is carried out under systematic monitoring and supervision.

Category I: Serious patients (those patients suffering from TB meningitis or disseminated TB or spinal TB or intestinal and genitourinary TB or bilateral/extensive pleurisy or pulmonary TB with extensive parenchymal involvement.)

Isonex (600 mg) and rifampicin (450 mg) and pyrazinamide (1500 mg) and ethambutol (1200 mg) are given on alternate days (under supervision) for 2 months followed by isoniazid and rifampicin on alternate days for 4 months.

Category II: (This group comprises sputum positive patients who have either relapsed or failed or defaulted). They are treated by

Isoniazid (600 mg) + rifampicin (600 mg) + pyrazinamide (1500 mg) + ethambutol (1200 mg) and streptomycin. All these drugs are given in combination on alternate days for two months followed by HRZE for one month and HRE for five months.

Category III: (Sputum negative or extrapulmonary not serious patients). This group is treated by giving HRZ for two months followed by HR for 4 months.

Role of Steroids in Tuberculosis: Steroids are added to TB treatment in following conditions:

1. Rapidly progressing infection: Pulmonary TB, tuberculous pneumonia and miliary tuberculosis and if patient shows toxic symptoms.
2. In endotracheal tuberculosis: To prevent bronchial stenosis.
3. In tuberculous meningitis: To prevent adhesions, arachnoditis and hydrocephalus.
4. In tubercular pleurisy and pericarditis and constrictive pericarditis.
5. To counter hypersensitive reactions to drugs during treatment.
6. In rapidly enlarging midiastinal lymph nodes.
   To prevent fibrosis in eyes and genitourinary tract during treatment of tuberculosis in these areas.

Steroids are not given in abdominal TB.

Chemoprophylaxis of Tuberculosis: It is given to

(a) Contacts of open cases.
(b) Neonate of mother suffering from tuberculosis.
(c) Immunocompromised patients.

INH + rifampicin are given.

Treatment during pregnancy: All drugs except streptomycin can be given and after delivery infant is given BCG along with INH for prophylaxis.

DRUGS USED IN LEPROSY

Leprosy is a disease caused by *Mycobacterium leprae*. It is common in India. It is of four types:

1. Lepromatous leprosy — infiltration, CMI absent and lepromin reaction –ve.
2. Tuberculoid leprosy (anaesthetic patch, lepromine +ve).
3. Indeterminate leprosy.
4. Dimorphic (border line) — bilateral, symmetrical polyneuropathy.

Classification of Drugs used in Treatment of Leprosy

Drugs effective against M. laprae: Sulphonamides–dapsone (DDS), acedapsone (DADDS) sulfoxone sodium, phenaxone derivatives, clofazamine.

Antitubercular drugs effective in leprosy: Ofloxacin, minocycline, rifampicin, clarithromycin, ethionamide and thiacetazone sulfidoxine.

Sulfones: These drugs resemble sulphonamides in chemistry as well as in pharmacolgical actions. They are bacteriosatic in nature.

These drugs are effective against:

(a) Bacteria which are sensitive to sulphonamides.

(b) *Mycobacterium tuberculosis.*

(c) *Mycobacterium leprae.*

Dapsone

Advantages

1. Cheapest.
2. It is slowly but completely absorbed from the gut.
3. It is cumulative in nature.
4. **Gets specifically concentrated in areas of skin affected by leprosy.**
5. It has enterohepatic circulation, therefore **effect is long lasting**.
6. It can be given orally and IM as repository.

Disadvantages

1. Absorption from gut is slow.
2. Certain **M. leprae** have become **resistant to sulfones**.
3. Action is antagonised by PABA.

Adverse reactions

1. Haemolytic anaemia specially in the **G6PD** deficient patients.
2. Liver and kidney damage.
3. Allergic reactions

All other preparations (sulfones) act by releasing DDS in the body.

Do not give to patients with Hb less than 7 gm%.

Acedapsone: It is a repository preparation of dapsone. It is given IM.

Efficacy lasts for 70–80 days.

Preparations and doses

1. Dapsone: 100 mg/day orally or intramuscularly.
2. Sulfetrone sodium 0.5 ml (250 mg) is given intramuscularly once a week.
3. Acedapasone: It is depot preparation (225 mg) and is given intramuscularly every 70–80 days.

Rifampicin: It is highly effective against leprosy.

Advantages

1. It is bactericidal and given in multibacillary leprosy.
2. It can be given orally.
3. In the recommended doses it produces only few toxic effects.
4. Decreases duration of treatment.

Dose: 600 mg on alternate day.

Disadvantages

1. It is expensive and bacterial resistance has been reported.
2. Produces hepatitis

Clofazimine: It is a weak bactericidal. Gets concentrated in reticuloendothelial tissues. Reddish black discolouration is major side effect. It is avoided in pregnancy.

Advantages

1. It is bactericidal.
2. It is effective against dapsone resistant leprae.
3. It has anti-inflammatory activity.
4. Does not produce serious toxicity.
5. Specially useful when intolerance occurs to DDS.

Minocycline in combination with clarithromycin (500 mg) given daily produces beneficial effects. Specially usedful in patients allergic to sulfones and with resistant strains.

Ethionamide and Prothionamide: Used when patient does not tolerate clofazimine.

Advantages

1. It is bactericidal.
2. Onset of action is quicker.

Disadvantages

1. It is expensive.
2. It is more toxic.

Chaulmoogra and Hydnocarpus Oils: These oils are less effective.

They are applied locally into the lesions by intradermal injections.

They are not popular any more.

Multidrug therapy reduces symptoms, decreases bacterial load, reduces duration of therapy and decreases emergence of resistance.

Dapsone and rifampicin are given in paucibacillary for 6 months.

Multibacillary dapsone, rifampicin and clofazamine are given for two years or till disease is inactive.

Nursing care

1. Nurses must reassure her patients.
2. Must check on their drug compliance.
3. Should observe for development of any adverse drug reactions.
4. Nonresponding cases should be referred to treating physician.

Lepra reaction: This reaction is produced during treatment with these drugs. It is characterised by acute excerbation of leprosy.

Thalidomide 100 mg three times a day is the drug of choice.

It is treated by clofazimine 100 mg three times a day.

Chloroquine 250 mg three times a day for at least two weeks.

If above two drugs fail to control lepra reaction steroids can be tried.

Prevention of leprosy: Dapsone can be given to contacts.

70

Drugs used in Malaria

Malaria is an infectious disease caused by *Plasmodium*. There are four types of these organisms *Plasmodium vivax* (**commonest**), *P. falciparum, P. ovale and P. malariae*.

Infection is introduced into a healthy individual through anopheline female mosquito bite. These parasites reach the liver through the bloodstream. They breed and multiply in the liver. This is called pre-erythrocytic stage. After multiplication they invade the bloodstream and invade RBC. Once in the red blood cells, they multiply and after variable intervals (24–72 hours depending upon the species) they burst out of the infected red cell. At this stage patient experiences chills and fever. Each parasite (merozoite) then invades another RBC and so the process goes on.

Some merozoites (liberated from RBC) form male or female gametocyte. Along with the human blood, gametes are taken up by the female mosquito during bite. These undergo multiplication and maturation in the stomach of the female mosquito from where they are regurgitated and deposited in man through mosquito bite.

Different drugs act at different stages of life cycle of malarial parasite.

Following drugs are used in malaria:

1. Quinine, bulaquine.
2. Chloroquine, hydroxychloroquine and amodiaquine.
3. Primaquine, pentaquin and pamaquine.
4. Mepacrine.
5. Proguanil, chlorproguanil and cycloguanil pamoate.
6. Pyrimethamine.
7. Mefloquine.
8. Sulfones, sulfonamides, tetracyclines and quinghaosu.
9. Arteether and artemether.

Treatment of malaria can be divided into following three headings:

(a) **Chemoprophylaxis or causal, true causal prophylactic agents.** Drugs given to suppress the occurrence of malarial infection in a healthy individual living or passing through an endemic area, **chloroquine.**

(b) **Suppressives of clinical attack:** Drugs given to kill malarial parasite after they have invaded the bloodstream from the liver and are multiplying in large numbers within the red cells (treatment of an acute attack of malaria). **Quinine, chloroquine, hydroxychloroquine and amodiaquine.**

(c) Radical cure agents: Drugs which eradicate parasite both from the liver as well as RBC, e.g. **primaquine and pyrimethamine**.

Quinine: It is an alkaloid obtained from cinchona bark. **It destroys the schizonts in the RBC. Sexual form of *P. vivax* and *P. malariae* are destroyed. Has no effect on sexual forms of *P. falciparum*.** Latent tissue phase and development of gametocytes are not affected.

Advantages

1. It is **useful to suppress as well as treat acute attack of malaria**.
2. It is highly effective **against chloroquine resistant strains of malaria**. It is a **life saving drug in these cases**.
3. **Resistance does not develop to this drug**.

In addition to antimalarial action quinine produces following pharmacological actions.

(i) It exerts **quinidine like activity** on the heart. It reduces contraction of myocardium and reduces conduction of impulses.

(ii) It has irritant action and is used as sclerosing agent in varicose veins.

(iii) It irritates gastric mucosa and produces nausea and vomiting.

(iv) It **reduces tone** of the skeletal muscles.

(v) It produces **contraction of the uterus** — was used to induce abortion.

Disadvantages

1. It is very bitter.
2. It does not produce radical cure.

Adverse reactions

1. Allergic reactions
2. It produces acute fatal reaction (called cinchonism) in high doses.
   This condition is characterised by ringing in ears, headache, nausea, deafness, vertigo, blurred vision and photophobia. Respiration is depressed, blood pressure falls and patient goes into coma.
3. It may produce hemolysis of RBC (specially in G6PD deficient patients).

Dose: 300–600 mg orally three times a day for 5–7 days.

Children–25 mg/kg/day is divided doses.

Uses

1. In malaria specially
   (a) **Cerebral malaria**
   (b) **Chloroquine resistant falciparum malaria.**
2. Myotonia congenita.
3. As sclerosing agent.

Bulaquine: It is a mixture of two drugs and is used for treatment as well as prevention of malaria: 25 mg/day for 5 days is given on 2nd day of chloroquine for complete cure.

Chloroquine: Anti-malarial actions same as quinine
1. It has **no effect against the tissue phase of malarial parasite.**

2. By inhibiting growth of the parasite in RBCs it only **suppresses clinical attack**. It does not protect patient against relapses.

3. It **takes at least 48 hours** for the action to manifest.

Other actions of chloroquine

1. It has **anti-inflammatory activity**.
2. It suppresses conduction in heart (**antiarrhythmic action**).
3. It gets concentrated in liver and makes it useful in the treatment of **amoebic hepatitis**.

Adverse reactions

1. Nausea and vomiting are very common.
2. When used for long-term it produces retinal damage.
3. Skin reactions.
4. Changes in ECG are produced.

Uses

1. For prophylaxis of malaria: 300 mg is given once a week in immune people and twice a week in nonimmune people (not living in endemic area). This treatment should start one week before entering endemic area and should continue for 4 weeks after leaving endemic area.
2. In the treatment of clinical attack — 1.0 g initially followed by 500 mg 6 hourly for 2 days. This produces radical cure in *P. falciparum*.

   In falciparum it can be given intravenously (300 mg in 200–500 ml of normal saline is given intravenously slowly as infusion).
3. In the treatment of amoebic hepatitis.
4. In treatment of **rheumatoid arthritis**.

Precautions: Injectiable preparation not to be given in children and G6PD deficient patients.

Amodiaquine: Actions are same as chloroquine but single dose a day is sufficient.

Hydroxychloroquine: It is claimed to be less toxic.

Primaquine

1. It is **effective against gametocytes** and suppresses latent tissue phase and **has sporonticidal action** in mosquitoes.
2. Used along with chloroquine it produces **radical cure in malaria**.
3. It produces causal prophylaxis but is not used for this purpose as it is toxic.

Adverse reactions

1. Abdominal pain and blood stained vomiting are frequent reactions.
2. It produces break down of RBCs in Negroes and G6PD deficient individuals (haemolytic effect).

Use: It is used along with chloroquine to give radical cure.

Pentaquine and Pamaquine are rarely used.

Mepacrine: It was extensively used during second world war. It is not used now.

Disadvantages

1. It is **less effective** than chloroquine in treating acute attack.
2. It is **more toxic** than chloroquine.

Adverse reactions

1. Nausea, vomiting and diarrhoea.
2. Yellow staining of skin and sclera.
3. Headache and fever.

Precautions: **It increases toxicity of primaquine. It should not be given with this drug.**

Uses

1. It was used to treat acute attack of malaria.
2. It is **useful in giardiasis and tapeworm infestation.**

Dose: 0.1 g/day.

Proguanil

1. It is useful in the causal prophylaxis of falciparum malaria.
2. Useful in preventing multiplication of parasite inside mosquito. This reduces spread of infection.

Disadvantages

1. It cannot be used to treat clinical attack as the action is slow to start.
2. Parasites can become resistant to it.

Adverse reactions

1. Nausea and vomiting.
2. In few cases hematuria may occur.

Chlorproguanil and Cycloguanil Pamoate: Both these drugs have longer lasting effect and are used for prophylaxis.

Chlorproguanil is given in the dose of 20 mg/week.
Cycloguanil pamoate 5 mg/kg is given IM. It gives protection for 3 months.

Disadvantages

1. Both these drugs produce deficiency of folic acid.
2. Malarial parasite develops resistance to these agents.

Pyrimethamine: It has action against tissue phase of malarial parasite during incubation period. It is gametocidal only to *P. falciparum*.

Advantages

1. When combined with DDS or a sulfonamide it is used to treat *P. falciparum* **resistant to chloroquine**.
2. Development of resistance is delayed.
3. Prevents transmission of malaria.
4. This combination is used even in **treating toxoplasmosis.**

Disadvantages

1. It cannot be used for clinical cure of malaria (because of slow action).
2. Resistant strains develop. It is used for prophylaxis.

Dose: 5 mg/week.

Adverse reactions

1. Megaloblastic anaemia.
2. Thrombocytopenia and agranulocytosis may occur occasionally.

Mefloquine: It is antimicrobial agent that acts on erythrocytic phase of malaria and has strong schizonticidal activity.

Advantages

1. It is highly effective against asexual form of parasites and against gametes of *P. vivax* and *P. malariae*.
2. It is **effective against multidrug resistant strains of *P. falciparum*.**

Disadvantage: Resistance is quick to develop therefore use restricted to reactant strains.

Adverse reactions

1. Abdominal pain.
2. Nausea and vomiting.

Uses: Second line treatment.

Sulphonamides are active against asexual blood forms but action is slow. Given in combination with pyrimethamine or proguanil or sulfadoxine these are highly **effective against *P. falciparum* resistant to chloroquine.**

Tetracyclines are effective against
(a) primary exo-erythrocytic stage of *P. falciparum*
(b) blood schizont

Action is slow therefore used in combination with other drugs to treat chloroquine resistant cases.

Quinghaosu: It is obtained from plant—Artemisia annua.

Artesunate is given as tablet or IV. It is effective against schizonts. It has quick effect.

Useful in treating severe malaria including **cerebral malaria and chloroquine resistant falciparum.**

Treatment of acute attack: **Chloroquine** 4 tabs given at once followed by 2 tabs 6 hours later and then 2 tabs are given daily for the next two days.

Chloroquine resistant malaria: Quinine 600 mg three times a day is given or
Metakelfin 1 tab twice a day.

For treating cerebral malaria

(a) Chloroquine 250–400 mg intramuscularly
(b) Quinine in the dose of 15 mg/kg given intramuscularly or even intravenously.

Drugs for radical cure

Radical cure is not necessary for individuals living in endemic area, it should be given only to those who leave endemic zone permanently. **Primaquine** is given in the dose of 15 mg/day for 15 days.

Mosquito repellants can be used for protection from mosquito bites.

Prophylaxis

1. Chloroquine 2 tab/week: Start one week before and for 4 weeks after leaving endemic area.
2. Mefloquine: 250 mg/week for chloroquine resistant strains, start one week before and for 4 weeks after leaving endemic area.
3. Doxycycline 100 mg daily start 2 days before journey and continue for 4 weeks after leaving endemic area.

Nursing care of patient of malaria

1. Question the patient about the unusual auditory sensations pertaining to VIII nerve irritation (ringing in the ears). These are caused by quinine.

2. Record urinary output of patients receiving quinine (as it causes renal damage).

3. Monitor patients for hypotension and respiratory depression.

Patients usually ignore anti-malarial drugs. Encourage patients to comply with drug regimens.

71

Drugs used in other Protozoal Infections

AMOEBIASIS

Amoebiasis is caused by *E. histolytica*. This infection is highly prevalent in India and is acquired through ingestion of contaminated food or water. Motile form of amoeba invades mucosa of gut and forms ulcers. Amoebae are carried to liver and other tissues and produce **hepatitis** and **amoebic abscesses**. **Motile** as well as **cystic** forms of amoeba pass in stool.

Dysentery and hepatitis characterise this infection. Some patients may not show any symptoms and act as carriers. Following drugs are used in this disease

1. **Drugs effective both in intestinal and extraintestinal amoebiasis — metronidazole, tinidazole**, ornidazole emetine and dehydroemetine.
2. **Drugs effective only in extraintestinal amoebiasis — chloroquine.**
3. **Drugs effective only in intestinal amoebiasis:** Iodochlorhy — droxyquin, diiodohydroxyquin, carbarsone and glycobiarsol, tetracycline, diloxanide furoate, emetine bismuth iodide and paramomycin.

Metronidazole: It is prodrug and its active metabolite inhibits protein synthesis in amoeba and anaerobic bacteria. It is effective against both intestinal and extra intestinal amoebiasis. It is also effective against anaerobic microbes.

Advantages

1. It kills amoebae.
2. It is also active against *Giardia lamblia* **and** *Trichomonas vaginalis*.
3. It is effective both in intestinal and extraintestinal amoebiasis.

Disadvantages

1. Ineffective in asymptomatic cyst passers (carriers).
2. Ineffective in chronic intestinal amoebiasis.

Adverse reactions

1. Nausea and vomiting
2. Headache, vertigo and ataxia.
3. Skin rashes.
4. Metallic taste in mouth.

5. It is mutagenic.

6. Peripheral neuropathy.

It interacts with alcohol and produces antabuse-like reactions.

Uses

1. Amoebic infections
2. *Trichomonas vaginitis*.
3. Giardiasis.
4. Ulcerative gingivitis.
5. In treatment of anaerobic infections (gynecological and colorectal surgery).
6. Dracanculosis (guinea worm) (niridazole is drug of choice).
7. Pseudomembranous colitis.
8. *H. pylori* infections.

Dose: 400 mg three times a day for 10 days.

Topical preparations are used in skin infections and acne.

Tinidazole: This resembles metronidazole in all respects except that

(a) It is better tolerated.

(b) It has longer half life.

Dose: 500–800 mg orally three times a day for 5 days.

Secnidazole is longer acting and can be given as single 2 gm dose for all conditions in which metronidazole is used.

Satranidazole twice as active as metronidazole. It is useful in giardiasis, amoebiasis and in anaerobic infections.

Uses

1. In intestinal amoebiasis.
2. In trichomonas vaginitis.
3. In leucorrhoea.

Emetine: It is an alkaloid obtained from ipecac.

Advantage: It is highly effective in destroying trophozoites.

Disadvantages

1. It has no effect against cystic forms.
2. It is toxic to heart.
3. It has to be injected.

Adverse reactions

1. It is highly irritant. It produces pain, tenderness and stiff muscles at the site of injection.
2. When given orally it produces nausea and vomiting.
3. It is **toxic to heart**. Arrhythmias and changes in ECG are produced. It produces fall in blood pressure.

Uses

1. In amoebiasis **not responding to metronidazole**.
2. In treatment of lung flukes and *Fasciola hepatica*.

Dose: 60 mg subcutaneously or intamuscularly at night for 7–10 days.

Dehydroemetine

Advantages

(a) It is less toxic than emetine.
(b) It can be given orally as well as IM.

Emetine Bismuth Iodide: It has 25% anyhydrous emetine and 20% bismuth. Adverse reactions are same as with emetine.

Dose: 60–200 mg/day given orally after meals.

Advantage: It is effective when given orally.

Adverse effects on gastrointestinal tract are less marked than with emetine.

Use: For intestinal amoebiasis.

Precautions in the use of emetine and emetine containing drugs

1. Emetine is cardiotoxic, therefore it should not be given to patients with cardiac problems.
2. To reduce the incidence of adverse effects of this drug patient should be kept in bed for at least 48 hours after start of the treatment.
3. ECG and BP should be taken before starting therapy and it should be repeated on 5th and 10th day of treatment.
4. These drugs should be given for limited period.
   Emetine should not be repeated before 3 months.
5. It is never given IV

Chloroquine: This drug has been described in detail in chapter on Drugs used in Malaria.

(i) It gets concentrated in liver and **kills the trophozoite forms of amoeba in the liver.**
(ii) It has **no effect on the intestinal amoeba** because it does not reach the site of action in the required concentrations.

Dose: 250 mg four times a day for 2 days followed by 250 mg twice a day for two weeks.

Uses

1. In amoebic hepatitis as an alternative to metronidazole.
2. In combination with carbarsone or diiodohydroxyquin, it is given in intestinal amoebic infections.

Diiodohydroxyquinoline (Diiodoquin): It is effective against motile as well as cystic forms of amoeba. It is used in intestinal amoebiasis.

Adverse reactions

1. Nausea, vomiting and diarrhea.
2. Few patients complain of headache and vertigo.
3. **Allergic symptoms** are seen in patients **sensitive to iodine**.

Dose: 600 mg thrice daily for 20 days.

Iodochlorohydroxyquinoline (Quiniodochlor, vioform)

1. It is useful in treating **carriers** but not useful during acute attack.
2. It also has antifungal activity.

Paromomycin (Humatin): It is poorly absorbed from gut. It is useful in both acute and chronic amoebic dysentery. Better drugs being available it is not used now.

Diloxanide Furoate is Amoebicidal

1. It is useful in acute as well as chronic intestinal amoebiasis.
2. It is **useful in carriers and cyst passers**.
3. It is given with metronidazole for cure of amoebiasis.

Disadvantages

1. It is either not effective or less effective in acute severe dysentery.
2. It is less effective than metronidazole or emetine.
3. It is **not effective in amoebic hepatitis**.

Adverse reactions

1. Nausea and vomiting.
2. Skin rashes.

Dose: 500 mg three times a day for 10 days.

Fumagillin: It is an antibiotic derived from Aspergillus fumigatus.

Advantages

1. It is effective against both **vegetative and cystic forms** of amoeba.
2. Resistance does not develop to this drug.

Disadvantage: Not effective in extra-intestinal amoebiasis.

Adverse reactions

1. Skin rashes.
2. Nausea, vomiting and diarrhea.

Phanquone

1. It is effective against **intestinal** as well as **extra-intestinal amoebiasis**.
2. It has **antibacterial** activity.

Adverse reactions

1. It colours urine.
2. It produces nausea and vomiting.

Dose: 150 mg twice daily for 5–10 days.

Treatment of amoebic dysentery

I. Acute intestinal amoebiasis

1. 400 mg of metronidazole given three times a day for 10 days controls amoebic dysentery and prevents spread of infection to liver.
2. Anti-diarrheal mixture is added to metronidazole therapy for better results. Tetracycline 250 mg 4 times daily is also added. If patient does not respond to this drug or condition is severe, patient should be hospitalised and treated with emetine for 3–4 days. This should be followed by emetine bismuth iodide 200 mg daily and diloxanide furoate for 10 days.

II. Subacute chronic amoebic dysentery is treated with emetine bismuth iodide 200 mg daily for 10 days or diloxanide furoate 500 mg three times daily for 10 days. This should be followed by chloroquine 600 mg base for 15 days.

III. Ameobic hepatitis is treated by metronidazole 800 mg three times daily for 10 days. Alternatively, chloroquine is given in the dose of 500 mg three times a day for 2 days followed by 250 mg twice a day for 2 to 3 weeks. Emetine 1 mg/kg SC or IM for 10 days.

Prevention

1. Avoid fecal contamination of water and food.
2. Cutting of nails is very important as the cysts may be transferred to food. Drugs are not used for prevention.

Drugs used for other protozoal infections

1. Drugs used in leishmaniasis.
2. Drugs used in trichomoniasis.

3. Drugs used in giardiasis.
4. Drugs used in trypanosomiasis.
5. Drugs used in toxoplasmosis.

LEISHMANIASIS

It is of two types:
1. Visceral called **kala-azar** and is prevalent in Bihar and Orissa.
2. Cutaneous is also called **oriental sore**.

A. **Antimony compounds and diamidines** are used for these conditions, e.g. **ethylstibamine, sodium stibogluconate, meglumine antimonate, urea stibamine, dihydroxystilbamidine and pentamidine.**

B. **Amphotericin B, ketoconazole, allopurinol and paramomycin.**

Antimony Compounds: Trivalent compounds of antimony though effective **are highly toxic. Pentavalent antimonials are used**. Ethylstibamine is used as 5% solution for intravenous injections.

Dose: 200 mg initially followed by 300 mg/day for 15 days. Sodium stibogluconate 500 mg is given for sensitivity test followed by 1.0 to 1.5 g daily or on alternate day. 12.0 gm is the total dose.

Urea Stibamine

Advantage: It is effective even in cases resistant to other antimonials.

Disadvantages
1. It needs to be given intravenously.
2. If the treatment is interrupted organisms develop resistance to this drug.

Dose: 50–200 mg on alternate day for 4 weeks.

Ethylstibamine: It is a mixture of four compounds. Ethylstibamine given as 2.5% or 5% solution either IM or IV on alternate days. Sodium stibogluconate is IV or IM.

Adverse Reactions of Antimonials: GIT — Nausea, vomiting, diarrhoea and metallic taste.

CNS: Giddiness, delirium and unstable body temperature
Renal: Hematuria
Gen: Muscular pain, blood dyscrasias and jaundice.

Diamidine Derivatives: **Hydroxystilbamidine** and **pentamidine** are usually used as they are less toxic. These are effective in treating **trypanosomiasis, pneumocystis carcarinician and fungal infections**.

Uses

Diamidines are used in:
1. Sleeping sickness (trypanosomiasis).
2. Chagas disease.
3. Leishmaniasis.

Pentamidine

Advantage: More effective but more toxic than antimony compounds.

Uses

(a) Given only in resistant cases of leishmaniasis.

(b) Prophylactically against *T. gambiense*.

(c) ADRs—nausea, vomiting and breathlessness.

Dihydroxystilbamidine: 250 mg/day for 10 days. It is given intravenously.

Adverse reactions

1. Headache, fever and allergic symptoms.
2. If given by rapid intravenous injection produces circulatory collapse.

Precautions

1. Urea stibamine undergoes chemical change if exposed to air. This should be avoided.
2. Fresh solution of ethylstibamine should be prepared for intravenous injection.
3. Sensitivity test should be done.
4. Medical kit should be ready to meet any emergency arising out of allergic reactions.
5. Intravenous injection should be made slowly.
6. Antihistaminics can be given along with these drugs to reduce adverse reactions.

Allopurinol: A drug found to be effective in treatment of hyperuricemia has been found to be useful in treatment of leishmaniasis. It is given in combination with other antileishmanials.

Amphotericin B: Given for treatment in endemic areas where antimonials may be ineffective.

Ketoconazole: Inhibits ergosterol synthesis in Leishmania and is also effective is cutaneous leishmaniasis.

Paramomycin: It is an amoebicidal drug which is also found to be effective in leishmaniasis. It is used alone or in combination with antimonials.

Oriental Sore

(a) Pentavalent arsenicals are given into the lesion.

(b) Sodium antimony gluconate and stibophen are given IV and IM respectively.

(c) Early stages of disease are treated by local infiltration of mepacrine.

(d) Dehydroemetine resinate is also used. It can be given orally.

(e) **Amphotericin B, rifampicin and ketoconazole** have also been used.

TRYPANOSOMIASIS

Following are the drugs used in treatment of sleeping sickness which is due to *T. rhodesiense* and Chagas disease which is due to *T. cruzi*.

Pentamidine, suramin sodium and tryparsamide, Mel B and malarsonyl potassium and amphotericin B.

Nitrofurazone has also been found to be useful.

Suramin Sodium: It is drug of choice for early disease but is not effective when infection reaches brain as it cannot cross BBB. Also effective against *O. volvulus*.

Pentamidine Isoethionate: It is useful for prevention of trypanosomiasis.

Tryparsamide: It is useful in treating encephalitic stage of this infection. One injection every six months prevents against *T. gamisian* but not *T. rhodesian*.

Adverse reactions

1. Nausea and vomiting.
2. Liver damage.
3. Dermatitis.
4. In occasional patient it may produce nitroid crisis.
5. Visual acuity is reduced.

Melarsoprol (Mel B): It is trivalent arsenic compound. It is effective in early as well as late stages of **encephalitic stage** of trypanosomiasis. It is less toxic than tryparsamide.

Adverse reactions

1. Vomiting and abdominal pain.
2. Neuritis.
3. Encephalitis.

Cautions

It should not be given in cardiac patients. Patients suffering from kidney malfunction.

Malarsonyl Potassium (Mel W): It is less effective as well as less toxic.

Uses

1. In treatment of guinea worm infestation.
2. In trypanosomiasis.

Nifurtimos and Benznidazole: Useful in chagas disease South American trypanosomiasis.

Advantages

1. It can be given orally.
2. It is effective against organisms resistant to arsenicals.
3. It is less toxic than other compounds.

TOXOPLASMOSIS

This infection is responsible for repeated abortions. It is treated by **pyrimethamine and sulfadiazine** given for 4–6 weeks. **Clindamycin** and **spiramycin** are also useful in this condition **atovaquone** is given in AIDS patient.

TRICHOMONIASIS

Trichomonas vaginalis is a common disease. Following drugs are used:
1. Metronidazole.
2. Furazolidine.
3. Locally acting agents, e.g. vinegar, boric acid and lactic acid povidone iodine.

Metronidazole (Flagyl): For details please refer Drugs used in Amoebiasis.

Dose: 200 mg three times a day given orally. Vaginal tablets contain 500 mg of this drug.

Tinidazole: 2.0 g as a single dose is sufficient.

GIARDIASIS

Metronidazole is highly effective. Other drugs which are used in this condition are **dehydroemetine** and **diiodohydroxyquinoline**.

72

Antiviral Drugs

There is paucity of drugs with antiviral activity. Viruses exist intracellularly and the drugs which enter the cell not only destroy virus but exert bad effects on the cell also.

Following drugs have been used to treat viral infections.

1. **Antiherpetic and antimegalovirus drugs:** Idoxyridine, acyclovir, famcyclovir, gancyclovir and forscarnet.
2. **Anti-influenza drugs:** Amantadine and rimantadine.
3. **Antiretroviral drugs.**
   (a) Nucleoside reverse transcriptase inhibitors: Zidovudine, didanosine, zalcitabine, stauvudine, lamivudine and abacavir.
   (b) Non-nucleoside retroviral durgs (NNTII): Nevirapine and efavirenz.
   (c) Protease inhibitors: Ritonavir, lovenavir, saquanavir, amprenavir and nelfinavir.
   (d) Miscellaneous or nonselective: Ribavarine and interferon.

Idoxyuridine

Uses

1. As eye drops in Herpes simplex keratitis. 0.1% solution is used every 2 hours.
2. It is given intravenously for treatment of encephalitis caused by Herpes simplex.

Adverse reactions

1. Leucopenia.
2. Thrombocytopenia.
3. Loss of hair from head.
4. Liver damage.

Adenine Arabinoside (Vidarabine)

1. It is used to treat ocular Herpes simplex (local application) and Herpes encephalitis.
2. It is given intravenously (15 mg/kg daily) to treat viral encephalitis.

Acyclovir: It is less toxic and more potent. It affords symptomatic relief but post-herpetic neuralgias can occur. **It is not effective against CMV.**

Advantages

1. It is effective against Herpes simplex of cornea, but not effective on skin.

2. It is also effective against Herpes zoster infections.

3. It is well tolerated and less toxic.

4. It can be given orally.

Famcyclovir used as an alternative to acyclovir.

Ganciclovir: Highly toxic drug. It is used to treat serious cytomegalovirus (CMV) infection of retina in AIDS patients.

Foscarnate sodium: Effective against influenza A and Lhasa fever. It is active in acyclovir resistant cases of CMV.

In syncytial viral infection of respiratory system it is given by nebuliser or an aerosol.

Advantage: Resistance is not reported.

Disadvantage

1. It is teratogenic and cannot be used during pregnancy.

2. Causes severe anemia and renal damage.

Trifluridine is used to treat Herpes simplex.

Amantadine: It is effective against influenza A and Rubella virus. It is basically used for prevention of infection due to influenza A virus.

Adverse reactions

1. Confusion, sleeplessness and difficulty in thought process.

2. It produces hallucinations.

Uses

1. For prevention of influenza A viral infection.

2. For treatment of Parkinsonism.

Dose: 100 mg twice a day.

Zanamivir and oseltamivir are better than amantadine.

Thiosemicarbazone (Methisazone): It is effective against vaccinia and smallpox viruses.

Dose: 1.5–3.0 gm/twice a day for 4 days.

Adverse reactions

1. Intense nausea is produced.

2. It is advisable to give antiemetic drug along with it.

ANTI-AIDS DRUGS

Zidovudine: It is active against AIDS

(a) It improve CD_4 counts and improves well-being.

(b) Prolongs duration of life.

(c) Decreases mortality, causes anemia and neutropenia.

Didanosine: Causes pancreatitis, headache, insomnia and hepatitis. It is given orally. Does not cause bone marrow suppression.

Zalcutabine: It is given orally. It produces dose related neuropathy, oedema of lower limbs and general malaise. Not preferred.

Lamivudine: It is used in resistant cases of **HIV** and also to treat **hepatitis B infection**. Unwanted effects are mild (headache and gut disorders).

Stavudine: It is given orally. It penetrates into CSF (55% concentration of plasma). Causes neuropathy, joint pains and pancreatitis.

Nevirapine: Prevents mother to baby transmission of HIV if given to mother during pregnancy. Can be given to neonate—rash may occur. It is given orally.

Efavirenz is given orally but **can cause fetal abnormalities** and CNS symptoms.

Protease inhibitors: Protease enzyme does not occur in human, hence **these drugs are more specific against virus**. All are given orally.

Nelfinavir and ritonavir are better absorbed if given with food and saquinavir given within 2 hours of food.

Adverse reactions

1. Insulin resistance leading to high blood sugar and hyperlipidaemia.
2. Buffalo hump.
3. Stevens-Johnson syndrome.
4. All increase concentration of benzodiazepines.

INTERFERONS

These are substances produced by the body. They vary from species to species. They are produced from infected leucocytes, fibroblasts and lymphocytes. They serve following functions in the body.

1. Inhibit multiplication of viruses.
2. Act as immune modulators.
3. Increase activity of natural killer cells and macrophages.

Adverse reactions

1. Leucopenia and thrombocytopenia.
2. General ill health.

Uses: As adjunct therapy in treatment

(a) of hairy cell carcinoma

(b) AIDS related Kaposi's sarcoma

(c) condylomata acuminata.

73

Antifungal Antibiotics

Fungal infections occur on skin and mucous membranes. Fungus thrives in moist warm environment. Fungal infections occur periodically, when the resistance of the body is lowered. These infections can spread inside the body (systemic fungal infections).

Classification of Antifungal Drugs

1. **Antibiotics:** Amphotericin B, nystatin, hamycin, natamycin and griseofulvin.
2. **Antimetabolites:** flucytosine.
3. **Azole:** Imidazole, clotrimazole, econazole, miconazole and ketoconazole.
4. **Trizoles:** fluconazole and itraconazole.
5. **Allylamine:** terbinafine.
6. **Miscellaneous:** Tolnafetate, undecyclic acid, benzoic acid, qudochlor, ciclopirox and olamines sodium.

LOCALLY ACTING ANTIFUNGALS

Nystatin: It is found to be effective against *Candida, Histoplasma, Blastomycoses, Trichophyton* and *Microsporum*.

Disadvantages

1. It is not absorbed when given orally.
2. It is highly toxic if given by injection.

Uses: Its use is **restricted to local application** and treatment of moniliasis vaginitis and mouth, skin, corneal and conjunctival candidiasis. It acts by inhibiting respiration and glucose utilisation by the fungus.

Adverse reactions: Oral administration produces nausea, vomiting and diarrhea.

Vaginal tablets contain 100,000 units of nystatin. Ointment contains 100,000 units per gram.

Other antifungal antibiotics which are useful for local application are **punarcin and hamycin**.

Punarcin: It is effective against *Aspergillus, Trichophyton*. 5% ointment is used for eye infections and 2.5% suspension is used for inhalation to cure fungal infections of the respiratory tract.

Hamycin: It is highly effective against Cryptococcosis, Blastomycosis, Histoplasmosis and Coccidiodomycosis.

Candida infection also responds to this drug.

Uses

1. In treatment of blastomycosis and *Trichomonas vaginalis*.
2. In treatment of vaginal candidiasis. It produces hepatic and renal toxicity.

Trichomycin and Candicidin: These are used against *Trichomonas* and *Candida* infections of vagina respectively.

Griseofulvin: It is effective against most dermatophytes. Its basic use is in treatment of ringworm infection of different regions (head, hands, skin and nails). **It is given orally to treat skin infections**.

Advantages

1. It is well absorbed if given with fatty meal.
2. Gets deposited in keratin and prevents these cells from getting infected.
3. Of all the antifungal antibiotics available, it is least toxic.

Disadvantages and adverse reactions

1. It is **ineffective against *Candida albicans* and other deep fungi.**
2. It takes 1–2 months before showing good effects.
3. It produces neural disturbances, e.g. peripheral neuritis, lethargy, fatigue and blurring of vision.
4. Produces gynaecomastia (enlargement of breasts in male).
5. Superinfection with *Candida albicans* may occur.
6. It is fungistatic.

Uses: For treating dermatophytes, e.g. ringworm of scalp, beard and groin, ringworm of nails (treatment given for 4–6 months). Ringworm infection of head, feet and nails.

Dose: 250 mg twice or four times daily orally.

Triazoles, itraconazole and fluconazoles cross BBB and have better tissue penetrability. These are less toxic than ketoconazole. These drugs are effective against *Dermatophytes, Microsporum, Cryptococcus, Blastomyces, Occidiodes, Nocarida* and *Candida*. These drugs are used locally in mixed infections.

TO TREAT SYSTEMIC FUNGAL INFECTIONS

Amphotericin B: It is **used to treat systemic fungal infections and leishmaniasis.**

Disadvantages

1. It has to be given intravenously.
2. It is very toxic (renal failure may occur).
3. Drug is not well distributed in the body.

Adverse reactions

1. Allergic reactions.
2. Hepatic and kidney damage.

3. It may produce hypotension and cardiac arrest.

4. Hypokalemia.

Uses

3% solution is used for local application. For intravenous administration 0.1 g/ml in 5% dextrose is used.

1. It is applied locally for treating candida infections.

2. Used for treating systemic Blastomycosis and other fungal infections.

Nursing care

Testing of sensitivity is done before administration. It is **photosensitive** therefore cover the bottle to protect against light.

Clotrimazole: It is effective but is even more toxic. It is given orally.

Used to treat systemic infections, e.g. *Candida, Aspergillus, Sporotrichum* and *Cryptococcus*. Locally used to treat skin and vaginal infections.

Miconazole

1. Tissue penetration is better.

2. In addition has antibacterial activity.

3. It produces prolonged remission.

Uses

1. In treating systemic infections caused by *Candida*.

2. Is used in treating mixed skin infections.

3. For systemic use it is given intravenously.

Ketoconazole: It is broad spectrum antifungal and is given orally. It is used to treat superficial and deep fungal infections.

Dose: 200–400 mg/day.

Vaginal tablets are also available.

Fluconazole: It has wider spectrum than ketoconazole. It is used in cryptococcal meningitis and Histoplasmosis.

Terbenafin: It is fungicidal, is drug of choice for Onychomycosis (nail). It us less toxic than ketoconazole.

Itraconazole: It has broader spectrum than ketoconazole and fluconazole, but does not cross BBB.

Flucytosine: It is useful in cryptococcal meningitis and systemic candidiasis.

ROLE OF KERATOLYTIC AGENTS IN TREATING FUNGAL INFECTIONS

Fungus buries down to the base of the keratin layer and therefore gets protected from contact with locally applied medicines. Keratolytics act by softening keratin and loosening cornified epithelium. Keratolytic agent promotes desquamation of stratum corneum, remove the offending fungi and helps in penetration of the drugs.

Benzoic acid is used with salicylic acid

1. Salicylamide (5%) is applied on scalp to treat *Tinea capitis*.
2. Whitfield's ointment contains both salicylic acid and benzoic acid and is used to treat rignworm infections.

Salts of fatty acids are used as antifungals.

Sodium Propionate: It is used as antifungal agent and also is added to doughs to retard spoilage in baked foods.

Undecylenic Acid: This is marketed as powder, creams, lotion, topical aerosole and ointment to treat fungal infections.

Zinc Undecylenate: This has two actions.

(i) Astringent action.
(ii) Antifungal effect against dermatophytosis, specially tinea pedis. Acidic medium increases its activity.

Ichthammol: It is black liquid.

It is used as 10% cream/ointment to treat resistant dermatomycoces.

Selenium Sulfide: It is effective against dandruff.

It is used as suspension to be applied once daily for 5 days.

Many antiseptic agents have antifungal effect and they are used, e.g. **crystal violet, brilliant green and potassium permanganate, phenol, resorcinol and thymol** are also used to treat fungal infections.

Tolnaftate: 1% solution is used in skin fungal infections.

74

Anthelmintics

Helminth means 'Worms'.

These are of two types:
(a) Nematodes — which have a cylindrical shape
(b) Platyhelminths which are flat.

Nematodes can be:
(a) Intestinal, e.g. *Ascaris, Ancylostoma duodenale, Necator americanus, Enterobius vermicularis.*
(b) Extra intestinal, e.g. *Wuchereria bancrofti, Loa loa, Dracunculus medinensis* and *Onchocerca volvulus.*

Platyhelminths are of two types:
(a) Cestodes or tapeworm.
(b) Trematodes or fluke worms.

Ascaris lumbricoides (Roundworm): Eggs are ingested through contaminated food. Ingested eggs hatch into larvae in the small intestine. These then migrate to the lungs and later migrate back to stomach and intestine. In intestine they grow to adult size. The infection remains intestinal unless perforation occurs. Eggs produced by adults are passed out in the feces. This infestation **causes anemia and allergic manifestations.**

Preventions

1. Purification of water.
2. Thorough cleaning of food specially vegetables.
3. Nails should be cut and hands thoroughly washed after toilet.

Necator americanus and Ancylostoma duodenale (Hookworm): Eggs are passed in the feces. Larvae are produced in the soil. These penetrate the skin (usually of the foot) and reach blood-stream and then to the lungs. Larvae are coughed up the trachea and are swallowed to reach intestine as adult worms. Worm attaches itself to the intestinal mucosa and sucks blood from the host producing iron deficiency anemia and constant diarrhea leading to disturbances of fluid and electrolytes.

Preventions

1. Proper disposal of fecal wastes.
2. Wearing of shoes.

Strongyloides stercoralis: Larva in the soil enters the host by penetrating the skin of foot. Adult worm burries itself beneath the mucosa of the small instestine. Larvae produced in the intestine penetrate to all parts of the body.

Symptoms: Abdominal tenderness, epigastric pain and diarrhea are the predominant symptoms. Extraintestinal symptoms depend on the tissue invaded.

Prevention: Same as with *Necator americanus*.

Enterobius vermicularis (Pin Worm): Ova passed in stools dry up and get airborne. These get ingested. Ova under nails too get ingested. From these ova larvae are produced in the intestine. Worms migrate through the anus, especially at night and may also reach genital tract in females producing itching in perianal region or perineal region. Secondary infections caused by scratching may occur. Salpingitis or peritonitis are occasional complications in females.

Preventions

1. Careful washing of hands.
2. Disinfection of toilets.
3. Cutting of finger nails.

In children tight underclothing prevents itching and reinfection.

Trichinella spiralis (Pork Roundworm): Ingestion of **infected meat** is responsible for this infection. Ingested larvae reach maturity in the intestinal tract. Fertilised females deposit larvae in the intestinal muscosa. Larvae are carried in the bloodstream. These penetrate skeletal muscles and the organs evoking inflammatory response resulting in following symptoms:

(i) Pain in the skeletal muscles.
(ii) Effects of damage to internal organs are determined by tissues penetrated by these larvae, e.g. pneumonitis in case of lung, heart failure and encephalitis in case of heart and brain respectively.

Preventions

1. Avoid purchase of infected meat.
2. Cook thoroughly.
3. Clean thoroughly and frequently the utensils used to process raw meat.

Wuchereria bancrofti (Filariasis): It is transmitted by flies, mosquitoes and mites. Larvae are deposited by these insects in the skin of man. Microfilariae are produced by the fertilised females which migrate to the lymphatics and bloodstream and develop into worms which lodge in lymphatic vessels and nodes producing symptoms.

Inflammation is produced in areas where the microfilariae or adults are lodged. Lymph nodes of that area get enlarged, lymphatics get blocked which produce gross swelling of the area (**elephantiasis**).

Taenia saginata and *T. solium* (beef **and pork tapeworm**). The infection is caused by ingestion of raw or inadequately cooked **meat** from infected animals. The head (scolex) of the worm attaches itself to the intestinal wall and grows a variable number of segments. Each segment is capable of forming a long worm.

T. solium invades tissues (muscles, liver or brain).

Symptoms

1. Mild abdominal symptoms.
2. Weight loss.
3. Symptoms and signs of extraintestinal tapeworm infection vary with tissues involved.

Prevention: Thorough cooking of meat prevents infections.

Schistosoma haematobium and S. mansoni: Infection is transmitted from snails to man by way of the contaminated bathing water. Larvae enter through skin and reach blood and lymphatics. They first move to the lungs, then to liver, where they mature in the portal veins. The mature adult worms mate and move to areas of the large and small intestines and baldder producing eggs that are eliminated in stools and urine.

Symptoms: An itching rash called swimmer's itch develops as a reaction to larvae which die in the skin. About 1–2 months later fever, chills, headache and other allergic and inflammatory symptoms may occur. Heavy infestation causes abdominal pain and diarrhea. Engorgement of organs occurs due to venous pooling.

Prevention

1. Control snails.
2. Stop swimming in contaminated waters.

Infestation by worms is highly prevalent in India and is responsible for general ill health due to anaemia.

Drugs used: **Vermicides** are drugs which kill worms while **vermifuge** are agents which expel worms from the body:

Clinical classification of anthelmintics

1. **Roundworm—(*Ascaris lumbricoides*):** Mebendazole, pyrantel pamoate, bephenium hydroxy-naphthoate, piperazine, tetramisole, thiabendazole, diethylcarbamazine.

2. **Hookworm—(*Necator americanus, Ancylostoma duodenale*):** Piperazine, mebendazole, pyrantel pamoate, bephenium hydoxynaphthoate, thiabendazole, tetrachlorethylene and bitosanate.

3. **Whipworm**—mebenbazole, thiabendazole, bephenium hydroxynaphthoate and hexylresorcinol.

4. **Tapeworm**—niclosamide, mepacrine, chloroquine, paromomycin, dichlorophen and mebendazole.

5. **Pinworm**—(thread worm, vermicularis): vipyrynium (pyrvinium piperazine), tetracycline, gentian voilet, pyrantel pamoate.

6. ***Schistosomiasis***—lucanthone, hycanthone, trivalent antimony compounds such as antimony dimercaprosuccinate. Tartar emetic, stibophen, amphotalide, niridazole, metrifonate dichlorovas, oxamniquine, praziquantel.

7. ***Strongyloids stercoralis***—thiabendazole, viprynium.

8. ***Trichnella spiralis***—Adult worms—thiabendazole, methyridine, piperazine.

9. *Diphyllobothrium latum*—fish tape worm—paromomycin, niclosamide, dichlorophen.

10. *Hymenolepsis nana*—paromomycin, niclosamide and dichlorophen.

Larvae—manifestations of disease are treated symptomatically, **cortisone** may give considerable symptomatic relief.

Piperazine Citrate:
It is available in the form of 250 mg tablets and syrup containing 100 mg/ml. It is effective against roundworm and threadworm. Worms get paralysed and release their hold on the lumen of bowel and are removed by peristaltic movements. Parasites expelled in stool remain alive but paralysed.

Dose: For round worm: 3 g/day for 2 days. For threadworm 75 mg/kg/ day in two divided doses for 2 days.

Advantages

1. Highly effective—90% cure rate.
2. It is least toxic and it is employed for mass treatment.
3. It is well tolerated and safe in pregnancy but **contraindicated in epilepsy and renal failure**.

Adverse reactions: Nausea, dizziness and urticaria.

Not to be given in patients of jaundice, renal and liver diseases.

Nursing care
Saline purgative be advised after piperazine treatment.

Bephenium Hydroxynaphthoate (Alcopar):
It is effective against *Ascaris lumbricoides, Necator americanus, Ankylostoma duodenale* and *Strongyloides* species.

Advantages: It can be **used in mixed roundworm and hookworm infestations. No purgative is required.**

A single dose of treatment is effective in *A. duodenale* but repeated administrations are required for *N. americanus*.

Can be given to children, elderly and during pregnancy.

Dose: 2.5 g of drug is contained in 5.0 g sachets, should be given on empty stomach twice a day.

Adverse reactions: It has very low toxicity.

(i) Nausea and vomiting.
(ii) Headache, cramping, abdominal pain and diarrhoea. It can be given in mixed infections where piperazine citrate is contraindicated.

Thiabendazole:
It is effective against multiple infestations. It is **drug of choice for whipworm (*Trichuris trichuria*), *Strongyloides sterocralis* and *Trichinella spiralis*. Roundworm, hookworm and threadworm** also respond to this drug.

It is drug of choice in cutaneous larvae migrans.

Doses

1. In ascariasis and ancylostomiasis: 25 mg/kg is given after dinner and the same dose is repeated after breakfast.

2. In threadworm: 25 mg/kg twice a day and repeated after 7 days.

3. In strongyloid infections: 25 mg/kg twice a day for 5 days.

4. In trichuriasis: 25 mg/kg twice a day for 7 days.

Adverse reactions

1. Allergy.

2. Hypoglycemia.

3. Disturbances of colour vision.

4. Nausea, vomiting and diarrhea are common.

Precautions

(a) Caution should be exercised in patients of liver and kidney dysfunction, malnutrition and anaemia.

(b) It should not be given to pregnant and lactating mothers or to children below 15 years.

Mebendazole: It is effective against most worms. It is polyanthelmintic vermicide but is slow acting may take 2–3 days for clearance of worms from the intestine.

In trichuris: It is drug of choice: 100 mg twice daily for 3 to 4 days.

In roundworm and hookworm: 100 mg twice a day for 3 days.

In oxyuriasis : 100 mg single dose is sufficient. It is also found to be **useful in mixed infestations**.

Adverse reactions

1. Mild gastrointestinal symptoms.

2. Allergic reactions: Including photosensitivity and Stevens-Johnson syndrome.

3. **It is contraindicated during pregnancy** and in patients with ulcers in gastrointestinal tract.

Albendazole (Zentel): It is a broad spectrum anthelmenitic.

It is used as a single dose for treating **mixed infestation** with ascariasis, oxyuriasis, ankylostomiasis and trichuriasis produces 96% cure rate.

Dose: 10 mg/kg/day for 4 weeks in treatment of hydatid cyst.

Tetramisole/Levamisole: Available in the form of tablets containing 50 or 150 mg. It is effective against roundworms and hookworms. 2.5 mg/kg is given once in roundworm infestation. It is also used as **immunostimulant**.

No toxic effects are seen in short-term therapy.

Pyrivinium Pamoate or Viprynium (Vanquin): It is a red coloured compound and is available as 50 mg tablet or suspension (10 mg/ml). It is useful in treatment of *Oxyuris vermicularis* and *Strongyloides stercoralis*.

Dose: 250 mg once or 5 mg/kg once. If necessary it can be repeated after 2 weeks.

Adverse reactions

1. Nausea and vomiting.

2. Urine gets coloured therefore patient should be informed about it.

Pyrantel Pamoate: It produces spastic paralysis of worms. It is polyanthelmintic vermifuge.

It is effective against ascaris, hookworms and enterobius. It is poorly absorbed from the gut, hence it is devoid of systemic adverse reactions.

Single dose is effective (10 mg/kg) for ascariasis and for hookworm same dose is given for 3 days. 11 mg/kg single dose in oxyuriasis is sufficient. 11 mg/kg for 3 days is required in *N. americanus* infections.

Its analogue **oxantel** is used in trichuriasis.

Adverse reactions

1. Nausea, vomiting and diarrhea.
2. It is toxic to central nervous system and liver if given in high doses.

Precautions

Caution should be exercised when this drug is given to patients with malnutrition or anaemia and liver malfunction.

It should be avoided in patients allergic to this drug.

It **antagonises the effect of piperazine citrate**. The two should not be combined.

Oxytetracyclines: Oxytetracycline is **effective in oxyuriasis**. It is costly and produces adverse reactions hence not used.

Diethylcarbazine: It is the only drug for filariasis uses.

Diethylcarbamazine Citrate: It is available as 500 mg tablet. It is effective against microfilariae of all filarial worms namely *W. bancrofti, W. malayi, Loa loa* and *O. volvulus*. Adult worms of *W. malayi* and *Loa loa* are also killed.

Dose: 2–3 mg/kg three times a day for 2–3 weeks. It can be repeated after 3–4 weeks.

In *O. volvulus* infection if eyes are involved, the recommended dose is 25 mg/kg for 3 days and the dose is increased every 4th day. It is also given in tropical eosinophilia.

It is also effective against *Ascaris lumbricoides*, but is not preferred as better drugs are available.

1. Tropical eosinophilia.
2. Loiasis.
3. Filariasis.

Adverse reactions

1. Anorexia, nausea and vomiting.
2. Headache.
3. General weakness.

Praziquantel: Single dose of this drug is found to be useful. It is effective against

(a) All species of *Schistosomiasis haematobium, japonicum* and *mansoni*.
(b) Liver, lung and intestenal flukes.
(c) Cysticircosis.
(d) Cestodes.
(e) Taeniasis.

Advantages: It can be given orally. Adverse reactions are mild. Single doe (40 mg/kg) is effective for *S. hematobium* and 60 mg/kg for *S. mansoni* and *S. japonicum*. 10 mg/kg in taeniasis.

Produces high cure rate (80–90%).

Niridazole: It is available as 500 mg tablet. It gets concentrated in portal blood where it acts against *Schistosoma*.

It is effective against *S. haematobium* and *Dracunculus medinesis* but not very effective against *S. mansoni* and *S. Japonicum*.

Dose: 20 mg/kg/day in 2 equally divided doses for 7–10 days.

Adverse reactions: Abdominal symptoms like nausea, vomiting and diarrhea.

If treatment is prolonged then it produces ECG changes and central nervous system effects like confusion, insomnia and sometimes convulsions.

Niclosamide: It is available as 500 mg tablet. It is effective against all four types of tapeworms. Worms are killed therefore identification of scolex in stool is not possible. Saline purgative after this drug is recommended specially in the case of *T. solium*. **Ova are not affected and autoinfection is possible.**

Patient should be instructed to thoroughly chew the tablets before swallowing.

Dose: 2.0 gm single dose.

Advantage: It is safe and causes mild GI disturbances.

Lucanthone: It is marketed in the form of 250 mg tablet. The metabolite of this drug is active against *Schistosomaisis* (*S. haematobium* and *S. mansoni*). It is not effective against *S. japonicum*.

Dose: 5 mg/kg three times daily for 7 days. It can be repeated after 3–4 weeks.

Adverse reactions

1. Nausea and vomiting.
2. Loss of appetite.
3. Insomnia and restlessness.

Children tolerate this drug better than adults.

Antimonials: Trivalent antimony compounds, e.g. potassium antimony tartrate and stibophen are used in *Schistosomiasis*.

Stibophen: It is available as solution (300 mg in 5 ml) for intramuscular injection.

Dose: 300 mg/5 ml/day IM for 5 days.

Adverse reactions

1. Joint pains
2. Fever
3. Albuminuria
4. Thrombocytopenia

This drug should not be given in:
1. Malnourished patient.
2. Tuberculosis.
3. Fever.
4. Cardiac, renal or hepatic insufficiency.

Potassium Antimony Tartrate (Tartar Emetic): It is effective against all three types of *Schistosomiasis*.

Dose: Treatment is started with 8 ml of 0.5% solution of this drug given intravenously.

This dose, if tolerated, is repeated on alternate days till the total of 500 ml of 0.5% solution is given.

Adverse reactions

1. Cough and dyspnoea.
2. Cardiac effects like tachycardia and hypotension.
3. Anaphylactoid reaction may occur.

Contraindications: Severe hepatic or cardiac or renal disease.

Antimony Sodium Dimercaptosuccinate: It is as effective as stibophen but is less toxic.

It is given in the dose of 40 mg/kg in five doses at weekly intervals.

Bithionol: It is drug of choice for treating **liver fluke and lung fluke infections**.

Adverse reactions

1. Mild gastrointestinal upsets.
2. Headache, dizziness.
3. Allergic rashes.

Dose: 30–40 mg/kg orally on alternate days for 10–15 doses.

Dichlorophen: It is effective and safe drug for the treatment of **tapeworm infestation**. It is devoid of adverse reactions and no prior preparation of patient is required.

Dose: 70 mg/kg is given on an empty stomach in the morning without prior dietary restrictions or purgatives.

Breakfast is served 2 hours after this drug. Dose may be repeated next morning.

Emetine Hydrochloride: It can be used in *Fasciola hepatica*. It is very toxic and therefore rarely employed for this purpose.

Metrifonate: This drug **is effective in *S. haematobium* and *S. mansoni*** infecting urinary tract. Also **effective against *Ascaris*, hookworm and whipworms**.

Advantages

1. Highly effective. It produces 90–95% cure rate.
2. It is cheap.
3. It produces mild adverse reactions.

Dose: 5–15 mg/kg orally 3 times at interval of 2 weeks.

Niridazole

1. It is highly effective against guinea worm which is spontaneously expelled or easily removed after treatment. It is used in treating *S. Haematobium, S. mansoni* and *S. japonicum infections.* It produces 70–100% cure rate.
2. It is given to **treat amoebiasis** not responding to other drugs.

Dose: 25 mg/kg/day for 10 days.

Adverse reactions

1. Anorexia, nausea, vomiting and diarrhea.
2. Headache and dizziness.
3. Arthralgia and myalgia.
4. Sweating and palpitations.
5. Urine may become yellow brown with unpleasant smell.
6. T-wave changes and ST depression occur in ECG.

Precautions

It should be used with caution in the elderly and very young children.

Paromomycin (Humatin): It is effective against tapeworms. It is also used in treating intestinal amoebiasis.

Adverse reactions: Nephrotoxicity, ototoxicity and CNS toxicity are produced hence not commonly used.

Oxaminquine: It is effective against *S. mansoni*. Dose varies from area to area. It is well tolerated.

Dichlorovos: It is organophosphorus compound. It is available in granular form that causes slow release. It is effective against

(a) Trichuris.
(b) Hookworms.
(c) Roundworms.
(d) Schistosomes.

It is given as single dose to a 12 hourly **fasting patient**. Patient is **not allowed food for 2 hours after** this drug.

Ivermectin: Often used in veterinary medicine.

Single dose is effective in treating **onchocerciasis**. Also useful in **scabies**.

Advantages

(a) Single dose treatment
(b) It can be used for prevention of onchocerciasis
(c) **Kills microfilare but has no effect on female parasites hence microfilare reappear in 3 months.**
(d) It can be given orally.

Nursing care of patients receiving anthelmintic drugs

1. Verify the causative organism through laboratory reports.

2. These patients usually suffer from anaemia, fluid electrolyte imbalances and malnutrition. General supportive care may be needed prior to anthelmintics.

3. Pinworm infestations usually affects all members of the family. Therefore, all family members should be treated simultaneously.

4. Before piperazine is administered, epilepsy and renal impairment should be ruled out.

5. Tetrachlorethylene must not be administered in presence of roundworm infestation. Before administering this drug nurse must check the laboratory reports to rule out ascariasis. The patient must be given fat free diet for 48 hours before giving this drug.

6. Patients receiving hexylresorcinol should be warned against chewing the tablet.

Antiseptics and Disinfectants

75. Antiseptics and Disinfectants

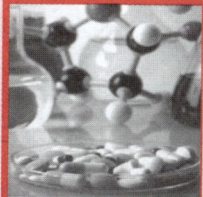

75

Antiseptics and Disinfectants

Antiseptics prevent or treat infections when applied locally. These drugs have bactericidal action and they are effective in killing all microorganisms in vegetative as well as spores states. It is desirable that these agents.

  (i) Should not irritate the tissue.

 (ii) Should have broad spectrum of activity.

(iii) Should not lose their activity in presence of necrotic material, pus or serum.

(iv) Should not stain clothes.

   Disinfectants are used to make the instruments or gloves free of microbes. This term is applied for antiseptics used for **non living**. These agents should not have corrosive activity.

Alcohol: Alcohols (ethyl, isopropyl) act by precipitating proteins of the microbes. 70% ethyl alcohol has greater efficacy than 100% alcohol. It hardens the skin owing to its astringent action. This action is responsible for its use in prevention and treatment of bed sores.

Disadvantages

    1. It is ineffective against spores.

    2. It is not effective against viruses.

Uses: For sterilisation of skin before injection and surgery.

Isopropyl Alcohol: It is more effective than alcohol. It is used for sterilisation of skin and catgut. Concentration: 72–100%.

Halogens

Iodine: It is used as tincture iodine and Mandl's paint.

Advantages

    1. It is highly effective against bacteria, fungi and certain viruses.

    2. It kills amoeba

    3. Higher concentrations and longer duration is required to kill spores.

    4. Its action is increased by alcohol.

Disadvantages

1. It is irritant and painful.
2. It delays healing.
3. It stains skin.

Uses

1. For cleaning unabraided skin before surgery.
2. Applied for treating ringworm.
3. For purification of non drinking water; 5 drops of iodine solution are added to a liter of water. It is allowed to react for 15 minutes.

Preparations available

1. Tincture iodine contains 10% iodine.
2. Weak iodine solution contains 2% iodine.
3. Mandl's paint is used for application on throat.
4. Non staining iodine ointment is also available.
5. Lugol's iodine is meant for oral use.
6. Povidone — iodine (betadine). It is used for disinfection of skin before surgery. It is available as solution, ointment and gel.

If iodine containing preparations meant for external use are accidentally taken orally severe irritation of the gastric mucosa is produced which may lead to coma and death. **Iodine toxicity is treated by administering 5% sodium thiosulfate.**

Iodophores: These are iodine carriers.

Advantages of Iodophores: They are less irritant than other iodine preparations and are used for disinfecting.

Chlorine: It is **effective against bacteria, viruses and amoebae**. Effective concentration is 0.25% parts per million (ppm). Concentrations over 1.0 ppm produces poisoning characterised by metabolic acidosis and irritation. Toxicity of chlorine is treated symptomatically.

Preparations available are **chloramines, sodium hypochlorite, halozone and chlorinated lime. Eusol** which is often used in hospital practice consists of **chlorinated lime** and **boric acid**.

Hydrogen Peroxide: IP solution of this agent is expressed in volumes. A-20 volume solution yields 20 volumes of oxygen from 1 volume of hydrogen peroxide.

1. It is used as antiseptic-cum-cleansing lotion. Oxygen that is liberated, mechanically removes the tissue debris.
2. It is used to clean root canals.

Potassium Permanganate: It is common antiseptic disinfectant used in household set up. It oxidises the material and renders it ineffective.

Uses

1. In the concentration of 1:1000 it is used for mouth washes, gargles and vaginal douches.
2. For urethral irrigation 1:5,000 is employed.

3. It is used for treatment of fungal infections such as athlete's foot.

4. Crystals of potassium permanganate are applied on the snake bite.

Phenol (Carbolic Acid): It is one of the oldest disinfectants, was first used by Lister. It acts by denaturing of the protein in microbial cells.

Advantages

1. It is highly effective against bacteria and fungus.

2. In addition to antiseptic effect it produces local anaesthesia.

Disadvantages

1. It is not effective against spores and viruses.

2. Its activity is reduced in presence of organic matter.

3. It loses its activity if combined with alcohol or glycerine.

4. It is highly irritant and may cause tissue necrosis.

5. It is readily absorbed and produces toxic symptoms.

Toxicity: If taken orally it produces **severe ulcers** in mouth, esophagus and stomach. **Shock** may supervene. Death may occur due to respiratory failure.

Toxicity is treated symptomatically. **Glycerine** and **alcohol** reduce its efficacy and toxicity.

Uses

1. It is applied on dog bitten area of skin and snake bites.

2. It is used to disinfect excreta.

3. Along with glycerine it is used as ear drops to relieve pain and itching of otitis media.

4. It is used as antipruritic agent (to treat itching).

5. It is used along with **camphor** for relieving pain of exposed tooth pulp.

6. It is added to calamine and sold as phenolated calamine lotion. This is used to treat insect bites, chicken pox eruptions and similar conditions.

Cresol is another phenolic compound.

Lysol is cresol in soap solution.

It is disinfectant commonly used in hospital practice.

Advantages

1. It is more effective.

2. It is less toxic.

It is used as 2% solution.

Thymol

Disadvantages

1. It does not dissolve in water easily (poor solubility).

2. It is highly irritant.

3. Its efficacy is reduced in presence of proteins.

Hexachlorophene: It is commonly used in toilet soaps and tooth pastes. By allowing a residue on the skin a cummulative antibacterial effect is produced.

Advantage: It is less irritant.

Disadvantages: It has short spectrum of activity. It is less effective against gram-negative bacteria.

Uses

1. It is used as deodorant.
2. Constant use of soaps containing hexachlorophene reduces the incidence of pyogenic skin infections.
3. It is used in the **treatment of carbuncles and seborrhic dermatitis**.

Adverse reactions

1. Local application may lead to allergic dermatitis in these individuals.
2. It gets absorbed when applied to abraded skin. On absorption it produces
   (a) Neurotoxicity
   (b) Cardiovascular collapse
   (c) Convulsions
   (d) Death due to respiratory failure.

Concentration used: 12%.

Boric Acid: Boric acid as well as sodium borate (borax) have been in use as home remedies.

It is a weak bacteriostatic but is nonirritant.

1. 2% solution is used for mouth washes, eye as well as skin lotions.
2. Occasionally used for bladder and vaginal washes.
3. Borax in glycerine is used as throat paint.

Benzoic Acid: This acid has antifungal as well as antibacterial activity.

Uses

1. 0.1% is used as preservative in foods.
2. Also used to test functioning of liver.

Salicylic Acid

1. It has bacteriostatic activity.
2. Antifungal activity.
3. It is a keratolytic agent, that is it produces break down of keratin.

Uses

1. In treatment of chronic skin ulcers.
2. For treatment of parasitic skin diseases.
   Benzoic acid has greater fungicidal activity while salicylic acid is more potent keratolytic agent. Combination of the two therefore is more useful.
3. As it is toxic it is **not used as food preservative**.

Formaldehyde (40% Formalin)

1. As formalin (weaker solution) it is used to preserve specimens in pathology department.
2. It is effective against bacteria, viruses and fungi.
3. Effective against *Mycobacterium tuberculosis*.
   This makes it useful for sterilisation of sputum and excreta of tuberculous patients.
4. It is used for dressing of **root canals**.
5. Formaldehyde in gaseous form is used for sterilisation of objects which can be destroyed by solution.

Disadvantages

1. Solution of this drug is extremely irritant.
2. On ingestion acute poisoning is produced characterised by abdominal pain, vomiting, diarrhoea and renal failure. Toxicity is treated symptomatically.

Gluteraldehyde: It has the following advantages over formaldehyde.

1. It is more potent.
2. It is less irritant.
3. Does not destroy lenses, rubber or plastic materials.
4. It can be used to sterilise respirators.

Anionic Surfactant

Detergents: Soft soaps

1. Soaps contain potassium or sodium hydroxide that are efficient germicidal agents.
2. These are mainly effective against gram-positive bacteria and Mycobacteria.

Disadvantages

1. Produce dryness of skin.
2. These are effective against limited number of bacteria — narrow spectrum.
3. Do not act in hard water.

Cationic Surfactants

Benzalkonium Chloride and Cetrimide: They are broad spectrum. These agents act against gram-positive as well as gram-negative bacteria.

Disadavantages

1. These are relatively ineffective against spores, viruses and fungi.
2. These are inactive in presence of acids.
3. These are less effective in presence of cotton and rubber.

Uses

1. Tubing made of polythene and nylon can be sterilised. 1:1000 solution is used for the purpose.
2. 1:8000 solution is used for steilising napkins.
3. 1:4000 solution is used for steilisation of the surgical instruments.
4. 0.5 percent sodium nitrite is added to reduce rusting of instruments.

Tween 80

1. It is an emulsifying agent — used in preparation of creams and ointments.
2. It is added to insecticides with a view to improve their functioning.

Gentian Violet: It is effective against gram-positive organisms, against whipworm and strongyloides parasite.

Disadvantages

1. It stains skin.
2. It is toxic.

Dose: 1 to 4 mg/kg is given intravenously as 1% solution.

Acriflavine and Proflavine: These are effective against gram-negative as well as gram-positive organisms.

Disadvantages

1. It stains skin.
2. It delays wound healing.

Uses

1. 2% solution is used in vaginitis.
2. 1:1000 is applied on infected wounds and burns.

Heavy Metals

Silver nitrate.

Uses

1. It is used as 1% eye drops in conjunctivitis and ophthalmia neonatorum.
2. Stick is used to remove warts.
3. 10–20% solutions are used for application to buccal ulcers and posterior pharyngeal granulations.

Mercurochrome: It is weak antiseptic. 1–2% solution is used on wounds, 0.1% solution of mercuric chloride is used as hand lotion or to disinfect instruments. Ointment of ammoniated mercury is used in dermatology for treatment of fungal infections.

Zinc Oxide/Zinc Sulfate: Zinc oxide is added to calamine lotion. Calamine too is zinc oxide with ferric oxide which gives it flesh colour. These drugs possess astringent as well as antiseptic activity.

Ethylene Oxide: This gas is explosive and is mixed with nitrogen or carbon dioxide before use. 30% is used for sterilisation of factories, and **heart lung machines** and **respirators**. It kills bacteria, spores and viruses.

HEAT

It is an effective way of sterilisation. It can be applied in two ways:
(a) Dry heat.
(b) Wet heat.

Dry heat is used as:

(i) Flame: Tips of forceps and inocculating wires are sterilised by putting them into direct flame for some time.

(ii) Hot air: Laboratory glassware and instruments are sterilised by keeping in oven.

(iii) Inceneration: This term is applied to procedure of burning things to ashes, e.g. dead bodies are burnt to ashes. This is a healthy way of disposal. In clinical practice this procedure is applied for disposal of solid dressings and pathological material.

Wet Heat

1. **Boilling:** This procedure removes gram-positive as well as gram-negative bacteria, **spores however are resistant.**

2. **Steam.**

Advantages: It can penetrate and reach areas which are otherwise unaccessible. Steam at high pressures is used to sterilise **culture media**, **dressing packs**, **surgical instruments** and certain pharmaceutical preparations.

Disadvantages

1. Sharp instruments turn blunt.

2. Endoscopes cannot be sterilised by this procedure.

3. Steam destroys the instruments by damaging the cementing substance.

FILTRATION

This is commonly employed for cleaning water in the remote areas of our country. In clinical practice this procedure is adopted for **cleansing human serum albumin**.

RADIATION

1. **Infra red rays** are used to sterilise syringes.

2. **Ultraviolet rays** are used for sterilisation of surfaces. Ionization radiation or gamma rays from cobalt 60 are used to sterlise syringes and equipment made of plastic (disposable syringes, heart lung machines, catheters).

Glassware should not be sterilised by gamma rays.

ANTISEPTICS AND DISINFECTANTS IN CLINICAL PRACTICE

1. For hands use soaps, followed by wash with chlorhexidine.

2. Disinfection of skin before injection.

   70% alcohol is applied, or isopropyl alcohol is used. This removes 80–90% of bacteria on skin. Alcohol should be **dried before giving prick**.

3. Disinfection of skin before surgery.

   Rub alcohol for 2 minutes. Tincture iodine is applied and removed by alcohol. **Antiseptic should dry off before giving incision.**

4. Wounds

Savlon which is a combination of **chlorhexidine and cetrimide** is used in dirty wounds.

5. Glass syringes to be boiled for at least 5 minutes.

6. Stainless steel and sharp insturments are put in the phenol.

Nursing care in handling antiseptics or disinfectants

1. Hydrogen peroxide

   (i) Store in tightly closed dark containers.

   (ii) Warn patient about the discomfort caused by this agent.

   (iii) Patient should be advised to protect eyes.

2. Potassium permanganate

   (i) Warn against staining properties of this drug.

   (ii) Dissolve crystals completely before using it.

   (iii) It is not effective against fungal infections.

3. Heavy metals (mercurochrome, silver nitrate, etc.)

   (a) Warn against discomfort produced by silver nitrate cream on burns.

   (b) Administer analgesics before application of silver nitrate on burns.

   (c) Caution patients to store these drugs with proper care. Keeping them away from children.

4. Iodine

   (a) Use freshly prepared iodine solutions.

   (b) Do not apply dressings to areas treated by iodine compounds.

   (c) Warn against accidental ingestion of this drug.

5. Alcohol

   (a) Not to be used for disinfecting metallic substances.

   (b) Glass instruments should be thoroughly cleaned before emmersing in alcohol solutions.

   (c) Do not apply alcohol to abraded or open skin areas.

   (d) Use alcohol rubs to cool, clean, dry and toughen skin **(bedsores)**.

6. Phenols

   (a) Avoid direct contact with phenols. Do not use these compounds near the eyes.

   (b) **Too frequent applications of phenol will produce painless burns.**

   (c) Hexachlorophene should not be applied on abraded skin.

INSECTICIDES

These agents are used to kill insects.

Insects carry and spread various diseases, e.g. malaria is spread by mosquito bite and cholera by flies, etc.

Dichlorodiphenyltrichloroethane (DDT): It was discovered during second world war. DDT gets stored in fatty tissues of organisms that ingest it. It is highly effective in the treatment of pediculosis. It is applied in the form of powder on skin for the treatment of lice. It does not irritate skin. It is not effective against scabies.

Adverse reactions

1. Reversible liver damage.
2. Infertility.
3. Increased infant mortality.

Lindane (Gama Benzene Hexachloride): Used to treat scabies.

Advantages

1. It has quicker onset of action.
2. Absorption by mammals is poor.

Adverse reactions

1. Skin rash on local applications.
2. Headache, nausea and vomiting if it gets absorbed.
3. Chronic exposure produces fatal aplastic anemia.
4. Serious liver and kidney damage is produced.

ORGANOPHOSPHORUS COMPOUNDS

Malathion and parathion are commonly used for spraying of farms. For toxicity and details please refer ANS.

Anticancer Drugs

76. Anticancer Drugs

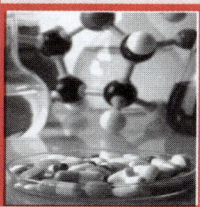

76

Anticancer Drugs

Cancer is responsible for 20% of all the deaths in the western world. In India too the incidence of cancer is on the increase.

Classification of anticancer drugs

(i) **Alkylating agents**, these are **cell cycle independent drugs**.

   (a) Nitrogen mustard cyclophosphamide, fosamide, mechlorethamine, melphalan and chlorambucil.

   (b) **Alkyl sulphonates**—busulphan.

   (c) **Triazenes**—dacarbazine.

   (d) **Nitrosoureas**—carmustine, lomustine and methyl lomustine.

   (e) **Ethylenimines and Methylmelamines**—hexamethylamine, thiotepa.

(ii) **Anti-metabolites:** These drugs act on **S phase** of the cycle.

   (a) Purine analogs.

   (b) Pyrimidine analogs.

   (c) Folic acid analogs.

(iii) **Antibiotics:** Dactinomycin, doxorubicin.

   (a) Vinca alkaloids—vincristine

   (b) Taxus alkalid—paclitaxel

   (c) Epipodophyllotoxins—etoposide.

(iv) **Hormones and other related substances.**

(v) **Miscellaneous agents.**

   (a) Enzymes—L-Asparaginase.

   (b) Biological response modifiers—TFN-α.

Properties of anticancer drugs

1. Anticancer drugs kill a constant fraction of cells rather than a fixed number.

2. Objectives of using anti-neoplastic drugs is to achieve complete remission. However, complete remission does not mean cure but denotes complete regression of all evidence of cancer.

3. Anti-neoplastic drugs are usually given in combination as in acute lymphocytic leukemia.

Disadvantages

1. All drugs used in cancer are toxic to normal tissues.
2. Cells that rapidly multiply, e.g. bone marrow, gastrointestinal tract and reproductive cells are highly sensitive to the damaging effect of these drugs.
3. Bone marrow depression is a common adverse reaction of these drugs.

Selection of the anti-neoplastic drug depends on

(a) Type of cancer.

(b) Pharmacological and pharmacokinetic factors of the drug.

(c) State of heart, liver and kidney functions of the patients.

Alkylating Agents: These drugs produce reactive intermediates of carbonium ion that forms alkylate guanine residues resulting in cross-linking or scission of DNA or abnormal base pairing.

All these drugs have cytotoxic and radiomimetic actions.

Nitrogen Mustards

Mechlorethamine

Uses

1. Generalised Hodgkin's disease.
2. Lymphomas.
3. Carcinomas of bronchi, ovary, and breast (other agents are better).

Adverse reactions

1. Severe nausea and vomiting.
2. Suppression of bone marrow.
3. Vesication and thrombophlebitis occur at the injection site.

Dose: 6 mg/m^2 intravenously. Solution should be freshly prepared before each administration.

Cyclophosphamide: It is most commonly used alkylating agent.

Advantages

1. It has greater selectivity for neoplastic tissues.
2. Thrombocytopenia is less common.
3. It can be administered through all routes (PO, IM, IV).

Uses

1. Hodgkin's disease.
2. Lymphomas.
3. Multiple myeloma.
4. Acute and chronic leukemias.
5. Neuroblastoma.
6. Cancer of ovary, breast and lung. This drug is combined with methotrexate and fluorouracil and is used to treat breast cancer when axillary nodes are involved.

7. It is a potent immunosuppressant and is used to prevent rejection of transplants.

8. It is also used in rheumatoid arthritis and nephrotic syndrome.

Adverse reactions

1. Nausea and vomiting.
2. Alopecia (loss of hair from head).
3. Severe hemorrhagic cystitis (administration of cysteine MESNA and sufficient water intake reduces this incidence).
4. It predisposes to cancer of urinary bladder.

Nursing care

Advise patient to take more of water.

Dose: 75–280 mg/m² intravenously daily for 10 days.

Melphalan

Advantages

1. It can be given orally and is less irritant locally.
2. Nausea, vomiting and alopecia are less common.

Uses

Multiple myeloma, breast cancer and malignant melanoma.

Adverse reactions

1. Bone marrow suppression is common.
2. Infection, diarrhea and pancreatitis are common complications.

Dose: 10 mg daily for 7 days or 6 mg daily for 2 weeks. After a gap of 4 weeks, maintenance dose of 2–4 mg is followed.

Ifosfamide: It is related to cyclophosphamide but has a longer half-life.

Uses

1. Carcinoma of bronchus, breast, testes, bladder, head and neck.
2. Osteogenic sarcoma.
3. Lymphomas.

Adverse reactions

1. Hemorrhagic cystitis (**Mesna** irrigation be given along with it to prevent this complication).
2. Nausea, vomiting, anorexia.
3. Leukopenia.
4. Nephrotoxicity.

Advantage: Causes lesser incidence of vomiting than cyclophosphamide.

Dose: 1.2 gm/m² IV over 30 min for 5 days.

Chlorambucil: It is shortest slowest acting and least toxic among all nitrogen mustards.

Use: It is the drug of choice for chronic lymphocytic leukemia and Hodgkins disease.

Adverse reactions

1. Nausea, vomiting and gastrointestinal discomfort and hepatitis.
2. Dermatitis.
3. Bone marrow suppression.
4. Pulmonary fibrosis.

Dose: 0.1–0.2 mg/kg daily orally for 3–6 weeks.

Busulfan (Myleran)

Advantages

It is more active against myeloid cells. Its pharmacological action is limited to bone marrow.

Uses

1. Drug of choice for chronic granulocytic leukemia.
2. Polycythemia vera.
3. Myelofibrosis with myeloid metaplasia.

Adverse reactions

1. Bone marrow suppression, thrombocytopenia is very common.
2. Nausea, vomiting and diarrhoea are less common.
3. Pulmonary fibrosis and gynaecomastia.
4. It precipitates gout, should be given along with allopurinol.
5. Hepatotoxicity is common.

Melphalan: It is drug of choice is multiple myeloma.

Carmustine and Lomustine: Cross BBB and are useful in treating brain tumors and meningeal leukaemias.

Adverse reactions

1. Causes bone marrow depression 3–6 weeks after starting treatment.
2. Carmustine causes renal damage.

Folic Acid Analogs: These drugs block synthesis of substances essential for synthesis of nucleic acid bases.

Methotrexate: This drug inhibits dihydrofolate reductase, the enzyme responsible for conversion of dihydrofolic acid to tetrahydrofolic acid. It is well absorbed when given orally.

Uses

1. In the treatment of acute lymphocytic leukaemia in children.
2. It is the drug of choice for treatment of choriocarcinoma—produces cure in most cases.

3. It is also given to treat Burkitt's lymphoma.
4. Mycosis fungoides.
5. Epidermoid cancer of head and neck areas.
6. Severe psoriasis.
7. For immunosuppression in steroid resistant asthma, Crohn's disease and transplant rejection.
8. Osteosarcoma.

Adverse reactions

1. Megaloblastic anaemia, thromocytopenia and leucopenia.
2. Stomatitis and diarrhoea.
3. Hemorrhagic enteritis.
4. Reversible hepatic dysfunction.

Dose: 2.5 mg daily or 150–500 mg/m^2 of body surface area IM at monthly intervals.

Fluorouracil: In the body it is converted to its active form 5-fluoro-2-deoxyuridine.

It prevents formation of thymine. It is relatively a less toxic drug.

Uses

1. It is used as a palliative therapy in stomach, breast, colon, rectum and ovarian cancers.
2. In inoperable cases of tumors of rectum and colon, it is often combined with radiotherapy.
3. It is applied to skin to treat cases of basal cell carcinoma and premalignant skin keratosis.
4. It is given through artery for the tumors of head and neck.

Adverse reactions

1. Anorexia, nausea and diarrhoea.
2. It destroys alimentary epithelium.
3. Causes bone marrow suppression.
4. Cerebellar toxicity.

Dose: 1 gm on alternate days for 6 days followed by 0.1–0.6 mg/kg/day for 4 days.

Cytarabine (Cytosine Arabinoside): It is the most active single drug available for treatment of acute myeloid leukaemia. It inhibits pyrimidine synthesis.

Uses

1. Acute myeloid leukaemia in adults.
2. Non-Hodgkin's lymphoma.
3. It is used as an immunosuppressant.
4. It is given in combination with thioguanine and adriamycin to treat acute lymphoblastic leukemias.

Adverse reactions

1. Suppression of bone marrow.
2. Nausea, vomiting and diarrhea.
3. Cerebellar ataxia.

Dose: 150 mg/m^2 intravenously daily for 5–7 days.

6-mercaptopurine and 6-thioguanine: Mercaptopurine is used for maintaining remission in **acute lymphocytic leukemias, chronic granulocytic leukemia** and **choriocarcinoma**. **Azathioprine** is a derivative of mercaptopurine and is used for suppressing immune responses.

Adverse reactions

1. Bone marrow suppression is the main adverse reaction.
2. Anorexia, nausea and vomiting.
3. Hepatic damage is produced. It is advisable to assess liver function tests in these patients routinely.
4. Produces hyperuricosuria.

Nursing care

Maintain urine of the patient on alkaline side.

Uses

(a) Acute lymphocytic leukemia
(b) Chronic granulocytic leukemia.
(c) It is especially effective in acute myeloid leukemia.
Thioguanine: No advantages over mercaptopurine.
Azathioprine is used as **immunosuppressant** in organ transplantation and **haemolytic anaemia**.
Nitrosourea: penetrates BBB and is useful in brain cancers.

Nursing care

1. Monitor clinical and laboratory tests for adverse drug reactions.
2. If the patient is likely to receive methotrexate assess his renal functions.
3. Patient on methotrexate should not receive **salicylates, tetracycline, chloramphenicol, phenytoin** or **sulfonamides**.
4. During methotrexate therapy the urine of the patient should be maintained on alkaline side.
5. Folinic acid can be given to counter adverse reactions of methotrexate.
6. MESNA should be given to patients on cyclophosphamide.
7. Patients receiving cyclophosphamide should take lots of fluids (2–3 litres) to avoid cystitis.
8. Patient must void off urine before going to bed.

NATURAL PRODUCTS

Vinca Alkaloids: There are two important anticancer alkaloids of this plant.
(a) Vinblastine.
(b) Vincristine.

Two of these alkaloids differ in their use and adverse reactions and there is no cross resistant between two, though they are chemically related.

Vinblastine: Acts by inhibiting mitosis: spindle toxic. It is not absorbed when given orally and is given IV.

Uses

1. Hodgkin's disease.
2. Lymphomas resistant to alkylating agents.

3. Choriocarcinoma resistant to methotrexate.

4. Neuroblastoma.

5. Cancer of breast.

6. In metastatic testicular tumors, it is given along with **bleomycin** and **cisplatin**.

Adverse reactions

1. Suppression of bone marrow.

2. Anorexia, nausea, vomiting and diarrhea.

Dose: 0.1 mg/kg once a week for 12 weeks.

Vincristine: It is one of the drugs used in MOPP regimen for Hodgkin's disease. It is **neurotoxic and causes alopecia.**

Uses

1. Acute lymphocytic leukemia.

2. Non-Hodgkin's lymphomas.

3. Neuroblastoma.

4. Wilm's tumor.

5. Rhabdomyosarcoma.

6. Brain tumors.

7. Hodgkin's disease.

8. Cancers of breast, kidney and those of reproductive systems.

Adverse reactions

The toxicity is manifested on two systems.

1. Peripheral nervous system.

2. Autonomic nervous system.

(a) Paresthesia, loss of deep tendon reflexes, neuritic pain, muscle weakness and double vision.

(b) Severe constipation, abdominal pain, paralytic ileum. Even bowel obstruction may occur.

(c) Alopecia.

(d) Fluid overload, hyponatremia and hemodilution are produced due to decreased ADH release.

Dose: 2 mg/m^2 of body surface per week IV.

Precautions: Caution has to be exercised in patients already suffering from peripheral neuropathies, e.g. diabetes mellitus.

Paclitaxel (Taxol) and Docetaxel: Isolated from the bark of *Taxus breifolia*. Inhibit mitosis.

Uses

1. Ovarian, esophagus, head neck cancer—as a first line of treatment.

2. Metastatic breast cancer refractory to cisplatin or doxorubicin.

Adverse reactions

1. Myelosuppression neutropenia (reversible)
2. Alopecia.
3. Neuropathy and myalgia.
4. GIT disturbance.
5. Bradycardia.

Nursing care

Before administration treat with dexamethasone and H_1 and H_2 blockers.

Docetaxel

It is like taxol but has longer half of life and adverse reactions are same as of taxol.

Dose: 100 mg/m^2 IV every 3 weeks.

Etoposide

It is semisynthetic drug and is given orally or IV. It acts by inhibiting DNA topoisomerase II that leads to damage.

Uses

1. It is used in combination with other drugs in treatment of testicular tumors that persist even after proper surgery and radiotherapy.
2. In treatment of lung cancer.
3. In treatment of certain lymphomas and leukemias.

Adverse reactions

1. Bone marrow suppression is the major draw back.
2. Temporary hypotension occurs when this drug is given intravenously.
3. Nausea and vomiting and alopecea.

ANTIBIOTICS

Bleomycin: This was isolated from *Streptomyces penuceticis*. It has a **radiomimetic** effect. It acts by inhibiting DNA repair.

Uses

1. It is used for palliative treatment of squamous cell carcinomas of head, neck, skin, esophagus and genitourinary tract.
2. It is given along with vinblastin and cisplatin to treat testicular tumors. This combination has successfully induced significant number of complete remissions.
3. Lymphomas resistant to other durgs.

Adverse reactions

Maximum toxicity is exerted on lungs and skin.

1. It produces **pneumonitis** leading to pulmonary fibrosis (incidence 10%).

2. On the skin it produces pruritic erythema, ulceration, vesiculation, hyperpigmentation and hyperkeratosis.

3. Alopecia, nausea and vomiting also occur.

4. Fever.

Dose: 10–20 units/m^2 of body surface area given intravenously or intramuscularly once or twice per week.

Precautions

This drug produces anaphylactic reaction. Sensitivity tests should be carried out before giving full dose.

Dactinomycin (Actinomycin D): It is produced by *Streptomyces parvullus*. It inhibits the synthesis of DNA dependent RNA.

Uses

1. Wilm's tumor.
2. Rhabdomyosarcoma.
3. It is also used in choriocarcinoma resistant to methotrexate.
4. Metastatic testicular carcinomas.

Adverse reactions

1. Suppression of bone marrow.
2. Irreversible cardiomyopathy.
3. Nausea, anorexia and vomiting.
4. Alopecia and other skin manifestations.

Dose: 0.5 mg/m^2 daily for 5 days. It is given by slow intravenous infusion.

Daunorubicin (Rubidomycin): It inhibits topoisomerase II in mammalian cell. It adversely affects function and structure of mitochondria.

Uses

1. It is used for producing remission in acute leukemias in adults.
2. Given for treatment of **acute lymphocytic leukemias** and **lymphoblastic lymphosarcoma** in children.

Adverse reactions

1. **Suppression of bone marrow** is the major drawback.
2. Alopecia, nausea, vomiting and diarrhoea.
4. It produces acute as well as delayed cardiac toxicity in the form of changes in ST segment, arrhythmias and cardiomyopathy.

Dose: 60 mg/m^2/day intravenously for 3 days, repeat weekly.

Doxorubicin (Adriamycin): It resembles daunorubicin in its mode of action.

Uses

1. It is the drug of choice in treatment of metastatic thyroid carcinoma.
2. It is used along with other agents in the treatment of cancers of ovary, breast and lung.
3. It is highly effective in the treatment of osteogenic sarcoma and neuroblastoma.
4. Hodgkin and non-Hodgkin's lymphomas.
5. Acute lymphoblastic leukemias.

Adverse reactions: These are same as with daunorubicin but are **more severe**.

Dose: 60–75 mg/m^2 given intravenously at 21 days interval.

Mithramycin (Plicamycin): It is derived from *Streptomyces plicatus*. If acts by inhibiting RNA synthesis.

Uses

1. It is used to treat advanced embryonal tumors of testes.
2. To treat **hypercalcemia** secondary to metastatic disease.
3. In Paget's disease it gives relief to patient from bony pains.

Adverse reactions

1. It induces bleeding tendencies.
2. Anorexia, nausea, vomiting and diarrhoea.
3. Hepatotoxicity and nephrotoxicity.
4. Nausea and vomiting.

Dose: 25–30 ug/kg daily IV for 8–10 days.

Mitomycin: It is obtained from *Streptomyces caespitosis*.

Uses

1. It is used for palliative therapy of adenocarcinoma of the stomach and the pancreas.
2. It is useful against certain cancers of colon, breast, head and neck.
3. It is used in treating granulocytic leukemia.
4. It is applied locally on superficial transitional cell carcinomas of urinary bladder.
5. It is injected into the hepatic artery to treat metastatic disease confined to liver.

Adverse reaction

1. Bone marrow suppression thrombocytopenia.
2. Anorexia, nausea, vomiting and diarrhoea.
3. Lung toxicity—pneumonia.
4. Neurological effects.
5. Renal failure and liver damage.

Dose: 2–10 mg/m^2 is given through intravenous infusion every 6–8 weeks.

ENZYMES

Asparaginase: It kills cancer cells by depriving them of their nutrition. Its use is limited in the treatment of **lymphoblastic leukemia** not responsive to other agents. It is not used in solid tumors.

Advantages

1. It causes minimal damage to bone marrow.
2. Anorexia, nausea and vomiting are not common features.
3. Alopecia is not a problem.

Disadvantage: It produces serious allergic reactions.

Adverse reactions

1. Liver damage occurs in about 25% cases.
2. Hemorrhagic pancreatitis is produced in about 5% cases.
3. Causes deficiency of clotting factor.
4. Anaphylactic reaction.

Dose: 50–200 IU/kg is IV given intramuscularly for 28 days.

HORMONES AND THEIR ANTAGONISTS

Adrenocorticosteroids: These drugs inhibit GI phase of mitosis, i.e. they are cell cycle dependent.

Uses

1. In acute lymphocytic leukemia in children these drugs are used along with other agents.
2. They are used during radiation therapy to control edema of mediastinum, brain (cerebral oedema) and spinal cord.
3. They are used to give symptomatic relief from pain and fever. They induce the feeling of well-being in the patient.
4. Prednisone is one of the drugs in the MOPP regimen for Hodgkin's disease.
5. They are used temporarily to treat **hemorrhagic symptoms due to drug** induced **thrombocytopenia**
6. To treat **bone marrow depression** secondary to radiotherapy and chemotherapy.

Adverse reactions

1. Sodium and water retention along with potassium loss.
2. Psychosis.
3. Exacerbation of diabetes, hypertension and peptic ulceration.
4. Precipitation of glaucoma and epilepsy.

Estrogens: These are female hormones and used to treat prostatic cancer.

Adverse reactions

These are usually dose-related.
1. Nausea and vomiting.
2. Sodium and water retention.
3. Aggravates chronic cystitis, mastitis, uterine fibrosis, migraine and endometriosis.
4. In males produces loss of libido and gynaecomastia.

Disadvantage: It may take 8–12 weeks before effectiveness of hormonal therapy can be satisfactorily assessed.

Dose: Stilbestrol 5 mg/day three times a day orally initially and then reduced to 1.0 mg TDS.

Progestogens: Megestrol and medroxyprogesterone are used in endometrial neoplasms and renal tumors.

Tamoxifen: **It is antiestrogen.** Tamoxifen is used in the palliative treatment of advanced cancers of the breast in patients with **estrogen dependent tumor** and the results are better when metastasis has occurred in soft tissues rather than in the bone. It has cardioprotective activity.

Adverse reactions

1. Hot flushes.
2. Nausea and vomiting.
3. Blurring of vision.
4. Thrombocytopenia.

Dose: 20–40 mg orally in two divided doses.

Androgens: These drugs are used in breast cancer.

Dromostanolone and Testolactone: Dromostanolone and testolactone are given intramuscularly (100 mg three times a day).

Adverse reactions: Virilization is the disturbing effect.

Uses: Prostatic cancer and advanced breast cancer.

Flutamide and Cyproterone: It is an androgen blocker is used in advanced prostatic cancer.

Fluoxymesterone: It is an orally active androgen is used in breast carcinoma.

Leuprolide Geserelin: It is a gonadotropin releasing hormone (GnRH) agonist.

Mitotane: It acts selectively on the adrenal cortex and is useful for treating carcinoma of this gland.

Adverse reactions

1. Anorexia, nausea and diarrhoea.
2. Somnolence and lethargy.
3. Dermatitis.
4. Adrenocortical insufficiency.

Precautions: Prednisolone (5 mg/day) and a mineralocorticoid such as fludrocortisone (0.1 mg/day) should be given along with it.

Octreotide: It is analogue of **somatostatin** and is used to treat **vipomas, carcinoid syndrome** and **glucogonamas.**

Streptozotocin: It has been used to treat metastatic pancreatic islet cell carcinoma and Hodgkin's disease.

Adverse reactions

1. Hepatic and renal damage.
2. Rarely bone marrow suppression is produced.

TOPOISOMERASE INHIBITORS

Topotecan

Uses

1. Refractory colorectal cancer.
2. Cancer of head and neck.
3. Malignant glioma.

Adverse reactions

1. Bone marrow suppression. Most significant is neutropenia.
2. Vomiting, diarrhoea.

MISCELLANEOUS AGENTS

Hydroxyurea: It acts in S phase of the cell cycle.

Uses

1. **Chronic granulocytic leukemia** not responding to busulfan.
2. **Malignant melanoma**.
3. Recurrent metastatic or **inoperable cancer of ovary**.
4. Carcinomas of head and neck.
5. Acute granulocytic leukemia.

Adverse reactions

1. Bone marrow suppression.
2. Alopecia, hyperpigmentation, erythema of hand and face.
3. Nausea, vomiting and diarrhoea.

Procarbazine: It can be given orally.

Uses

1. **Hodgkin's disease** is highly effective.
2. **Oat-cell cancer** of the lung.
3. **Multiple myeloma**.
4. **Malignant melanoma**.
5. **Brain tumors**.

Adverse reactions

1. Anorexia, nausea and vomiting.
2. Neurotoxicity.
3. Bone marrow suppression.
4. Dermatological toxicity.

Precautions

1. Foods rich in tyramine (chocolates and cheese) should be avoided.
2. Alcohol should be avoided by these patients as interaction produces **disulfiram type of reaction**.

Aminoglutethimide: It is used to treat.

1. Cushing's syndrome.
2. Ectopic ACTH secreting tumors.
3. Metastatic breast cancer.

Adverse reactions

1. Skin rashes (generalised muscular types).
2. Nausea and anorexia.
3. Somnolence, ataxia, nystagmus and lethargy. Bone marrow is not suppressed.

Dacarbazine

Uses

1. It is the main drug for treatment of malignant melanoma.
2. Hodgkin's diseases.
3. Various sarcomas.

Adverse reactions

1. Nausea and vomiting are initially troublesome but they tend to disappear as treatment continues.
2. Bone marrow suppression is produced.
3. Flu-like syndrome.
4. Neurotoxicity, skin reaction and hepatotoxicity.

Cisplatin

Uses

1. It is especially effective in **metastatic testicular tumors**.
2. It is also useful in **metastatic ovarian tumors**, advanced bladder carcinoma, cervical cancer, head and neck cancers and lung cancer.

Adverse reactions

1. Nausea and vomiting.
2. Nephrotoxicity (prevented by hydration and diuresis).
3. Anaphylactic reactions.
4. Hypomagnesemic tetany.
5. Loss of hearing.
6. Peripheral neuropathies.

Nursing care

1. Most of the drugs used in treatment of cancer produce adverse reactions of the following types:
   (a) Anorexia, nausea and vomiting.
   (b) Irritation of gastrointestinal tract which produces symptoms of diarrhoea, ulceration of intestinal bleeding.
   (c) Bone marrow suppression.
   (d) Alopecia.

(e) Cardiac, pulmonary, liver and kidney toxicity, cystitis and hyperuricemia are associated with only few drugs.

2. Monitor patient for major adverse reactions.

3. Monitor laboratory data for evidence of toxicity (leucopenia, anaemia and thrombocytopenia).

4. Intravenous administration should be done with care to avoid leakage.

5. Patients receiving busulphan must receive allopurinol prophylactically to avoid hyperuricemia.

6. Anorexia, nausea and vomiting lead to weight loss and generalised weakness. These symptoms can be avoided by looking after his nutrition.

7. A clean and comfortable environment, free of smell is important. Do not serve foods, not liked by the patient at the time of chemotherapy.

8. Antiemetics should be given to stop vomiting.

9. Stomatitis can be treated by mouth washes with hydrogen peroxide and nystatin oral suspension.

10. Suppression of bone marrow is treated by giving antibiotics (which do not add to bone marrow suppression). Amphotericin B, miconazole and cotrimoxazole are used to treat fungal infections and erythropoietin.

Vitamins

77. Vitamins

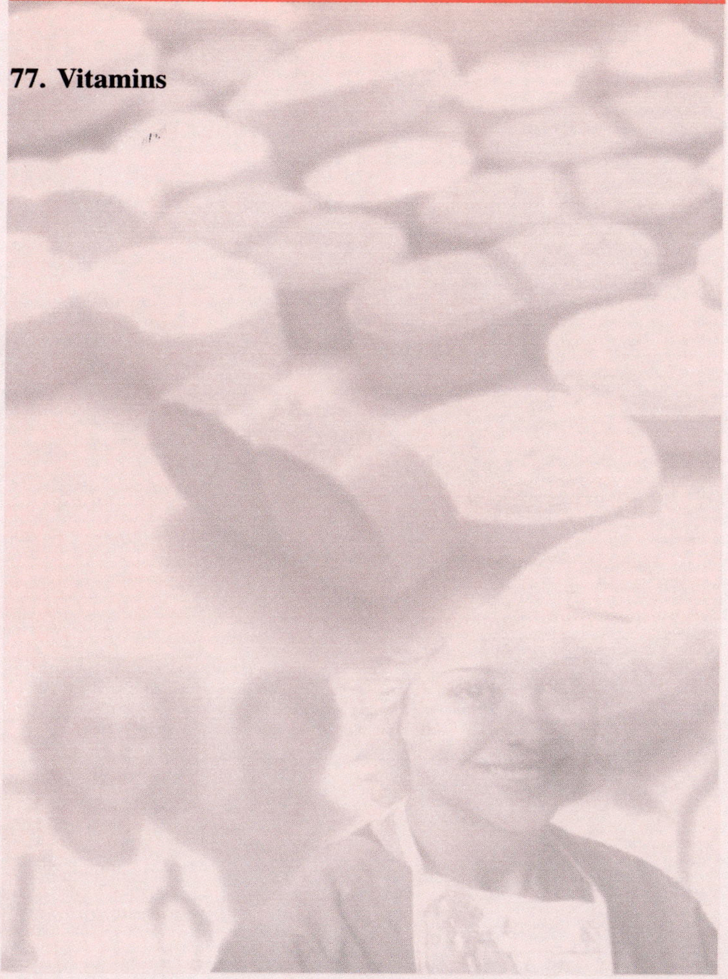

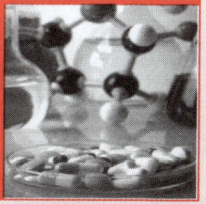

77

Vitamins

These are substances essential (vital) for the normal well-being of the individual and required in very small quantities.

Deficiency of any vitamin results in ill health. It is therefore essential to know their functions, symptoms due to their deficiency and their toxic reactions.

Toxic reactions of these agents have gained special status as they are misused by public.

Vitamins can be classified into two groups:

(a) Fat soluble vitamins A, D, K and E.

(b) Water soluble vitamins B group and C.

Fat soluble vitamins require presence of bile (thus it is essential that **liver and gallbladder** should be functioning normally), there can be deficiency of vitamins A, D, K and E in bile obstruction, cirrhosis and of all vitamins in **malabsorption syndrome**.

Fat soluble vitamins get stored in the body. It therefore, takes a few months before their deficiency manifests. Taken for long duration they produce **toxicity** as they accumulate in the body.

Vitamin A (Antixerophthalmic Vitamin): It is present in carrots, milk, cheese, butter, eggs and liver. Fish liver oils are rich in this vitamin.

Physiological Functions

(a) It is essential for maintenance of structure and functions of cornea and retina

(b) It is an essential catalyst for oxidation — reduction in epithelial cells and retards epithelial malignancy.

(c) It is a component of rhodopsin that is required for adaptation of eye to darkness, hence in its deficiency there is night blindness.

Signs and symptoms of deficiency

(a) Eyes: Dryness of cornea and conjunctiva (xerophthalmia), Bitot's spots and **night blindness**.

(b) Skin: Due to destruction of sweat glands the skin is **dry and rough**.

(c) Gut: Diarrhea.

(d) Renal system: Increase in incidence of renal stones.

(e) Miscellaneous: Abortions and sterility.

Uses

1. For prevention of vitamin A deficiency.
2. For cure of deficiency of vitamin A.

Dose: For prophylaxis — 4500 IU/day in individuals and 6000 IU/day during pregnancy, for cure 30,000 units/day till patient recovers.

Toxic effects: It accumulates in body and can cause toxicity:
1. General malaise and anorexia.
3. Hepatosplenomegaly.
4. Painful tender swellings over bone.
5. Signs of increased intracranial pressure.

Vitamin D

D_2 = Calciferol, ergocalciferol

D_3 = Cholecalciferol (formed in skin)

Milk, egg, yolk and liver are rich sources of this vitamin.
It is synthesised by skin on exposure to ultraviolet irradiation.
It is activated in the liver and further activated in the kidneys.

Actions

1. It increases absorption of calcium and phosphorus from intestine.
2. It helps in deposition of calcium in bone.
3. It reduces excretion of calcium in the urine.

Deficiency of this vitamin produces rickets in children and osteomalacia in adults. These conditions are characterised by **noncalcification** and **decalcification** of the osteoid tissue, respectively.

Its deficiency is produced in the following conditions:
(a) Malabsorption syndrome.
(b) Alcoholic cirrhosis.
(c) In growing children not exposed to sun.
(d) Phenytoin.

Requirement — 400 IU/day.
Toxicity due to hypervitaminosis D

It produces hypercalcemia which manifests as:
(a) Generalised malaise.
(b) Drowsiness, nausea, abdominal pain, thirst and constipation.
(c) Anorexia.
(d) Renal stones.

Vitamin K: Please refer haematology.

Vitamin E (The Tocopherols): It was recognised as an anti-sterility vitamin in rats.

It is present in soya bean oil and germ oil. 90% of tocoferol exists as alpha tocoferol.
Daily requirement: 10–30 mg.

Physiological functions: It has antioxidant activity prevents body against damaging effect of free radicals.

Peripheral neuropathy associated with spinocerebellar degeneration is produced during its deficiency.

Uses: Empirical use in neuralgias, skin diseases, anti-aging and intermittent claudication.

WATER SOLUBLE VITAMINS

Vitamin B Group: **Thiamine (B_1), folic acid and cyanocobalamin (B_{12})** are important constituents. **Pantothenic acid, inositol, biotin and para-aminobenzoic acid** are less important as their deficiency has not been reported clinically.

Thiamine (B_1): Deficiency of this vitamin occurs quite commonly in areas of famine and results in beriberi. This disease is characterised by peripheral neuritis (dry type) or congestive cardiac failure (wet type). Whole grains and eggs are rich source of this vitamin.

Physiological Functions

(a) Acts as coenzyme in carbohydrate metabolism.
(b) Participates in decarboxylation of alpha ketoacidosis.

Requirement of this vitamin depends on the amount of carbohydrate consumed –0.4 mg of B_1 is required for every 100 caloreis of carbohydrate consumed.

Uses

1. It is used to treat beri-beri.
2. It is given in diabetes mellitus associated with neurological symptoms.
3. Alcoholic polyneuritis responds to this vitamin.

Allergic reactions may occur, specially on parenteral adminstration.

Riboflavin (Vitamin B_2): It is light labile. It is present in milk, green leafy vegetables, yeast, egg and meat.

Physiological Functions: It is converted in the body to active compound — flavine adenine dinucleotide which is coenzyme. It is required for tissue oxidation in processes of cellular energy.

Daily requirement: 2 mg.

Dose: 5–10 mg/day in deficient states.

Nicotinamide: (Nicotinic Acid Amide) Vitamin B_3

Physiological functions: It is converted to nicotinamide adenine dinucleotide (NAD) or its phosphate (NADP). These act as coenzymes for proteins catalysing oxidation reduction processes.

Deficiency of this vitamin leads to **pellagra** which constitutes 3D-dementia, dermatitis and diarrhea. It occurs in malnutrition as well as in undernutritional subjects. People eating maize usually develop pellagra.

Patient of pellagra usually suffers from other deficiencies also. He should be given supplements of vitamins B_{12} and B_6.

Adverse reactions: Nicotinamide does not produce adverse reactions, but nicotinic acid, which is converted to nicotinamide in the body causes peripheral vasodilatation producing severe flushing and itching in the upper part of the body.

Pyridoxine (Vitamin B$_6$ — Pyridoxal and Pyridoxamine): It is present in liver, yeast and cereals. It is converted to pyridoxal in the body.

Physiological Functions

(a) It is essential for metabolism of amino acids.

(b) It is involved in carbohydrate as well as fat metabolism. Deficiency of this vitamin can be induced by certain drugs (INH).

Its deficiency produces microcytic hypochromic anaemia, mental irritability and convulsions and burning soles of the feet.

Uses

1. It is used in vomiting during pregnancy.
2. It is given along with INH to prevent development of peripheral neuritis.
3. It can be given in microcytic hypochromic anemia along with other haematinics.
4. It can be tried in homocystinuria.
5. **It reduces effect of levodopa.**

Pantothenic Acid: Deficiency of this vitamin produces neuromuscular degeneration and adrenocortical deficiency.

Uses

1. It has been found useful in few cases of postoperative paralytic ileus, rheumatoid arthritis and streptomycin toxicity.
2. It is applied on burns.

Biotin: Deficiency of this vitamin produces symptoms of seborrheic dermatitis, lassitude, anorexia and paresthesias.

Vitamin B$_{12}$ (Cyanocobalamin): Occurs mainly in animal products — eggs, milk, liver and fish.

Physiological Functions: It is essential for

(a) Cell growth.

(b) For **maintenance of normal myelin in CNS.**

(c) For normal metabolic functions of folate.

(d) For formation of DNA.

Deficiency produces:

(a) Megaloblastic anemia

(b) Neuritis with central scotomas

(c) Effects optic, peripheral and cranial nerves.

Folic Acid (Pteroylglutamic Acid): Rich sources of folic acid are yeast, liver, kidney and leafy green vegetables.

Daily requirement—100–200 mg/day.

Physiological Functions

(a) It is essential for one—carbon transfer reactions necessary for DNA synthesis.
(b) It is essential for synthesis of thymidylic acid—precursor of DNA.
(c) Stimulates haemopoiesis but does not prevent neurological symptoms associated with pernicious anemia.

Use: Megaloblastic anemias not associated with neurological symptoms.

Adverse reactions: Allergic symptoms.

REST OF THE VITAMINS BELONGING TO B GROUP

Choline and Methionine: Choline and methionine are called lipotropic factors and are used in cirrhosis.

Para-aminobenzoic Acid: It can produce toxic hepatitis, hyperglycemia, crystalluria, leucopenia and agranulocytosis.

Ascorbic Acid (Vitamin C): This vitamin occurs in fresh fruits (citrus fruits are rich) and green vegetables. Potatoes contain small amounts.

Physiological Functions

1. It is essential for synthesis of collagen.
2. Helps in formation of haemoglobin.
3. It is essential for tissue metabolism bones and teeth.
4. Wound healing suffers in its deficiency.

Deficiency of this vitamin was common in sailors on long voyages because sailing ships did not normally carry fresh fruits. Scurvy is characterised by weakness, anaemia, bleeding into skin and muscles. Bleeding from gums may be the first sign.

Vitamin C is easily destroyed by heating.

Normal body stores are about 1500 mg. Scurvy will develop in about 3 months if there is no intake.

Requirements: 30 mg/day

Uses of ascorbic acid

1. For acidification of urine to eliminate certain poisons.
2. For prevention and cure of scurvy.
3. For treatment of methaemoglobinaemia.

Dose: 500 mg/day.

Adverse reactions: Mega doses can lead to kidney stones.

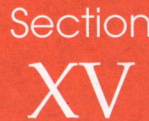

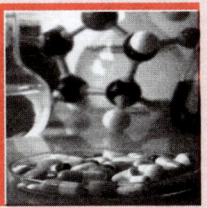

Heavy Metals
and their Antagonists

78. Heavy Metals and their Antagonists

78

Heavy Metals and their Antagonists

In ancient systems of medicine (Unani and Ayurveda) metals are often dispensed. Patients are not aware of the toxicity that can arise with use of these drugs.

Nursing staff must keep in mind that these drugs too can produce toxicity. Metals are sometimes employed for homicidal purposes. Individuals can suffer metal toxicity due to ingestion or as occupation hazard.

ARSENIC POISONING

Arsenic salts are used:

(a) To treat trypanosomiasis.

(b) As insecticide, herbicide and fungicide.

(c) For homicidal purposes.

Acute poisoning of this metal produces symptoms that resemble cholera.

GIT: Irritation, vomiting, watery diarrhea and liver damage.

Kidney: Damage of capillaries in glomeruli and renal tubules resulting in oliguric proteinuria and haematuria.

Chronic toxicity

(a) Peripheral neuropathy (stock and glove distribution)

(b) Muscular weakness of limbs

(c) Skin: Small doses produce cutaneous vasodilatation, necrosis and sloughing of skin. Hyperkeratosis in palms and soles. Cancer can occur.

Treatment of acute poisoning

1. Correction of electrolyte and fluid imbalance.

2. **Dimercaprol:** 3 mg/kg IV every 4 hrs until abdominal symptoms disappear

3. Suitable antibiotics

4. Haemodialysis is done if the above fails.

Treatment of chronic poisoning: Dimercaprol is given.

435

LEAD

It is distributed in air, water and dust. Toxicity occurs as occupational hazard.

Acute toxicity of lead produces paresthesiae, muscle cramps and weakness. Haemolytic crisis produces severe anaemia and haemoglobinurea. Lead **encephalopathy** occurs in children if lead levels in blood are very high. Epileptic fits and visual distrubances are produced in this condition.

Chronic toxicity of lead mainfests in the **gums, atrophy or contractures of skeletal muscles**. Abdominal **colic** is produced. Severe **anaemia** is produced.

Treatment of lead poisoning

Intravenous **penicillamine** is given. In lead encephalopathy — in addition **sodium calcium edetate** and BAL are given intramuscularly. After the acute phase is over **oral penicillamine** is continued till the blood lead concentration falls. Diet low in calcium is given to mobilise lead from bone to blood and this subsequently will help the chelators.

Chelating agents are not helpful in toxicity due to tetraethyl lead.

MERCURY

Acute toxicity was seen in patients being treated with organic mercurials.

Local application of mercurochrome may produce allergy in certain patients. Severe gastrointestinal irritation, electrolyte disturbances and peripheral circulatory collapse are produced during toxicity. Cardiac arrhythmias are produced which prove fatal.

It is treated by giving **dimercaprol**.

Acetyl pencillamine has been found to be more effective.

Chronic mercury poisoning produces: CNS irritability, tremors, headache, easy fatigability, stomatitis, and dermatitis.

Dimercaprol is an effective treatment for this condition.

SILVER

Toxicity due to silver is termed as **argyria**. There is bluish black discolouration of the skin.

GOLD

Please refer chapter on Gout and Rheumatoid arthritis.

ANTIMONY

Toxic effects resemble those of arsenic. **Dimercaprol** protects against toxic effects of organic forms but it is less effective against inorganic antimonial compounds.

BISMUTH

Chronic poisoning may lead to fever, gastrointestinal disturbances, urticaria, stomatitis, nephritis and nephrosis. **Dimercaprol** is used for its treatment.

CADMIUM

Acute toxicity of this metal produces gastrointestinal irritation and circulatory collapse. Cadmium when inhaled produces dyspnoea, cyanosis and vertigo. Chronic toxicity produces anosmia, colouration of teeth and adrenal damage. Chelating agents (EDTA and BAL) are not recommended for its treatment. **Calcium gluconate is found to be useful**.

COPPER

If taken orally it produces vomiting, diarrhea, colicky pain and shock. Kidney functions are impaired.

Treatment consists of giving egg albumin and tannic acid orally. **Penicillamine** is drug of choice. **Dimercaprol** is given parenterally.

COBALT

Disodium calcium EDTA is used to counter its systemic toxicity.

CHELATING AGENTS

Certain organic compounds are capable of combining with metals. This combination produces stable, soluble, nondissociable complexes called chelates. Chelating agents have been found to be of value in treatment of **metallic poisoning, hypercalcemia and Wilsons's disease**.

Dimercaprol (BAL-British Anti-Lewisite): This drug was developed during second world war to serve as an antidote for aresenic containing war gas-lewisite.

In **lead poisoning** it is given along with EDTA.

In **Wilson's disease** it promotes the efficacy of penicillamine.

Dose: 2.5 mg/kg IM is given at 4 hrly intervals for 2 days then twice a day for 1 day and then once a day till treatment demands.

Adverse reactions

1. Vomiting, tremors.
2. Rise of blood pressure.
3. Convulsions.

It is not used in iron toxicity.

ETHYLENEDIAMINETETRA-ACETIC ACID (EDTA)

It is available as:

(a) Disodium EDTA

(b) Sodium calcium EDTA

Calcium salt is used for treating **lead toxicity** while disodium EDTA is employed for treating **hypercalcemia, corneal opacities and in treatment of burns due to calcium hydroxide**.

Doses: In acute lead poisoning Na_2 Ca EDTA is given by slow IV infusion in the dose of 40 mg/kg twice daily.

This dose is repeated after 2–3 days.

PENICILLAMINE

It is obtained by the hydrolysis of benzyl penicillin. It **chelates copper, mercury, zinc and lead** and facilitates their excretion in the urine. It also combines with cystine and in cystinuria it prevents the formation of urinary calculi.

Uses

1. Wilson's disease.
2. Lead poisoning.
3. Cystinuria.
4. **Rheumatoid arthritis.**

Adverse reactions

1. Allergic episodes.
2. Anorexia, nausea and vomiting.
3. Renal damage.

ACETYL D-PENICILLAMINE

This drug is highly effective in **mercury poisoning.**

DESFERRIOXAMINE

It is obtained from *Streptomyces pilosus*. It is useful in preventing absorption of **iron** from gastrointestinal tract. **Iron of haemoglobin is not removed.**

Uses

1. Iron toxicity.
2. Haemosiderosis.

Dose: 1 gm followed by 500 mg 4 hourly. Total dose 6.0 g/day. In acute condition 1–2 g in 5% dextrose solution is given intravenously.

Adverse effects

Hypotension

Skin rashes

Gastrointestinal irritation.

Role of a nurse in heavy metal toxicity

Heavy metals are used in Ayurvedic and Unani Medicines. These drugs can produce toxicity. Lead is introduced into the body through lead painted utensils. Use of lead toys and such utensils must be reduced.

Nurse involved in industrial health can educate masses in prevention of toxicity due to heavy metals. If nurse in the causality suspects metal poisoning she must initiate treatment at the earliest.

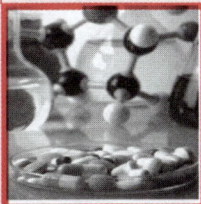

79

Immunity

The ability of the body to resist infection, or immunity, depends to a greater extent on the presence of antibodies. Antibodies are formed when the body is invaded by foreign agent. Antibodies either kill the organism (antigen) or make it easier for the polymorphonuclear leucocytes to phagocytose it. It is one of the **defence mechanisms** of the body.

Generation of antibodies is slower when the antigen enters the body initially (first time) but on subsequent exposures there is rapid synthesis of antibodies.

When the antibodies are already present in the body against the organism, infection does not set in easily but if the level of antibodies is low individual becomes susceptible to infection. This is seen in AIDS (Aquired Immuno Deficiency Syndrome).

Immunisation confers ability to resist infection. In healthy individuals this is done by stimulating his own defence mechanisms to generate antibodies (**active immunisation**) while in patients or individuals with certain diseases or of patients with poor nutritional status this is achieved through administration of antibodies (**passive immunisation**).

PASSIVE IMMUNISATION

Patient is injected with antibodies which have been produced by either another patient during the course of infection or by an animal which has been purposely infected with the specific organism.

Antibodies generated against a toxin are called **antitoxins**. For example, a patient of diphtheria is likely to die because of the effects of toxins produced by this organism. It is possible to prevent mortality in this patient by passively immunising the patient with antitoxins.

Passive immunisation is required in infections due to *C. diphtheria, C. tetani* and *C. welchii*.

Antibodies in animals are produced by repeatedly injecting an animal with toxin in small doses and animal produces antitoxin to it. By bleeding the animal it is possible to obtain life saving antitoxins.

Antibodies are normally present in the gamma globulin fraction of the blood. If large number of donor plasma is pooled, the collective sample is rich in antibodies particularly those which are active against viral infections, e.g. **measles, rubella (German measles), poliomyelitis, infectious hepatitis and smallpox.**

Doses

(a) In case of tetanus: 1500–3000 IV of antisera are given either SC/ID soon after injury.
(b) Gas gangrene: 10,000 IU or prophylactically or 30000–750000 IU therapeutically.

(c) Diphtheria: 500–3000 IU units given soon after exposure.

(d) Botulinum: 10,000 units given every 3–4 hrs.

(e) Rabies 40 IU/Kg body weight given IM within 24 hrs of bite and 400 IM around the wound.

Reactions to passive immunisation

1. Allergy

For passive immunisation serum obtained either from animal or human being is injected, it is likely to produce allergic reactions. These reactions may be of two forms:

(a) Acute anaphylactic shock: It may result in death if not attended promptly and correctly. It is therefore important to prevent its occurrence or to diagnose the condition at the earliest. Watch closely all patients whom you have injected with foreign serum for at least half an hour after the injection. Anaphylactic shock may cause **hypotension and bronchospasm**. Any patient who complains of feeling unwell immediately after an injection of foreign serum should be suspected of having developed or likely to develop anaphylactic reaction.

Treatment must be started immediately. This consists of 0.5 to 1.0 ml of 1: 1000 **adrenaline** subcutaneously **(noradrenaline will not help)** or IV injection should be made slowly — the entire amount should be injected in 5 to 10 minutes. Intravenous injection of hydrocortisone hemisuccinate (100 mg) is added.

(b) Serum sickness: This is an allergic reaction like anaphylactic shock but occurs on 10th to 14th day after vaccination. This reaction is charcterised by **high fever, polyarthritis, itching** and **enlargement of lymph nodes**. It is treated by giving antihistaminics and **corticosteroids**.

Precautions to be taken during passive immunisation

1. It is advisable to **test the sensitivity of the patient before giving full dose** of the vaccine.

   This is done by injecting 0.01 ml of 1: 1000 dilution of serum in normal saline ID or putting solution into eye while control (saline) is put in the other eye. In sensitive individuals lacrimation and conjunctivitis develops.

2. **Never inject serum into any patient without having an ampoule of adrenaline (1:1000) at hand.**

SERUM HEPATITIS

This condition is produced when the given serum or the syringes and needles used during administration are contaminated with hepatitis virus. **Human gamma globulins** do not produce this complication. Hence, use of human serum is declining and human gamma globulins are being used now.

GAMMA GLOBULINS

These are proteins synthesised by the B-lymphocytes. These are also called immune serum. These are used for prevention as well as treatment of various infections.

Adverse reactions

1. Allergic reactions
2. Joint pain and nausea.

Uses

1. For prevention of measles and rubella.
2. For treating infective hepatitis.
3. For prevention of smallpox and vaccinia.
4. For preventing complications of mumps and poliomyelitis.

Nursing care in prevention of serum hepatitis

Use of disposable sets may be encourged.

Syringes and needles must be sterilised by boiling for at least 5 minutes.

DOSES OF VARIOUS ANTITOXINS

Tetanus immunoglobulin — 250 IU intramuscularly.

Anti-D (rho) immunoglobulin (human) injection of 250 ug intramuscularly is given within 72 hours of delivery. This prevents complications during next delivery.

ACTIVE IMMUNISATION

In this techinque patient's immune mechanisms are stimulated so that he generates his own antibodies.

Advantages

1. The effect of acute immunisation lasts longer that is the immunity or protection against that infection lasts longer.
2. Adverse effects of passive immunisation do not occur.

Types of acute immunisation
1. Killed organisms.
2. Living organisms (live vaccine).
3. Substances derived from and similar to toxins produced by bacteria.

Killed organisms: Killed organisms continue to provoke antibody response but do not cause infection. Examples of this type of vaccines are **pertusis, typhoid and paratyphoid, cholera and plague.**

Living organisms (BCG, smallpox, yellow fever, measles, poliomyelitis and rabies) are also used.

In case of living organisms there is always a possibility that the patient may develop **infection**. To overcome this difficulty the microbes are treated in a way that they lose their virulence but retain their antigenecity. This is done in two ways.

1. Organisms are grown generation to generation in a culture medium that they lose virulence, e.g. BCG (Bacille Calmette Guerin).
2. Such organisms are used which are non-infected in human but have antigenicity, e.g. smallpox virus from cow is used for this purpose.

Microbes are treated in such a way that they lose virulence (attenuated) but retain antigenicity, e.g. measles.

Substances Derived from Bacterial Toxins: **Exotoxins of diphtheria and tetanus** are responsible for fatalities. It is possible to immunise patients with substances derived from these toxins. Immune system of the patient is stimulated to produce antibodies which act against and neutralise toxins.

Diptheria, tetanus and whooping cough vaccine (DPT) —triple antigen is given in 3 doses of 0.5 ml each at the interval of 4 to 6 weeks. Last dose (0.5 ml) is given in the 3rd to 4th year of life.

ACTIVE IMMUNISATION PROGRAMMES

Immunisation of the child at the proper age reduces infant and child mortality. Booster dose is required for diphtheria, pertusis and tetanus. Following immunisation programme is recommended.

Age	Vaccines
At birth –2 months	BCG, OPV and HBV
2 months	OPV, DPT, HBV and *Haemophilus* type b
4 months	OPV, DPT and *Haemophilus* type b
6 months	OPV, HBV and MMR
15–18 months	DPT (booster), Typhoid, *Meningococcus*
4–6 years	OPV, DPT (booster)
10–12 years	DT (booster)

Adults	
Hepatitis A	One dose in endemic area
Influenza	Single dose in high risk patients and the elderly
Meningococcal	During epidemics—single dose.
Rabies	Pre-exposure—3 dose given IM or ID on 0, 7 and 21 or 28 days
	Post-exposure—5 doses given IM. On days 0, 3, 7, 14 and 28
Cholera	Two doses in endemic areas

Precautions in active immunisation

1. There is increased risk of poliomyelitis consequent on immunisation if the dose has been given in an ailing child.
2. Vaccines which contain living organisms should **not be given to a patient on corticosteriod therapy.**
3. Live virus vaccines should be **avoided during pregnancy**.
4. Vaccines containing living microbes should be avoided in patients of agammaglobulinemia.
5. Patients allergic to eggs and chicken should not receive vaccines containing viruses grown on those media.

Nursing care

1. Vaccines must be properly stored.
2. Nurse must maintain chart of immunisation and inform mother regarding next dose.
3. She must not give active immunisation and live vaccines to immunocompromised patients and those on steroids.
4. Tetanus is the commonest vaccine used in adults. Sensitivity reactions are known to occur to this toxin. Care should be exercised in this direction.

5. Avoid live virus vaccines in pregnant women and specially live vaccines during first trimester.
6. All health care individuals should be immunised against hepatitis B, measles, rubella, inflenza and varicella.

Immunoglobulin: It is obtained from human plasma and is given in immunodeficiencies such as measles, hepatitis and auoimmune hemolytic anemia.

Peptides: Thymic factor is used to enhance T-lymphocytic functions. Various preparations are available.

IMMUNOSTIMULANTS

Cytokines: These regulate immune system. These include

(a) Interferon alpha

(b) Colony stimulating factors

(c) Interleukins (IL$_2$)

Interferon alfa stimulates production of macrophages, T-lymphocytes and natural killer cells. Also used for its antitumor activity in melanoma and renal cell carcinoma.

IFN — β is used in multiple sclerosis and IFN — gamma in granulomatous disease.

Colony Stimulating Factors (CSFs): These naturally occuring glycoproteins stimulate multiplication, differentiation and actions of neutrophils, monocytes and macrophages. These are:

Granulocyte macrophage-colony stimulating factor (GM-CSF).

Uses

In aplastic anemia and AIDS

Granulocyte CSF (G-CSF):

(a) Increases neutrophil production.

(b) Enhances phagocytic and cytotoxic activities of neutrophils.

(c) **Use:** For correcting neutropenia of AIDS patients during zidovudine therapy.

Sargramostim and filgrastim are synthetic preparations of GM-CSF and G-CSF respectively.

Use: Used to overcome bone marrow suppression during cancer chemotherapy.

ADRs: Pleural and pericardial effusion with sargramostim. Splenomegaly and bone pains with filgrastim.

Synthetic Agents

Levomasole: Increases T cell mediated immunity.

Uses

1. Hodgkins disease.
2. Rheumatoid arthritis.
3. As adjuvant drug in colorectal cancer.

Isoprinosine: Increases natural killer cell cytotoxicity. Not useful in AIDS.

IMMUNOSUPPRESSANTS

1. Inhibitors of T cell population.

(a) Muromonab-CD3

(b) Anti thymocyte globulin

2. Non specific inhibitors of B cells and T cell proliferation.

(a) Cyclosporine and tacrolimus.

(b) Steroids.

(c) Azathioprine, cyclophosphamide and methotrexate.

Muromonab-CD3: It is obtained from mouse monoclonal antibody.

Actions

1. Inhibits participation of T cells in immune response.
2. Depletes circulating T cells in minutes.

Use: It is used to prevent acute rejection in renal, hepatic and cardiac transplants.

Adverse reactions: Anaphylactoid reaction.

CNS effects.

Antithymocyte Globulin: It is obtained from horses and is given to treat acute allograft rejection

RHO(D) Immune Globulin: It is given within 72 hrs of miscarriage or delivery. It suppresses maternal reaction to RBC of Rh + ve baby. This helps in reducing complications in subsequent pregnancies.

Glucocorticoids: Prednisone and prednisolone are used as single or in combination with other immunosuppressants to treat autoimmune diseases and prevent graft rejection.

Actions

1. Inhibt T cell proliferation
2. Inhibit synthesis of cytokines — IL_1, IL_2, IL_6 and alpha interferon. Produce many adverse reactions hence their use is curtailed.

Cyclosporin and Tacrolimus: Tacrolimus is macrolide antibiotic while cyclosporin is decapeptide antibiotic.

Actions

1. Inhibit proliferation of lymphocytes
2. Prevent synthesis of IL_2

ADRs: Renal and hepatic toxicity is present.

Uses

(a) In kidney, liver and heart transplants

(b) Autoimmuno diseases

(c) Graft versus host syndrome.

Sicrolimus: It is used in heart and kidney transplant.

CYTOTOXIC AGENTS

These drugs inhibit cell replication and cell metabolism. The non specificity of action results in their adverse reactions hence not preferred **for details refer Cancer Chemotherapy.**

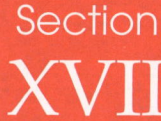

Radioactive Isotopes and Biological Effects of Radiation

80. Radioactive Isotopes and Biological Effects of Radiation

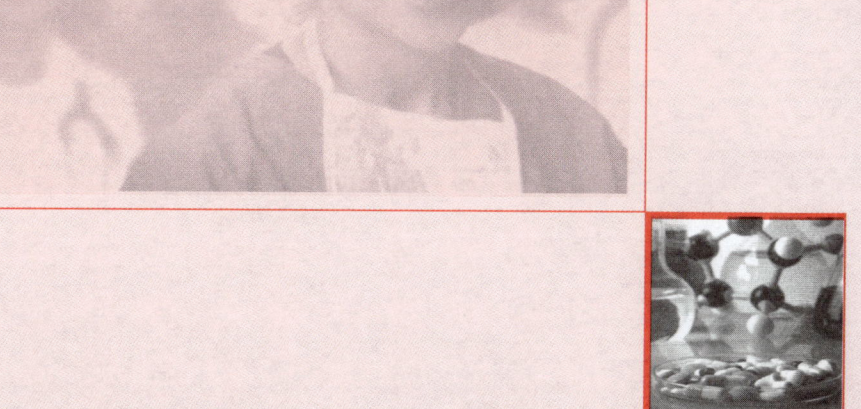

80

Radioactive Isotopes and Biological Effects of Radiation

Radioactive element has physical property of emitting radiations.

Radioactive isotopes can emit the following types of rays:

1. Alpha rays.
2. Beta rays.
3. Gamma rays.

Alpha rays have poor penetrability while **beta rays** are moderately strong and are used to destroy the tissues. **Gamma rays** have greater penetrability and are usually employed for diagnostic purposes.

Radioactivity of an isotope lasts for a fixed time after which it ceases to be active and becomes a stable element. This is called **radioactive decay**. The time taken for reduction of the activity to half of its zero hour value is known as its **half-life**.

The distribution of a radioactive element in the body follows the body distribution of the stable isotope. Body is unable to differentiate between stable and radioactive element.

Radioactivity in the body is detected by G.M. counters or scintillating counters.

Diagnostic uses of radioactive isotopes in medicine

1. For differentiating hot (thyrotoxic) from cold (cancerous) nodule in thyroid.
2. Uptake of I^{131} by the thyroid gland indicates the degree of its function.
3. Distribution of I^{131} in body helps in tracing the spread of malignant thyroid and also its treatment.
4. Labelled compounds (i.e. compounds tagged with radioactive isotope) are utilised to study absorption, distribution and metabolism of the concerned compound (experimental).

For treating diseases

1. I^{131} with half-life of 8 days is used to treat thyrotoxicosis.
2. I^{131} also used for treating metastasis from thyroid cancer
3. I^{125} with half-life of 60 days is used for thyroid cancer.
4. Radioactive **gold and cobalt** are used for treatment of ovarian and uterine malignancies.
5. P^{32} is used in the treatment of polycythemia vera.
6. Tantallium is used for treating cancer of bladder.
7. Au^{198} with half-life of 2.7 days is used to treat abdominal tumors, ascitis and pleural effusion due to malignancies. It is also given to treat carcinoma cervix.

Hazards of Radiation: Radiation produces two major effects on the cell.

Acute effects

1. Fast multiplying cells of gastrointestinal tract, bone marrow and reproductive system are inhibited or destroyed.
2. Radiation produces following adverse reactions.
   (i) Severe diarrhea and vomiting leading to dehydration. Absorption of nutrients is likely to suffer as gut flora is killed producing deficiency of vitamins B and K. Superinfections by fungus become easier.
   (ii) Bone marrow is depressed which results in aggranulocytosis. The resistance of the body falls. Patient is likely to catch infections.
   (iii) Reproductive system is adversely affected, sperm count in males is reduced.

Delayed Effects of Radiation

1. Radiation produces mutagenic change in the cell. Due to the mutagenic changes brought about by radiation chances of development of cancer are increased.
2. Aging process sets in earlier — cataract and degenerative manifestations of age are manifested.
3. It brings about the genetic change in the cell. Fertility is reduced.

Treatment of Radiation Toxicity: As yet there is no drug that can give either protection or cure against hazards of radiation.

Protection against radiation

The effect of radiation being irreversible, it is necessary to protect individuals employed in radiodiagnosis and radiotherapy departments. This is achieved through following means.

1. Use personal monitoring — film badges containing radiosensitive plates. This helps in detecting the degree of exposure to radiation. Individual can be removed from the exposure area after specified period.
2. Proper shielding by wearing lead apron.

Protection to patient

1. Dose required should be calculated correctly. Minimum effective dose should be given.
2. Increase the distance between the source of radiation and the individual.
3. Patient receiving radioactive substance should be kept away from the rest.
4. Radioactive isotopes should not be used in children or the younger population.

Section

XVIII

Enzymes

81. Enzymes

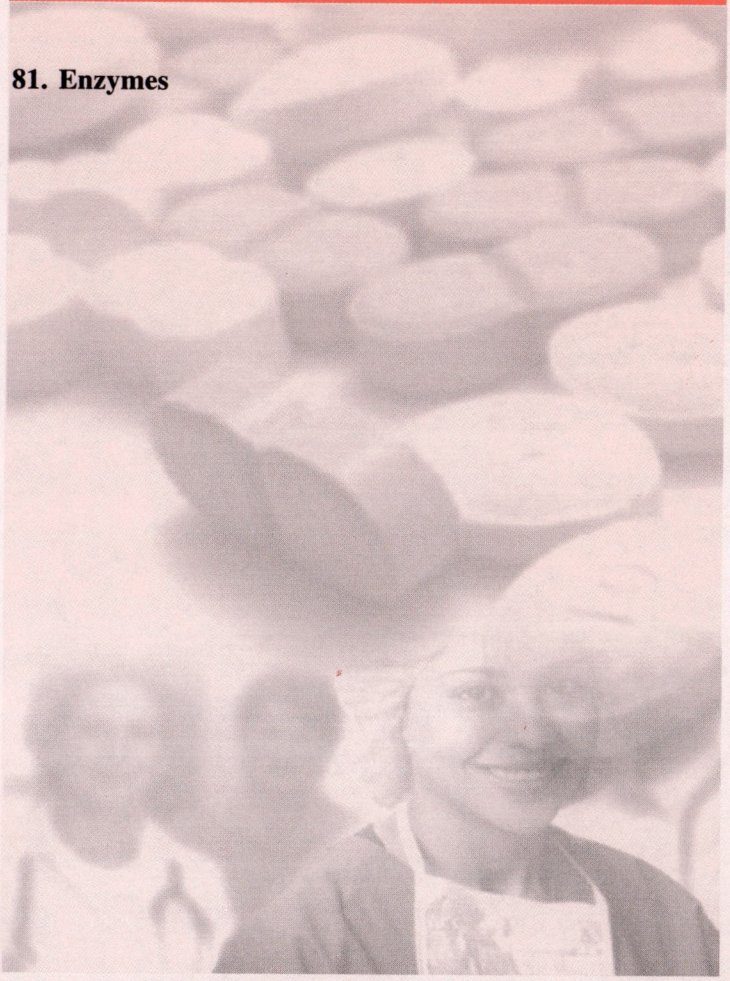

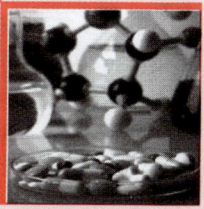

Enzymes

Enzymes play vital role in the body. Few drugs act through either stimulation of enzymes or by inhibiting them. Enzymes per se can also be used as drugs.

Disadvantages of enzymes as drugs
1. They produce allergic reactions.
2. They cannot be given orally. Therefore, parenteral therapy becomes essential.

Uses

(i) **Pancreatin, disastase, pepsin and papain** participate in digestion. These enzymes are used in therapeutics to promote digestion.
(ii) **Fibrinolysin, thromboplastin, urokinase** participate in coagulation process (for details regarding these enzymes please refer haematology).
(iii) Other enzymes used therapeutically are:

Hyaluronidase: This enzyme is also known as 'spreading factor'. It breaks down the ground substance and helps spreading fluids through intercellular spaces. This helps in quicker absorption of drugs and fluids.

Dose: 150 units.

Disadvantages

1. It produces allergic reactions.
2. It helps in spreading infection.
3. It may aid in spread of malignant cells.

Trypsin: It is obtained from the pancreas of ox. It destroys proteins. It does not require a cofactor for this activity.

Uses

1. It is instilled into closed cavities to liquefy clots.
2. It is applied locally on chronic suppurative wounds to remove the dead tissue.

Adverse effects

1. When applied locally it produces burning sensation.
2. Intramuscular injection of this enzyme produces intense pain at the site.

Precautions

1. It should not be given to patients with asthma or other allergic conditions.
2. It should not be administered to patients with hepatic or renal insufficiency.
3. **It should never be given intravenously**.

Chymotrypsin: It is obtained from bovine pancreas. It has same actions as trypsin.

Uses: It is used as anti-inflammatory agent. It is applied locally or given orally for this purpose.

Alpha Chymotrypsin: It is used in eye for dissolving the suspensory ligament of the lens. This is needed during surgery for extraction of dislocated lens.

Adverse reactions

1. It increases the intraocular tension for short duration.
2. Loss of vitreous may result.
3. Rarely retinal damage may be produced.

Collagenase: Removal of dead tissue is essential for healing.

It is applied on wounds and burns to remove the dead tissue.

Poisoning and its Treatment

82. Poisoning and its Treatment

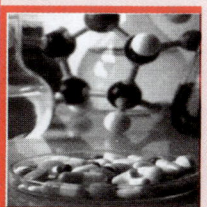

82

Poisoning and its Treatment

Poisoning can occur due to:
   (a) Chemcials used in industry or at home.
   (b) Animal toxins such as snake bites.
   (c) Drugs.
   (d) Consumption of toxic plants.

Role of nurse in domiciliary practice

1. Brief history should be taken.
2. (i)   Remove the individual from the polluted environment.
   (ii) In case of organophosphorus poisoning remove contaminated clothing and wash skin.
   (iii) In cases of acid or alkali burns — wash skin with water for at least 5 minutes.
   (iv) Eyes should be washed with water with lids held apart.
3. (a)   Patent airway should be maintained.
   (b)   Give artificial respiration if necessary.
   (c)   Maintain adequate circulation.
4. In case poisoning has occured due to ingestion: give 1–2 glasses of milk, beaten eggs or flour or starch suspension orally to dilute and adsorb the poison (this can only be done in conscious patient).
5. Attempt to induce vomiting **in conscious patient** by tickling the fauces or by giving him hypertonic salt solution. **This should not be done in patients with convulsions or patients who have ingested a corrosive substance (acid or alkali) or volatile substances (petroleum distillate).**
6. Control convulsions by diazepam (5–10 mg). Repeat after 15 minutes if necessary.
7. Collect vomitus for analysis.
8. Make arrangements to shift the patient to hospital if above fails.

Nursing measures in hospital practice

1. Wash skin in case of organophosphorus poisoning and in burns due to acid or alkali.
2. Maintain patent airway and support respiration and circulation.
3. Gastric lavage or emesis should be considered if the patient is conscious has consumed poison orally and has reached hospital within 3 hrs.

4. Administer specific therapy if available.

5. Increase rate of excretion of poison through kidneys by administering IV fluids and diuretics.

6. Symptomatic treatment of convulsions or shock should be given.

7. Collect laboratory samples for identification and determination of poison — this helps in treatment as well as in legal cases.

MANAGEMENT OF ACUTE INTOXICATIONS

Drugs can produce acute and chronic toxicity that has been discussed in earlier chapters. In addition large number of poisons which are not used therapeutically but are encountered in environment, as they are used in household, industry or farm are misused for purposes of **suicide** or **homicide** or may be **accidentally** consumed by the children. The acute poisoning by all agents need immediate attention.

Prevention of poisoning

1. Patients should be instructed to keep medicines in locked cabinets out of reach from children.

2. **Do not store poisonous medicines with other medicines.**

3. Label all stored medicines and materials.

4. Do not put eatables or cleaning material in the medicine store or cupboard.

Nursing care of patient of acute poisoning

Gastric lavage is performed with the patient lying on left side and with his head down. A rubber tube is passed into stomach and 4 ounces of tap water is repeatedly pushed through this tube and withdrawn.

Gastric lavage should not be performed in the following conditions:

(a) If more than 2 hours have elapsed after ingestion of poison and 30 minutes after corrosive agents (acids or alkalis).

(b) It should not be done if patient has consumed **kerosene, paint thinner or spot remover.**

(c) If patient is not conscious (coma, stupor or delirium are all contraindications).

(d) If convulsions are present.

1. **Emesis:** This procedure is adopted only in the conscious patients. **Contraindications to emesis are same as of gastric lavage.**

2. **Ipecac syrup** 15–20 ml is given by mouth. Dose can be repeated after 15–20 minutes if the first dose fails.

   Apomorphine is preferred, as it is quick acting. 6 mg is given IM in children and dose of 0.05 mg/kg IM is given. Action of this drug can be reversed by nalorphine in the dose of 0.1 mg/kg IM.

3. **Adsorbents:** If the poison is identified, gastric lavage can be carried out using specific adsorbents which help in removal and detoxification of the poison, e.g. **phosphate is used to remove iron. Ammonium nitrate or ammonium hydroxide is used for formaldehyde and sodium thiosulfate to detoxify iodide.** Potassium permanganate is given in alkaloidal poisoning. For longer lasting effect, these agents are left in the stomach. **Activated charcoal** if properly prepared and properly stored is found to be effective in various poisons (**except alcohol or caustics**).

4. **To increase the excretion of toxic substances:** Toxic effects of the drugs can be reduced by promoting their metabolism or their excretion through the kidney.

(i) By increasing the volume of urine the toxicant too gets excreted. For this action give diuretics, e.g. 25% solution of mannitol or 40 mg IV frusemide.

(ii) Change of pH of urine affects excretion of drugs. Barbiturates are better excreted in alkaline urine and amphetamine in acidic urine.

5. **Specific antidotal therapy**
   (a) Antisera for venoms and toxins.
   (b) **Ethyl alcohol** for **methyl alcohol**.
   (c) **Atropine** with **PAM** for anticholinesterase organophosphorus compounds.
   (d) **Epinephrine** for anaphylaxis.
   (e) **Naloxone** for **morphine and other opiates.**
   (f) **Oxygen** for **carbon monoxide.**
   (g) **Amyl nitrite** for **cyanide.**
   (h) **Physostigmine** (0.5–2 mg IV) for **atropine.**
   (i) **Flumazenil** 0.2 mg IV initially and after 30 seconds for treatment of **benzodiazepines**.
   (j) **Glucagon** (50–150 ug/kg IV) for **insulin.**
   (k) **Calcium gluconate** (0.2–0.5 mg/kg) for **calcium channel blockers.**
   (l) **N-acetylcysteine** (140 mg/kg followed by 70 mg/kg) for **acetaminophen.**
   (m) **BAL** (5 mg/kg) for **arsenic, gold and mercury.**
   (n) **Vitamin K** for **warfarin sodium** and other oral anticoagulants.

6. **Symptomatic therapy:** It sustains the patient during the period of detoxifiction. Symptomatic treatment is given for:
   (a) Pain
   (b) Vomiting and diarrhea
   (c) Correcting fluid and electrolyte imbalance.
   (d) Shock: This condition is produced by barbiturates and other CNS depressants and should be treated by re-expansion of the plasma volume rather than vasopressors (for details refer CVS).
   (e) Coma
   (f) Convulsions: Oxygen should be administered between convulsions. If the toxicant is not a CNS depressant diazepam can be effectively used.

DIALYSIS

Peritoneal dialysis is easy but less effective. Hemodialysis is effective but expensive. It is useful in removal of **lithium, barbiturates, alcohol, chloral hydrate, methanol, barbiturates, meprobamate, ethinamate, methaqualone, paraldehyde, aspirin, phenacetin, propoxyphene, imipramine, arsenic, mercury, lead, sodium, lithium, calcium, magnesium, fluorides, iodides and heroine.** Benzodiazepines are nor removed by dialysis.

Hemoperfusion: It is effective in removing drugs that are highly protein bound and have a small apparent volume of distribution.

Cyanide Toxicity: Cyanide is highly toxic. Death due to this radical occurs in minutes. Treatment of cyanide poisoning:

1. **Amyl nitrite** is given for 30 seconds every two minutes.

2. Sodium nitrite (300–500 mg) is given intravenously.

3. Slow infusion of **sodium thiosulfate** (12.5 g in 50 ml) is given after the first two. Entire amount of this drug must go in 10 minutes.

4. If **cobalt edetate** is available it can also be used.

Dose: 600 mg IV.

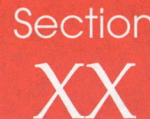

Drug Interactions

83. Drug Interactions

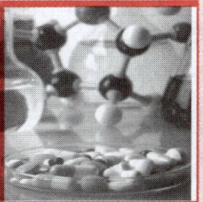

83

Drug Interactions

Why Study Drug Interactions

1. Patients commonly receive more than one drug.
2. Patients are often given to self medication because many drugs can be bought without prescription, e.g. analgesics, cough mixtures, vitamins and haematinics. In fact in our country practically all drugs (except narcotics) can be purchased without medical prescription.
3. Drugs may interact with each other in such a way as to produce effects that may not be predictable from a knowledge of their actions separately.

Thus the knowledge of drug interactions is necessary for safe drug therapy.

Physician combines drugs with a view to obtain greater advantage but these combinations can sometimes produce fatal results.

This chapter highlights few of these interactions. It is not possible to enumerate all in this book. The stress is laid on those combinations which are common and produce serious problems and should be avoided.

I. Drug Interactions in vitro: Many drugs are inactivated rapidly when added to incompatible fluid.

Erythromycin remains active for four hours when added to dextrose but lasts for 24 hours in normal saline.

Salts of weakly acidic drugs (**penicillin, ampicillin, heparin, erythromycin, hydrocortisone, sulfonamides, barbiturates, methicillin and novobiocin**) cannot be added to dextrose, levulose or fructose solution as they get precipitated. Isotonic saline solution is suitable for all above metioned drugs. Noradrenaline alone is unstable in this medium but addition of ascorbic acid makes this fluid compatible for this drug.

Noradrenaline can be added to dextrose alone.

No drug can be added to blood, plasma, solutions of sodium bicarbonate and mannitol.

Following is the list of drugs which cannot be combined in the same perfusion bottle, i.e. these drugs should not be combined together in the same syringe and injected.

1. Penicillins precipitate out tetracyclines and inactivates gentamicin. Therefore, cannot be combined.
2. Tetracyclines precipitate out penicillin, sulfonamides, cephaloridine, hydrocortisone and sodium chloride, it cannot be given with any drug containing calcium as it gets inactivated.
3. Heparin (a highly acidic drug) precipitates catecholamines, tetracyclines and aminoglycosides.
4. Long acting insulins with regular insulin.

1. Drugs cannot be added to blood, solutions of amino acids or fat emulsions
2. The addition of more than one drug to a solution of dextrose or normal saline should be avoided if possible.
3. IV fluids should be examined before and after the addition of a drug. Look for foreign matter or precipitate. If these are found the bottle should be discarded and sister in-charge or physician on duty informed about it.
4. Add drugs to solutions just before infusion.

II. Interactions at the Site of Absorption

(a) Drugs that affect the motility of the intestine may increase or decrease absorption. **Atropine, propantheline, benzhexol** and **morphine** decrease motility. The stay of other drugs in ileum is prolonged resulting in increased absorption but delayed onset of action.

(b) Two drugs taken together may interact in GIT. **Calcium, magnesium, aluminium** and **iron salts** interfere with absorption of **tetracycline** as they form complexes which do not get easily absorbed.

(c) One drug may alter the pH of the stomach in a direction that may adversely affect the absorption of the second drug, e.g. **sodium bicarbonate** reduces absorption of **iron** and **tetracycline.**

(d) Presence of bentonite in PAS impairs the absorption of rifampicin whereas absorption of griseofulvin is reduced by phenobarbitone.

(e) Desferrioxamine and iron interaction is a desirable one in iron toxicity as the former drug reduces the absorption of iron.

(f) Orally given broad spectrum antimicrobials potentiate effect of oral anticoagulants as these reduce gut flora required in synthesis of vitamin K.

(g) Phenytoin hampers absorption of folic acid.

III. Drug Interactions at the Transport or Storage Site: Most of the drugs get bound to plasma proteins. One drug may displace the other from its binding site and increase the level of free drug in plasma. Liberation of free drug in excess leads to toxicity. There are many examples of this type of drug interactions. Few are mentioned here.

(a) Tolbutamide is displaced by Bishydroxycoumarin, phenylbutazone and salicylates, thereby increasing hypoglycemic activity.

(b) Warfarin sodium (oral anticoagulant) is displaced from its binding sites by phenylbutazone, oxyphenbutazone and clofibrate. Hemorrhagic tendencies are increased.

(c) Bile pigments are displaced by sulphaphenazole, sulphamethoxyridazine and salicylates. Displacement of bile pigment results in jaundice.

(d) Imipramine reduces antihypertensive effect of guanethidine.

IV. Stimulation of Drug Metabolism: These drugs are called enzyme inducers: **Chloral hydrate, barbiturates, phenytoin, griseofulvin, DDT** (dicophane) and **alcohol**.

Drug given in combination with any one of the above mentioned drugs will have short duration of action and the effect will be reduced. **On withdrawal of the enzyme inducer serious toxicity can set in**.

In contrast to above certain drugs inhibit drug metabolism enzymes, e.g. metabolism of tolbutamide is reduced by bishydroxycoumarin, disulfiram and chloramphenicol. This leads to development of serious hypoglycemia. Metabolism of phenytoin is inhibited by INH, phenylbutazone, disulfiram and chloramphenicol.

Role of nurse

It is important for the nurse to remember few common drug interactions and she must warn her patient against self medication.

Metabolism of alcohol is inhibited by disulfiram, chlorpropamide, metronidazole and griseofulvin. All these drugs produce severe flushing, diarrhea and hypotension. Except for disulfiram, all other drugs are commonly used. Nurse must instruct her patients not to take alcoholic drink during ingestion of these drugs.

V. Interaction at Sites of Action (Receptors):
Many drugs act on a specific part of the body (e.g. receptor) and get selectively concentrated where they act. Drug is actively taken up by the receptors. If the receptor site is occupied by another drug that has greater affinity, this cannot take up a second drug for which it has lower affinity.

Acetylcholine combines with receptors in the neuromuscular junction and produces contraction of skeletal muscle, d-tubocurarine combines with the same receptors. Acetylcholine given after tubocurarine fails to produce muscle contraction. Proparanolol combines with β receptor sites in the heart and prevents isoprenaline from producing tachycardia.

This type of interaction is of clinical utility, e.g.

1. **Naloxone** is taken up by receptor sites in the brain in preference to morphine and it displaces morphine and other opiates from these sites. Thus naloxone is used to treat patients suffering from morphine toxicity.
2. Use of **beta blockers** in hypertension and cardiac arrhythmias is based on this principal. It reduces the activity of sympathetic system on heart.
3. **Atropine** is used in cases of mushroom poisoning producing cholinomimetic effects.
4. **Diuretic** and **digoxin**. This interaction is important because these drugs are often combined and this can produce cardiac arrhythmias. Diuretics like thiazides, frusemide and ethacrynic acid induce potassium depletion, thus increasing excitability of the heart making digitalis very much more liable to irritate cardiac muscle and produce dangerous arrhythmias.

Potassium supplements prevent this complication (for details refer CVS).

VI. Interactions at Sites of Excretion:
If a drug changes the pH of urine it may increase or decrease the rate of excretion of drugs through kidney. **Sodium bicarbonate** given to the patient will cause increase excretion of **aspirin** and **phenobarbitone**. This is a double edged weapon. In an epileptic patient the use of sodium bicarbonate (as an antacid) will precipitate epileptic attack in a patient controlled by phenobarbitone while in toxicity of barbiturates sodium bicarbonate will save the life of patient.

Probenecid reduces excretion of **penicillin, indomethacin and riboflavin**. Excretion of amphetamine is increased in acid urine.

Summary of some important and potential interactions that nurse must remember:

1. Aspirin and phenylbutazone increase effects of warfarin, tolbutamide, chlorpropamide and methotrexate.

2. Sulphonamides increase effect of chlorpropamide.

3. Thiazides, frusemide and ethacrynic acid increase sensitivity of cardiac muscle to toxic effects of digoxin.

4. Barbiturates reduce effect of warfarin, phenylbutazone, phenytoin and griseofulvin. The dose of these drugs has to be increased in presence of barbiturates. Patient must be warned that stoppage of barbiturate will produce toxicity of these drugs.

5. **Rifampicin causes pill failure**.

6. Imipramine and amitryptyline antagonise the hypotensive action of adrenergic blocking drugs such as guanethidine and bethanidine.

7. Monoamine oxidase inhibitors produce hypertensive crisis if the patient consumes tyramine containing foods such as cheese, meat extracts and red wine.

8. Interactions with **alcohol**: Layman does not consider alcohol as a drug but alcohol acts with various drugs.

   (i) Drowsiness induced by barbiturates, antihistaminics, chlorpromazine, diazepam and antidepressants is worsened by alcohol.

   (ii) Alcohol given with any one of these drugs **(chlorpropamide, disulfiram, griseofulvin and metronidazole)** produces hypotension and other highly undesirable effects.

Keeping all the above points in mind, nurse must

1. Impress on her patient that he must never take any medicine on his own for any illness however trivial without first consulting his doctor.

2. If the patient has more than one medicine prescribed for him he must continue to take all tablets until such time as the doctor tells him to stop.

Index

Reader's Note